HIV

THIRD EDITION

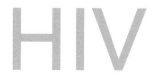

HIV

Third Edition

Howard Libman, MD, FACP

Associate Professor of Medicine
Harvard Medical School
Director, HIV Program, Healthcare Associates
Divisions of General Medicine and
  Primary Care and Infectious Diseases
Beth Israel Deaconess Medical Center
Boston, Massachusetts

Harvey J. Makadon, MD

Associate Professor of Medicine
Harvard Medical School
Director of Professional Education, The Fenway Institute
Division of General Medicine and Primary Care
Beth Israel Deaconess Medical Center
Boston, Massachusetts

AMERICAN COLLEGE OF PHYSICIANS   PHILADELPHIA

Associate Publisher and Manager, Books Publishing: Tom Hartman
Director, Editorial Production: Linda Drumheller
Developmental Editor: Marla Sussman
Production Supervisor: Allan S. Kleinberg
Senior Production Editor: Karen C. Nolan
Editorial Coordinator: Angela Gabella
Cover Design: Kate Nixon
Index: Nelle Garrecht

Printed in the United States of America
Printing/binding by Versa Press
Composition by ATLIS Graphics

ISBN: 978-1-930513-73-0

The authors and publisher have exerted every effort to ensure that the drug selection and dosages set forth in this book are in accordance with current recommendations and practice at the time of publication. In view of ongoing research, occasional changes in government regulations, and the constant flow of information relating to drug therapy and drug reactions, the reader is urged to check the package insert for each drug for any change in indications and dosage and for additional warnings and precautions. This care is particularly important when the recommended agent is a new or infrequently used drug.

Contributors

Edward P. Acosta, PharmD
Associate Professor of Clinical
  Pharmacology
Division of Clinical Pharmacology
Department of Pharmacology
  and Toxicology
University of Alabama at
  Birmingham School of Medicine
Birmingham, Alabama

Sigall K. Bell, MD
Instructor in Medicine
Harvard Medical School
Division of Infectious Diseases
Beth Israel Deaconess Medical
  Center
Boston, Massachusetts

Andrew Carr, MD
Professor of Medicine
University of New South Wales
Senior Staff Specialist, HIV,
  Immunology, and Infectious
  Diseases Unit
St. Vincent's Hospital
Sydney, Australia

Sonia Nagy Chimienti, MD
Assistant Professor of Medicine
Harvard Medical School
Director, Fellowship Training
  Program
Division of Infectious Diseases
Beth Israel Deaconess Medical
  Center
Boston, Massachusetts

David A. Cooper, MD, DSc
Scientia Professor of Medicine
National Centre in HIV
  Epidemiology and Clinical
  Research
University of New South Wales
Head, HIV, Immunology, and
  Infectious Diseases Unit
St. Vincent's Hospital
Sydney, Australia

Lisa A. Cosimi, MD
Instructor in Medicine
Harvard Medical School
Brigham and Women's Hospital
Boston, Massachusetts

Judith S. Currier, MD, MSc
Professor of Medicine
David Geffen School of Medicine
Center for Clinical AIDS Research
    and Education
University of California at
    Los Angeles
Los Angeles, California

Susan Cu-Uvin, MD
Associate Professor of Obstetrics
    and Gynecology
Brown Medical School
The Miriam Hospital
Providence, Rhode Island

Benjamin Davis, MD
Assistant Professor of Medicine
Harvard Medical School
Division of Infectious Diseases
Massachusetts General Hospital
Boston, Massachusetts

Bruce J. Dezube, MD
Associate Professor of Medicine
Harvard Medical School
Division of Hematology-Oncology
Beth Israel Deaconess Medical
    Center
Boston, Massachusetts

John P. Doweiko, MD
Assistant Professor of Medicine
Harvard Medical School
Division of Infectious Diseases
Beth Israel Deaconess Medical
    Center
Boston, Massachusetts

Gregory Fenton, MD
Instructor in Medicine
Harvard Medical School
Medical Director, Sidney Borum
    Community Health Center
Boston, Massachusetts

Jon D. Fuller, MD
Associate Professor Medicine
Boston University School of
    Medicine
Center for HIV/AIDS Care and
    Research
Boston Medical Center
Boston, Massachusetts

Joel E. Gallant, MD, MPH
Professor of Medicine and
    Epidemiology
Johns Hopkins University School
    of Medicine
Associate Director, Johns Hopkins
    AIDS Service
Baltimore, Maryland

John G. Gerber, MD
Professor of Medicine and
    Pharmacology (Retired)
Divisions of Infectious Diseases
    and Clinical Pharmacology
University of Colorado Health
    Sciences Center
Denver, Colorado

Eric P. Goosby, MD
Professor of Clinical Medicine
University of California at
    San Francisco School
    of Medicine
Chief Executive Officer, Pangaea
    Global AIDS Foundation
San Francisco, California

Camilla S. Graham, MD, MPH
Assistant Professor of Medicine
Harvard Medical School
Division of Infectious Diseases
Beth Israel Deaconess
    Medical Center
Boston, Massachusetts

Amita Gupta, MD, MHS
Assistant Professor of Medicine
Deputy Director, Center for Clinical
    Global Health Education
Division of Infectious Diseases
Johns Hopkins University School
    of Medicine
Baltimore, Maryland

Lisa R. Hirschhorn, MD, MPH
Associate Director, International
    Monitoring and Evaluation
Division of AIDS
Harvard Medical School
Boston, Massachusetts

Louise Ivers, MD, MPH
Instructor in Medicine
Harvard Medical School
Brigham and Women's Hospital
Boston, Massachusetts

Daniel R. Kuritzkes, MD
Professor of Medicine
Harvard Medical School
Director of AIDS Research
Brigham and Women's Hospital
Boston, Massachusetts

Matthew R. Leibowitz, MD
Assistant Clinical Professor
    of Medicine
David Geffen School of Medicine
Center for Clinical AIDS Research
    and Education
University of California at
    Los Angeles
Los Angeles, California

Howard Libman, MD, FACP
Associate Professor of Medicine
Harvard Medical School
Director, HIV Program, Healthcare
    Associates
Divisions of General Medicine and
    Primary Care and Infectious
    Diseases
Beth Israel Deaconess
    Medical Center
Boston, Massachusetts

Harvey J. Makadon, MD
Associate Professor of Medicine
Harvard Medical School
Director of Professional Education,
    The Fenway Institute
Division of General Medicine and
    Primary Care
Beth Israel Deaconess
    Medical Center
Boston, Massachusetts

Patrick W.G. Mallon, MBBCh, PhD
Lecturer in Medicine
School of Medicine and
    Medical Sciences
University College Dublin
Mater Misericordiae University
    Hospital
Dublin, Ireland

Kenneth H. Mayer, MD
Professor of Medicine and
    Community Health
Brown Medical School
Medical Research Director, Fenway
    Community Health Center
Division of Infectious Diseases
The Miriam Hospital
Providence, Rhode Island

Elizabeth A. McCarthy, MPH
Senior Policy Analyst
Consortium for Strategic HIV
  Operations Research
Clinton Foundation HIV/AIDS
  Initiative
Boston, Massachusetts

Megan O'Brien, PhD
Research Director
Consortium for Strategic HIV
  Operations Research
Clinton Foundation HIV/AIDS
Initiative
Boston, Massachusetts

Lori A. Panther, MD, MPH
Assistant Professor of Medicine
Harvard Medical School
Division of Infectious Diseases
Beth Israel Deaconess Medical
  Center
Boston, Massachusetts

Peter J. Piliero, MD
Associate Professor of Medicine
Albany Medical School
Division of Infectious Diseases
Albany Medical Center
Albany, New York

Raymond O. Powrie, MD
Associate Professor of Medicine
  and Obstetrics and Gynecology
Brown Medical School
Director, Division of Obstetric
  and Consultative Medicine
Women and Infants Hospital
Providence, Rhode Island

William Rodriguez, MD
Assistant Professor of Medicine
Harvard Medical School
Division of AIDS
Massachusetts General Hospital
Brigham and Women's Hospital
Boston, Massachusetts

Steven A. Safren, PhD
Associate Professor of Psychology
Harvard Medical School
Massachusetts General Hospital
Boston, Massachusetts

Jeffrey H. Samet, MD, MA, MPH
Professor of Medicine and Public
  Health
Boston University Schools of
  Medicine and Public Health
Chief, Section of General Internal
  Medicine
Boston Medical Center
Boston, Massachusetts

Paul E. Sax, MD
Associate Professor of Medicine
Harvard Medical School
Clinical Director, Division of
  Infectious Diseases and
  HIV Program
Brigham and Women's Hospital
Boston, Massachusetts

Marissa B. Wilck, MBChB
Instructor in Medicine
Harvard Medical School
Brigham and Women's Hospital
Boston, Massachusetts

Michael T. Wong, MD
Assistant Professor of Medicine
Harvard Medical School
Division of Infectious Diseases
Beth Israel Deaconess Medical
  Center
Boston, Massachusetts

Preface

The care of HIV-infected patients continues to evolve dramatically, with antiretroviral drugs becoming more readily available in developing countries over the past several years. What was previously a progressive disease manifested by opportunistic infections and neoplasms is now a treatable chronic medical condition in many patients around the world. However, the significant changes in management over the past decade have resulted in important challenges for clinicians. Drug resistance, long-term treatment complications, and barriers to implementing care in resource-limited settings are now common concerns.

In this third edition of *HIV*, all chapters have been thoroughly updated to reflect the current state of the art of clinical practice. New to this edition are chapters on global epidemiology, clinical considerations in developing countries, and antiretroviral treatment and barriers to implementing care in resource-limited settings. Written by a team of authors with established clinical, teaching, and research expertise, this text provides essential information for the care of HIV-infected patients. We have tried to indicate where uncertainty exists and to present a reasonable approach to management based on the medical literature and accepted standards of clinical practice.

We thank our talented authors for their informative contributions. We are indebted also to the American College of Physicians, especially Tom Hartman and his colleagues in the book division, for their wonderful support. Finally, we wish to acknowledge the staff and faculty of Beth Israel Deaconess Medical Center and Harvard Medical School. Their professionalism and commitment to care continue to inspire us.

We dedicate this book to our HIV-infected patients, who have taught us much about living with dignity. While encouraged with the progress that has been made over the four years since the publication of the last edition, we are cognizant that there is still much work to be done in improving the lives of HIV-infected patients and making antiretroviral drugs available to all those who are still in need worldwide.

Howard Libman, MD, FACP
Harvey J. Makadon, MD

Contents

Chapter 1

Transmission, Pathogenesis, and Natural History

I. Transmission
KENNETH H. MAYER, MD

II. Pathogenesis
SIGALL K. BELL, MD

III. Natural History
SIGALL K. BELL, MD

As the HIV epidemic emerged in the early 1980s, its diverse manifestations were described and categorized. HIV-infected patients are defined as having the acquired immunodeficiency syndrome (AIDS) if they have specific clinical conditions such as opportunistic infections (OIs) or malignancies indicative of significantly impaired immune function or a CD4 cell count of less than 200/mm^3 (Box 1-1). Since the onset of the epidemic, close to 60 million people have become infected with the virus, with almost 20 million people dying from its complications. Of the more than 40 million people with HIV infection today, 95% live in the developing world. Close to half of them are women, and more than 3 million are children under the age of 15. In 2005, AIDS was responsible for the deaths of more than 3 million people globally. By the beginning of 2006, more than 1 million Americans were living with HIV infection, and almost a half a million persons had died from its complications. More than 80% of people living with HIV infection in the United States were diagnosed as adults, with slightly more than half acquiring it from male homosexual contact and 31% from injection-drug use; 11% acquired HIV infection from heterosexual contact, and 2% were recipients of infected blood products.

Box 1-1.   Indicator Conditions for Case Definition of AIDS

- Candidiasis, esophageal
- Candidiasis of bronchi, trachea, or lungs
- Cervical cancer, invasive
- Coccidioidomycosis, disseminated or extrapulmonary
- Cryptococcosis, extrapulmonary
- Cryptosporidiosis, chronic intestinal
- Cytomegalovirus disease (other than liver, spleen, or lymph nodes)
- Encephalopathy, HIV-related
- Herpes simplex, chronic ulcer(s) or bronchitis, pneumonitis, or esophagitis
- Histoplasmosis, disseminated or extrapulmonary
- Isosporiasis, chronic intestinal

- Kaposi's sarcoma
- Lymphoma, Burkitt's
- Lymphoma, immunoblastic
- Lymphoma, primary (in brain)
- *Mycobacterium avium* complex or *M. kansasii*, disseminated or extrapulmonary
- *Mycobacterium tuberculosis,* any site
- *Pneumocystis jiroveci (carinii)* pneumonia
- Pneumonia, recurrent
- Progressive multifocal leukoencephalopathy
- *Salmonella* septicemia, recurrent
- Toxoplasmosis of brain
- Wasting syndrome, HIV-related

Box 1-2.   What We Know About HIV Transmission

- HIV transmission is a high-consequence, low-probability event (range <1/1000 to >1/10 exposures).
- Multiple cofactors may affect infectiousness and susceptibility.
- HIV can be transmitted as a cell-free or a cell-associated virus.
- Lower plasma HIV concentration is associated with a reduced risk of transmission.
- Drug-resistant HIV transmission is well documented.
- Being on antiretroviral therapy is not the same as being noninfectious.

I. TRANSMISSION
KENNETH H. MAYER

HIV transmission is a high-consequence but low-probability event that may be associated with a single exposure but usually occurs after repeated risk-taking behaviors (Box 1-2). There are multiple cofactors involved in HIV transmission, which explains why there is a high level of variability in estimates of the relative risk of infection for specific exposures. HIV may be transmitted as cell-free or cell-associated virus, and different factors may affect expression of viral concentrations in body fluids (e.g., blood, semen, cervicovaginal secretions). Although lower blood concentrations of HIV are associated with lower rates of transmission, antiretroviral drugs do not render HIV-infected persons noninfectious. In fact, the sexual transmission of multidrug-resistant HIV has been well documented, underscoring the need for clinicians to promote safer sexual behaviors among patients on antiretroviral therapy.

Biology

HIV is most often transmitted through sexual contact by rapidly binding to cells that are present in the cervical, vaginal, penile, urethral, and rectal mucosa (Table 1-1). The male foreskin contains abundant cells that can bind HIV. Thus, being uncircumcised is associated with increased risk for HIV acquisition and transmission. The exact mechanisms responsible for the sexual transmission of HIV in humans are not fully understood. In animal models, both cell-free and cell-associated HIV have resulted in infection after mucous membrane exposure. The cells that are the source of HIV transmission in the genital tract have one of two surface markers, CCR5 or CXCR4, that express the coreceptors for binding. HIV target cells include lymphocytes, monocyte/macrophage cells, and Langerhans' cells. Follicular dendritic cells may be particularly important, since after binding HIV on their surface membranes they internalize the virus and migrate via the lymphatics to distant sites, where propagation in submucosal lymphoid tissues can occur leading to viral dissemination.

Based on animal data, it is estimated that HIV results in an established systemic infection within 72 hours. During this critical period, antiretroviral drug therapy, also known as postexposure prophylaxis (PEP), has been recommended to prevent infection with the virus. The relative efficiency of

Table 1-1.   Efficiency Modifiers of HIV Transmission

	Infectiousness	*Susceptibility*
Sexually transmitted diseases	↑	↑
Genital tract inflammation (e.g., traumatic sex, douching)	↑	↑
Circumcision	↓	↓
Cervical ectopy	?	↑
Genetic profile (CCR5 mutation)	?	↓
HIV subtype (subtype A or C)	↑	NA
Monocytotropic strain	↑	NA
Acute infection	↑	NA
Advanced infection	↑	NA
Antiretroviral therapy	?↓	NA

NA = Not applicable.

HIV transmission after an exposure may be influenced by many factors. Persons with higher plasma viral loads and/or intercurrent sexually transmitted diseases (STDs) may be more likely to transmit HIV after contact with a susceptible host. HIV-seronegative persons who have inflammatory conditions that can increase the number of target cells in the genital mucosa that bind HIV are more susceptible to becoming HIV-infected. Ulcerative lesions, such as syphilis, chancroid, and genital herpes simplex virus (HSV) infection, are most likely to potentiate HIV acquisition and transmission. These infections afford portals for viral entry and recruit immunologically active cells that bind HIV and propagate the infection. Inflammatory STDs, such as gonorrhea, *Chlamydia trachomatis*, and trichomoniasis, have also been associated with increased HIV acquisition and transmission. They may act either by increasing the number of white blood cells in the genital tract or by the elaboration of cytokines and chemokines (chemical mediators of immune cell interactions) that upregulate HIV expression and increase genital HIV concentration. Other factors that may result in genital tract inflammation include douching, the use of irritating contraceptive gels, and traumatic sexual intercourse.

The amount of HIV in semen or cervicovaginal secretions may range from as high as 10 million copies/mL to an undetectable level. Generally there are 10 times as many HIV-RNA copies detected in the blood as in genital secretions. Patients with higher plasma HIV viral loads are more likely to have greater amounts of the virus in their genital secretions, but there is not a consistent correlation. Cells may traffic between the blood and the genital tract, but local factors such as STDs may result in a higher concentration of virus in the genital tract without necessarily causing the same upregulation of HIV expression in blood. Patients with acute HIV infection and patients with advanced HIV disease with high plasma viral loads often have increased HIV concentrations in their genital secretions and are more likely to transmit the virus to their partners.

Patients whose plasma HIV viral load is suppressed on antiretroviral therapy will tend to have a lower, but sometimes still detectable, concentration of the virus in the genital tract. Moreover, not all antiretroviral drugs penetrate genital secretions well. The reasons for this "blood-genital tract barrier" include differences in the pH of blood and genital secretions and in binding proteins. Protease inhibitors have been shown to achieve much lower levels in genital tract secretions than in the blood, while nucleoside reverse-transcriptase inhibitors tend to achieve comparable or even higher concentrations. Suboptimal adherence to antiretroviral therapy can result in the development of HIV drug resistance in the blood and genital tract. Thus, the benefits of antiretroviral therapy in slowing the spread of HIV have been debated. In some countries, such as Brazil and Taiwan, public health officials have argued that wider availability of antiretroviral drugs in conjunction with culturally nuanced prevention campaigns have been effective in reducing transmission. Others have pointed to the experience in the United States, where despite widespread availability of antiretroviral therapy, the number of new HIV infections has remained steady at 40,000 per year over the past decade.

The different tissues of the male and female genital tract have varying levels of susceptibility to HIV infection. The vaginal epithelium is stratified and multilayered and contains fewer cells containing HIV coreceptors than the endocervix, which has a thin layer, is highly vascular, and contains a much higher concentration of HIV-binding cells. Altered physiology of the endocervix, such as that resulting from *C. trachomatis* infection or the use of hormonal contraceptives, increases its susceptibility to HIV. The penile foreskin contains many cells that can readily bind and express HIV, resulting in increased viral acquisition and transmission in uncircumcised males. A recent randomized, controlled trial confirmed the protective effect of adult male circumcision. The oropharynx contains many fewer cells that can bind HIV, which may partially explain the relative inefficiency of oral exposure to the virus as a means of transmission. In addition, salivary secretions contain several compounds, such as secretory leukocyte protease inhibitor, that have been found to inhibit HIV transmission in vitro. Interestingly, however, rhesus macaques have been readily infected with simian immunodeficiency virus after an oral challenge, with evidence of viral replication in tonsillar and adenoidal tissues.

Other factors that affect the efficiency of HIV transmission include the specific characteristics of the infecting viral strain. HIV may preferentially replicate in monocytes (monocytropic strains) or CD4 lymphocytes (lymphocytotropic strains), but the virus is usually sexually transmitted by monocytropic strains. Epidemiologic and laboratory studies suggest that HIV subtypes A and C, which are most common where the epidemic is spreading most rapidly (sub-Saharan Africa and South and East Asia), may be more readily transmitted sexually than subtype B, which is the predominant strain in North America and Europe. This observation may partially explain the varying rates of transmission in different parts of the world. Additionally, systemic inflammatory conditions, such as tuberculosis and malaria, which are more prevalent in the developing world, may increase the amount of virus in the blood and genital tract. Local STD rates and different patterns of social and sexual behavior may also explain the varying rates of global HIV transmission.

Innate and acquired host factors may affect susceptibility to infection. Patients who are homozygous for a 32 base pair deletion mutation in the CCR5 coreceptor that binds HIV are more resistant to becoming infected with the virus than people who do not have it. This mutation, which is present in up to 3.6% of Caucasian cohorts studied, makes it harder for the monocytotropic form of HIV to infect cells. It is much less common in African and Asian populations, which may also explain the rapidity of

HIV spread in those parts of the world. Women have differences in vaginal microflora that may play a role in their susceptibility to HIV infection. For example, bacterial vaginosis, characterized by a paucity of hydrogen peroxide–producing lactobacilli and an increase in genital anaerobes, increases the risk for HIV infection, even in the absence of symptoms or signs of vaginitis. This condition appears to be more common in African and African-American women and may be responsible for potentiating the spread of HIV in these populations.

An immunologic response to HIV may occur in the absence of infection. In several cohorts of HIV-exposed but uninfected African commercial sex workers, evidence of mucosal antibody and cell-mediated immune responses was present. In another study, when sex workers reduced risk-taking behaviors, they had a decrease in mucosal antibodies, and some women became infected later after contact with a new partner. These data and studies of HIV-serodiscordant couples suggest that HIV may be most likely to spread after initial sexual encounters, and subsequent exposures may result in some level of acquired immunity. Understanding the immune responses of people who may be relatively resistant to infection may help in HIV vaccine development.

Epidemiology

Because multiple cofactors may alter the amount of virus in the blood and genital tract, the calculation of infection risk for each type of HIV exposure is imprecise. Moreover, much of the data used to generate per-contact risks have been based on cohort studies in which patients recall their level of risk during a preceding time interval, usually 3 to 6 months. It is important when patients ask questions about the likelihood of risk to reassure them that a one-time exposure to HIV is unlikely to result in transmission and to explain that the reason why the epidemic has become so widespread is because of people engaging in recurrent risk-taking behaviors.

Having noted the limitations of how risk calculations are obtained, certain principles have emerged. The likelihood of encountering an infected person's secretions and the amount of virus to which one is exposed play a role in determining the risk of becoming HIV-infected after percutaneous or sexual contact. Direct intravascular exposure to HIV is a highly efficient way of transmitting the virus, and percutaneous needle contact much less so. For example, shared needle use by injection-drug users is considerably more likely to transmit HIV than an occupational needle stick with a solid suture needle in a health care setting. The range of risk for people who share injection drug paraphernalia ranges from 0.6% to 3%, while the risk for a health care worker after having been exposed to a needle with HIV-infected blood is about 0.3% (Table 1-2).

Table 1-2.   Estimates of Per-Contact Risk of HIV Infection

	Risk
Needle-sharing	6/1000–30/1000
Occupational needle stick	1/300
Receptive anal sex	8/1000–30/1000
Receptive vaginal sex	2/1000–8/1000
Insertive anal or vaginal sex	3/10,000–10/10,000
Receptive oral sex	Unknown

Data sources summarized in Mayer KH, Anderson DT. Heterosexual HIV transmission. Infectious Agents and Disease. 1995;4:273-84.

This range overlaps with the level of risk for people who engage in un-protected receptive anal or receptive vaginal intercourse. Receptive anal intercourse has been estimated to be more than seven times as efficient in transmitting HIV compared to insertive anal intercourse. The risks of unpro-tected insertive anal intercourse and insertive vaginal intercourse are thought to be of a similar magnitude, with uncircumcised men being more likely than circumcised men to become HIV-infected after a comparable exposure.

Cofactors, such as a source patient with a high-plasma HIV concentra-tion or concomitant STD, can greatly increase the average per-contact risk. In the developed world, epidemiologic data have suggested that men are more likely to transmit HIV to their female partners than visa versa. But in several studies of HIV-serodiscordant couples in sub-Saharan Africa, the rates of male-to-female and female-to-male transmission were quite similar. The reasons for this difference may be because of the decreased prevalence of male circumcision and the higher prevalence of other STDs in some de-veloping countries. For anal intercourse, an insertive partner is less likely to acquire HIV from an infected receptive partner than vice versa. However, there are sufficient susceptible cells in the distal male urethra and foreskin and an abundance of HIV-infected cells and mucus secretions in an infected receptive partner that an insertive partner is still at some risk.

It is clear that receptive oral sex, either fellatio or cunnilingus, is a much less efficient way to acquire HIV, but there are well-documented case re-ports showing that oral exposure to ejaculate may result in viral transmis-sion. The relative efficiency of oral sex is below that of unprotected receptive vaginal intercourse (less than one case per 1000 exposures). In counseling patients who have concerns about oral sex, it is important to in-form them that, while the risk is lower than that of many other sexual ac-tivities, it is still possible to acquire HIV in this manner. Thus, it is preferable to avoid any oral exposure to semen or cervicovaginal secretions from a partner who is known to be at risk for, or infected with, HIV. Although HIV has been found in pre-ejaculatory secretions in very small concentrations, there are no reliable case reports of HIV transmission through exposure to pre-ejaculate.

Prevention

Treatment of Sexually Transmitted Diseases

There are several different ways that HIV transmission may be minimized (Figure 1-1). One approach is the aggressive diagnosis and treatment of STDs. In a study in the Mwanza district of Uganda, management of STDs in a region where the epidemic was still in an early stage resulted in decreasing HIV incidence in the communities. However, in a study in the Rakai district of Tanzania, periodic mass treatment of at-risk adults for STDs (using several broad-spectrum antibiotics) did not result in a decrease in HIV incidence. In this report, the HIV epidemic was already much more advanced (16% of the adult population infected), and there was a high prevalence of untreated HSV infection. Studies are underway to evaluate whether chronic HSV suppression with oral acyclovir may decrease HIV transmission or acquisition in HSV-infected persons.

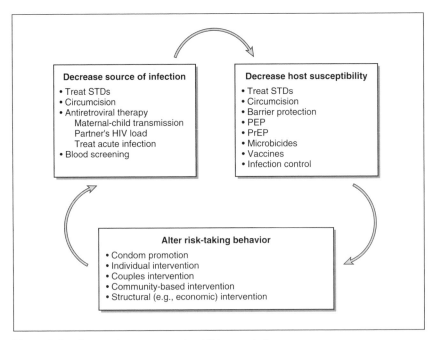

Figure 1-1.   Approaches to preventing HIV transmission.

Mother-to-Child Transmission

Another approach is the reduction of mother-to-child spread of HIV (see Chapter 11). The first study to demonstrate the utility of antiretroviral therapy in decreasing HIV transmission used zidovudine (ZDV) monotherapy in the mother starting in the 24th week of pregnancy through delivery and in the newborn until 6 weeks postpartum. It resulted in a decrease in the rate from 25.5% to 8.3%. Subsequent studies have indicated that shorter-course treatment for the mother at the time that labor begins and postpartum treatment for the infant are particularly important in reducing transmission. The level of the maternal plasma viral load has been an important predictor of the likelihood of HIV transmission. In a study in Uganda, a single dose of nevirapine (NVP) given to the mother when labor commenced and a single postpartum dose to the infant resulted in decreasing the rate of transmission from 25.1% to 13.1%. Other factors that may increase the likelihood of mother-to-child transmission include premature birth, chorioamnionitis, maternal genital tract infection, and premature rupture of the membranes. Postnatally, infants can acquire HIV infection through breast-feeding, particularly if breast milk is mixed with other types of nutrition. It has been postulated that mixed feeding in neonates may present more antigens to the immature gut, and inflammation may facilitate gastrointestinal HIV transmission. In the developed world, where women generally have access to antiretroviral therapy, obstetric care, and formula to feed their infants, HIV transmission rates are consistently less than 5%.

Antiretroviral Therapy and Postexposure Prophylaxis

The use of antiretroviral therapy to decrease the infectiousness of people living with HIV may also facilitate prevention of viral transmission. However, recent studies have suggested that in communities where the availability of antiretroviral therapy is not accompanied by a decrease in risk-taking behavior, HIV transmission may continue to occur at high levels. For example, among men who have sex with men in San Francisco, the rate of rectal gonorrhea has increased, and the incidence of HIV infection has risen. Moreover, because antiretroviral therapy does not sterilize the genital tract, there is the potential for transmission of resistant HIV strains. Surveillance at six different sentinel sites in the United States between 1995 and 2000 found that among newly HIV-infected patients, the rate of resistance to at least one drug increased from 3.5% to 14.1% (Table 1-3). Thus, if antiretroviral therapy is to have the beneficial impact of slowing the transmission of HIV infection, attention must be paid to continued risk-reduction counseling, as well as to monitoring of medication adherence.

An additional potential use of antiretroviral therapy is PEP (see Chapter 12). Animal data suggest that if PEP is to be beneficial it must be instituted

Table 1-3.   Transmission of Resistant Virus

	1995-1998 (%)	1999-2000 (%)	P Value
At least one drug	3.5	14.1	0.001
NRTI	2.7	8.2	0.03
NNRTI	1.3	7.1	0.007
PI	0.4	8.2	0.0001
≥2 Drug classes (MDR)	0.4	5.8	0.002

MDR = multidrug-resistant; NNRTI = non-nucleoside reverse-transcriptase inhibitor; NRTI = nucleoside reverse-transcriptase inhibitor; PI = protease inhibitor. (From Little SJ, Daar ES, Holte S, et al. Persistence of transmitted drug resistance among subjects with primary HIV infection not receiving antiretroviral therapy. 9th Conference on Retroviruses and Opportunistic Infections. Seattle; 24-28 February 2002. Abstract 95; with permission.)

within 72 hours of exposure and maintained for 28 days. The only clinical data supporting PEP comes from a retrospective case-controlled study from the era of ZDV monotherapy that suggested that the use of ZDV after needle-stick exposures among health care workers resulted in a five-fold decrease in the rate of HIV transmission. In general, two drugs (e.g., ZDV and lamivudine [3TC]) are used for occupational PEP in low-to-moderate risk exposures, with a third drug (e.g., efavirenz or lopinavir/ritonavir) added for higher-risk exposures.

Because of the effectiveness of occupational PEP and animal studies showing that antiretroviral therapy can be protective after mucosal challenges, health care workers are increasingly being asked to make these drugs available to persons who are exposed to HIV sexually or from sharing needles (nonoccupational PEP; see Chapter 12). In a cohort of Brazilian men who have sex with men, participants were given ZDV/3TC "starter packs" and instructed by study staff to practice safer sex but, if they did have unprotected contact with a known or suspected HIV partner, to start the antiretroviral drugs within 72 hours and use them for 28 days. Of the men in the cohort who had sexual risks, one-half used the antiretroviral drugs and the other half did not. There were ten acute infections in the group that did not use antiretroviral drugs compared with one infection in the group that did. Although not a randomized controlled trial, the Brazilian study suggests that the prompt use of antiretroviral drugs after a high-risk sexual exposure may be beneficial.

Given that the per-contact risk for HIV transmission without PEP is low, any use of antiretroviral therapy after a sexual or needle-stick exposure should be accompanied by risk-reduction counseling. Several studies have documented increased risk-taking behaviors in the United States as of late, particularly in men who have sex with men, because of the perception of HIV infection as a treatable condition. However, none of them has identified knowledge about PEP as a reason for increased risk taking.

Animal studies also suggest that providing antiretroviral drugs before a challenge with HIV, an approach known as pre-exposure prophylaxis (PrEP), may be protective. Several studies are underway to examine whether PrEP is safe and effective in humans. Concern has been raised that the perception that antiretroviral drugs prevent HIV transmission might lead to increased risk taking by some uninfected persons. Balancing it is the recognition that, unlike a vaccine or microbicide, which remains theoretical, PrEP, if efficacious, could be made available to patients today.

HIV Antibody Testing

The use of HIV antibody testing in the prevention of HIV infection in the United States is so well established that it seems almost routine. One important example is the screening of blood products. The transmission of HIV via infected blood in developed countries over the past two decades has been exceedingly rare. In other parts of the world, where the relative cost of screening is high, blood supplies may not be as safe. Another intervention for preventing HIV transmission is the recommendation that HIV antibody testing be performed in all pregnant women. The patient declining to be screened because of the perception of not being at risk or the obstetrician/gynecologist's failure to offer the test may be contributing factors for perinatal transmission.

The recent recommendations of the Centers for Disease Control and Prevention to include HIV antibody testing as part of the routine health care maintenance of healthy adults and adolescents may over time reduce the number of HIV-infected persons who are unaware of their serostatus. As these recommendations are implemented, the hope is that decreased HIV transmission will result through a reduction in risk behaviors and the institution of antiretroviral therapy in appropriate patients.

Vaccine Development

An ultimate goal of HIV prevention is to develop a safe and effective anti-HIV vaccine. At the present time, the search for a vaccine has been hindered by the lack of an appropriate animal model, as well as the cost of vaccine research using existing protocols. The chimpanzee immune system is closest to the human but does not develop AIDS when challenged with HIV. Rhesus macaques have an immune system that is reasonably homologous to humans, and they develop AIDS. However, one cannot automatically extrapolate results of monkey studies to humans.

An additional impediment to HIV vaccine development is the lack of consensus among researchers as to the best correlates of immunity to study in evaluating whether a vaccine candidate should undergo extensive field trials. Because HIV can infect animals and probably humans as either cell-free or cell-associated virus, it is not clear whether antibodies, cytotoxic

T-lymphocytes, or a combination of both are necessary to protect people against HIV. Antibodies are useful in binding free virus, whereas cytotoxic T-lymphocytes are more effective in eliminating cell-associated virus.

Several vaccine prototypes have been based on presenting subunits of the virus envelope in order to generate antienvelope antibodies. These antibodies have been shown to block infection in animal models when challenged with laboratory strains and some naturally occurring strains. However, researchers are concerned that such antibodies may not be effective against many HIV strains in newly infected populations. In addition, these antibodies generally do not prevent cell-associated HIV challenge. The largest vaccine trials to date, using a preparation called AIDSVAX based on the HIV gp120 envelope glycoprotein, were conducted in the United States, Canada, the Netherlands, and Thailand. Unfortunately, the results did not demonstrate its efficacy.

Researchers have more recently been involved in developing vaccines designed to generate cytotoxic T-lymphocytes. Several different vaccine vectors are being studied, including canarypox, Venezuelan equine virus, *Salmonella*, and other microbial platforms. These vaccines use an intact, but avirulent, biological organism which has had HIV antigens inserted into their genomes. These agents can then be presented to the human immune system in a way in which expressed antigens generate cytotoxic T-lymphocytes that recognize HIV-specific antigens. There have been T-cell responses to several of these vaccines, and vaccines using adenovirus have demonstrated responses of a sufficient magnitude to warrant the initiation of efficacy trials.

Additional studies are underway to evaluate the utility of giving both a subunit vaccine to produce antibodies and a cell-associated vaccine to produce cytotoxic T-cells, in order to have both arms of the immune system activated to prevent the transmission of cell-free and cell-associated virus. The use of "naked" DNA and interleukin-2 to optimize host immune responses is also being assessed.

Microbicide Development

Another approach to HIV prevention is the development of microbicidal drugs that can be used as lubricants during sexual activity (Table 1-4). Thus far, none of these compounds has been shown to be safe or effective, but several remain under investigation.

The best known microbicide is nonoxynyl-9 (N-9), which has been commercially marketed in several products as a spermicide and sexual lubricant. N-9 acts as a detergent, increasing the permeability of microbial cell membranes. In vitro, N-9 was found to inhibit a wide array of sexually transmitted pathogens including HIV. Unfortunately, several large clinical trials have now failed to demonstrate any protective activity of N-9 when used in vivo. It is possible that the failure of N-9 to protect women against HIV is related to its irritant properties. White blood cells and cytokines that

Table 1-4.   Microbicides Being Evaluated for Prevention of HIV Transmission

Mechanism of Action	Examples
Surfactant	• Nonoxynyl-9 • Belalkonium chloride • Chlorhexidine • C 31-G
Acid-buffering agent	• Buffergel • Acigel
Natural product	• Lactobacillus suppository • Cyanovirin
Inhibitor of viral entry	• Carageenan • PRO 2000 • Dextrin sulfate • Soluble CD4
Inhibitor of HIV replication	• Tenofovir • Fusion inhibitors • Integrase inhibitors

increase HIV expression are increased in the genital tract after exposure to the product. N-9 is not recommended as a preventive lubricant to prevent HIV transmission but in low concentrations is still marketed as a contraceptive gel.

Several other promising candidates that act by different mechanisms are currently being evaluated in clinical trials. An acidic vaginal pH has been associated with decreased transmission of STDs. However, semen is a base buffer and transiently raises pH after ejaculation during intercourse. One group of prospective compounds maintains the acidic environment of the vagina in the presence of semen. Certain microbes, particularly lactobacilli, produce organic acids in the vagina that are protective against HIV transmission and are being studied as a suppository. Another group of compounds inhibits HIV binding to mucosal surfaces, and several are being evaluated for efficacy. Other candidate compounds include antiretroviral drugs, such as tenofovir gel, which have been shown to protect animals from HIV transmission.

To demonstrate that vaccines or microbicides are effective raises some ethical and logistical dilemmas. No clinical researcher would ever want to have subjects become infected with HIV, but at the same time, to prove that a product works, new infections need to be identified in the control group. Researchers have to recruit large cohorts of high-risk people into these studies and provide state-of-the-art HIV risk-reduction counseling in order to minimize the likelihood of new infections. The more successful the staff are in counseling people to prevent HIV infection, the fewer seroconversions will occur and the harder it will be to prove that a specific product is effective. Thus, for many of the vaccine and microbicide studies, enrollment of 5000 to 10,000 people is necessary. The cost of each trial ranges from tens to hundreds of million dollars. These challenges have ensured a deliberative, but slow, developmental process.

Behavioral Approaches

The decision to engage in an HIV risk behavior is a complex one that may involve issues related to early life events, low self-esteem, contextual issues in relationships, interpersonal power dynamics, and substance use. Thus, no one behavioral approach will invariably lead to an adaptation of consistent safer sexual or drug-using practices (see Chapter 2). However, several studies have now indicated that the provision of individual counseling and/or small group sessions can be helpful in assisting people in moderating their risk. Good elements of risk-reduction programs include the ability of the counselor to approach the patient in a nonjudgmental manner to elicit a realistic assessment of the person's pattern of risk-taking behavior. Given the slow progress in vaccine and microbicide development, the role of the primary care provider in patient education, discussion of risk-taking behavior, initiation of risk-reduction counseling, and triage to appropriate prevention services is an essential part of HIV prevention.

KEY POINTS

- Because multiple cofactors are involved in HIV transmission, it is difficult to determine the absolute risk of infection for specific sexual exposures. However, relative risks have been estimated.
- Some of the factors that affect the efficiency with which HIV infection is transmitted are 1) the amount of virus in genital secretions, 2) the number of target cells that bind HIV, 3) the presence of STDs or noninfectious causes of genital tract inflammation, 4) the type of microflora that colonize the vagina, 5) specific characteristics of the infecting viral strain, and 6) physiologic events that increase exposure of the endocervix to HIV (e.g., use of hormonal contraceptives).
- A lower plasma HIV concentration is generally, but not always, associated with reduced risk of transmission. Local factors such as STDs may result in a higher viral concentration in the genital tract without an upregulation of HIV expression in the blood.
- Direct intravascular exposure to HIV carries the greatest risk of transmission. Shared needle use by injection-drug users is much more likely to transmit HIV than an occupational needle stick.
- While vaccine and microbicide development offer hope for HIV prevention, emphasis today must be placed on behavioral approaches and the appropriate use of PEP.

SUGGESTED READINGS

Blower SM, Aschenbach AN, Gershengorn HB, Kahn JO. Predicting the unpredictable: transmission of drug-resistant HIV. Nat Med. 2001;7:1016-20.

Centers for Disease Control and Prevention. HIV prevention through early detection and treatment of other sexually transmitted diseases. United States recommendations of the Advisory Committee for HIV and STD Prevention. MMWR. 1998;47(RR-12): 1-24.

Centers for Disease Control and Prevention. Prevention Research Synthesis Project. Compendium of HIV prevention interventions with evidence of effectiveness. March 1999: 1-57. Available at http://www.cdc.gov/hiv/pubs/hivcompendium.pdf.

Centers for Disease Control and Prevention. Updated U.S. Public Health Service guidelines for the management of occupational exposures to HIV and recommendations for postexposure prophylaxis. MMWR. 2005;54(RR-9):1-17.

Centers for Disease Control and Prevention. Antiretroviral postexposure prophylaxis after sexual, injection drug use, other nonoccupational exposure to HIV in the United States, Recommendations from the US Department of Health and Human Services. MMWR. 2005;54(RR-2):1-19.

Centers for Disease Control and Prevention. Revised recommendations for HIV testing of adults, adolescents, and pregnant women in health-care settings. MMWR. 2006; 55(RR-14):1-17.

DeGruttola V, Seage GR 3rd, Mayer KH, Horsburgh CR Jr. Infectiousness of HIV between male homosexual partners. J Clin Epidemiol. 1989;42:849-56.

de Vincenzi I. A longitudinal study of human immunodeficiency virus transmission by heterosexual partners. European Study Group on Heterosexual Transmission of HIV. N Engl J Med. 1994;331:341-6.

Dilley JW, Woods WJ, McFarland W. Are advances in treatment changing views about high-risk sex? [Letter]. N Engl J Med. 1997;337:501-2.

European Study Group on Heterosexual Transmission of HIV. Comparison of female to male and male to female transmission of HIV in 563 stable couples. BMJ. 1992;304:809-13.

Fleming DT, Wasserheit JN. From epidemiological synergy to public health policy and practice: the contribution of other sexually transmitted diseases to sexual transmission of HIV infection. Sex Transm Infect. 1999;75:3-17.

Fredman L, Rabin DL, Bowman M, Bandemer C, Sardeson K, Taggart VS, et al. Primary care physicians' assessment and prevention of HIV infection. Am J Prev Med. 1989;5:188-95.

Gerbert B, Bronstone A, Pantilat S, McPhee S, Allerton M, Moe J. When asked, patients tell: disclosure of sensitive health-risk behaviors. Med Care. 1999;37:104-11.

Gibson DR, Flynn NM, Perales D. Effectiveness of syringe exchange programs in reducing HIV risk behavior and HIV seroconversion among injecting drug users [Editorial]. AIDS. 2001;15:1329-41.

Grosskurth H, Mosha F, Todd J, Mwijarubi E, Klokke A, Senkoro K, et al. Impact of improved treatment of sexually transmitted diseases on HIV infection in rural Tanzania: randomised controlled trial. Lancet. 1995;346:530-6.

Gupta P, Mellors J, Kingsley L, Riddler S, Singh MK, Schreiber S, et al. High viral load in semen of human immunodeficiency virus type 1-infected men at all stages of disease and its reduction by therapy with protease and nonnucleoside reverse transcriptase inhibitors. J Virol. 1997;71:6271-5.

Heimer R, Khoshnood K, Bigg D, Guydish J, Junge B. Syringe use and reuse: effects of syringe exchange programs in four cities. J Acquir Immune Defic Syndr Hum Retrovirol. 1998;18 (Suppl 1):S37-44.

Janssen RS, Holtgrave DR, Valdiserri RO, Shepherd M, Gayle HD, De Cock KM. The Serostatus Approach to Fighting the HIV Epidemic: prevention strategies for infected individuals. Am J Public Health. 2001;91:1019-24.

Johnson AM, Petherick A, Davidson SJ, Brettle R, Hooker M, Howard L, et al. Transmission of HIV to heterosexual partners of infected men and women. AIDS. 1989;3:367-72.

Kamb ML, Fishbein M, Douglas JM Jr, Rhodes F, Rogers J, Bolan G, et al. Efficacy of risk-reduction counseling to prevent human immunodeficiency virus and sexually transmitted diseases: a randomized controlled trial. Project RESPECT Study Group. JAMA. 1998;280:1161-7.

Katz MH, Gerberding JL. The care of persons with recent sexual exposure to HIV. Ann Intern Med. 1998;128:306-12.

Kelly JA, Otto-Salaj LL, Sikkema KJ, Pinkerton SD, Bloom FR. Implications of HIV treatment advances for behavioral research on AIDS: protease inhibitors and new challenges in HIV secondary prevention. Health Psychol. 1998;17:310-9.

Lee TH, Sakahara N, Fiebig E, Busch MP, O'Brien TR, Herman SA. Correlation of HIV-1 RNA levels in plasma and heterosexual transmission of HIV-1 from infected transfusion recipients [Letter]. J Acquir Immune Defic Syndr Hum Retrovirol. 1996;12:427-8.

Leynaert B, Downs AM, de Vincenzi I. Heterosexual transmission of human immunodeficiency virus: variability of infectivity throughout the course of infection. European Study Group on Heterosexual Transmission of HIV. Am J Epidemiol. 1998;148:88-96.

Lollis CM, Strothers HS, Chitwood DD, McGhee M. Sex, drugs, and HIV: does methadone maintenance reduce drug use and risky sexual behavior? J Behav Med. 2000;23:545-57.

Macke BA, Maher JE. Partner notification in the United States: an evidence-based review. Am J Prev Med. 1999;17:230-42.

Marks G, Burris S, Peterman TA. Reducing sexual transmission of HIV from those who know they are infected: the need for personal and collective responsibility [Editorial]. AIDS. 1999;13:297-306.

Mayer KH, Klausner JD, Handsfield HH. Intersecting epidemics and educable moments: sexually transmitted disease risk assessment and screening in men who have sex with men [Editorial]. Sex Transm Dis. 2001;28:464-7.

Metzger DS, Navaline H, Woody GE. Drug abuse treatment as AIDS prevention. Public Health Rep. 1998;113 Suppl 1:97-106.

Mofenson LM, McIntyre JA. Advances and research directions in the prevention of mother-to-child HIV-1 transmission. Lancet. 2000;355:2237-44.

Needle RH, Coyle SL, Normand J, Lambert E, Cesari H. HIV prevention with drug-using populations—current status and future prospects: introduction and overview. Public Health Rep. 1998;113(Suppl 1):4-18.

Nicolosi A, Corrêa Leite ML, Musicco M, Arici C, Gavazzeni G, Lazzarin A. The efficiency of male-to-female and female-to-male sexual transmission of the human immunodeficiency virus: a study of 730 stable couples. Italian Study Group on HIV Heterosexual Transmission. Epidemiology. 1994;5:570-5.

Operskalski EA, Stram DO, Busch MP, Huang W, Harris M, Dietrich SL, et al. Role of viral load in heterosexual transmission of human immunodeficiency virus type 1 by blood transfusion recipients. Transfusion Safety Study Group. Am J Epidemiol. 1997;146:655-61.

Peterman TA, Stoneburner RL, Allen JR, Jaffe HW, Curran JW. Risk of human immunodeficiency virus transmission from heterosexual adults with transfusion-associated infections. JAMA. 1988;259:55-8.

Quinn TC, Wawer MJ, Sewankambo N, Serwadda D, Li C, Wabwire-Mangen F, et al. Viral load and heterosexual transmission of human immunodeficiency virus type 1. Rakai Project Study Group. N Engl J Med. 2000;342:921-9.

Royce RA, Seña A, Cates W Jr., Cohen MS. Sexual transmission of HIV. N Engl J Med. 1997;336:1072-8.

Ruiz MS, Gable AR, Kaplan EH, et al., eds. Institute of Medicine/Committee on HIV Prevention Strategies in the United States. No Time to Lose: Getting More from HIV Prevention. Washington, DC: National Academy Press; 2001.

Scheer S, Chu PL, Klausner JD, Katz MH, Schwarcz SK. Effect of highly active antiretroviral therapy on diagnoses of sexually transmitted diseases in people with AIDS. Lancet. 2001;357:432-5.

Shain RN, Piper JM, Newton ER, Perdue ST, Ramos R, Champion JD, et al. A randomized, controlled trial of a behavioral intervention to prevent sexually transmitted disease among minority women. N Engl J Med. 1999;340:93-100.

Stall RD, Hays RB, Waldo CR, Ekstrand M, McFarland W. The Gay '90s: a review of research in the 1990s on sexual behavior and HIV risk among men who have sex with men. AIDS. 2000;14 Suppl 3:S101-14.

STD Control Program and the HIV/AIDS Control Program, Public Health—Seattle & King County, Seattle, Washington, USA. Sexually transmitted disease and HIV screening guidelines for men who have sex with men. Sex Transm Dis. 2001;28:457-9.

Valleroy LA, MacKellar DA, Karon JM, Rosen DH, McFarland W, Shehan DA, et al. HIV prevalence and associated risks in young men who have sex with men. Young Men's Survey Study Group. JAMA. 2000;284:198-204.

Vernazza PL, Gilliam BL, Dyer J, Fiscus SA, Eron JJ, Frank AC, et al. Quantification of HIV in semen: correlation with antiviral treatment and immune status. AIDS. 1997;11:987-93.

Vernazza PL, Gilliam BL, Flepp M, Dyer JR, Frank AC, Fiscus SA, et al. Effect of antiviral treatment on the shedding of HIV-1 in semen. AIDS. 1997;11:1249-54.

Vittinghoff E, Douglas J, Judson F, et al. Per-contact risk of HIV transmission between male sexual partners. Am J Epidemiol. 1999;150:307-11.

Wasserheit JN. Epidemiological synergy. Interrelationships between human immunodeficiency virus infection and other sexually transmitted diseases. Sex Transm Dis. 1992;19: 61-77.

II. Pathogenesis

SIGALL K. BELL

Viral Entry and Replication

HIV is a cytopathic virus composed of a central cylindrical core of RNA surrounded by a spherical lipid envelope with glycoprotein (gp) surface markers. A number of HIV-specific antigens have been identified, including p24, gp120/160, and gp41. Successful infection of a cell requires docking and binding of HIV at two separate sites: the CD4+ receptor and a 7-transdomain chemokine receptor. Although numerous chemokine receptors are capable of serving this function, the most important of these are CCR5 and CXCR4. CCR5 is the principal coreceptor used by macrophage-tropic viral strains (R5 viruses) that predominate in early HIV infection. CXCR4 is the main coreceptor used by T-tropic viral strains (X4 viruses) that are often present in the later stages of HIV disease. Once HIV binds at the receptor/coreceptor complex, the virus fuses with the cell membrane and enters the cell. At the time of acute infection, HIV generally first encounters dendritic cells (DC) harboring the CCR5 coreceptor. DC-SIGN, an HIV-specific DC receptor, binds HIV at its gp120 domain without requiring direct infection of the cell. Infected and uninfected dendritic cells traffic to regional lymph nodes, where they present antigen and prime T lymphocytes for infection. Viral replication and dissemination ensues. The role of the gastrointestinal tract in early HIV infection is an area of active investigation. CD4+ T lymphocytes in the gut are rapidly depleted during early HIV infection with limited recovery even with treatment. Some long-term nonprogressors show reduced gut CD4 cell depletion, and early treatment of acute HIV infection may abrogate gut CD4 cell loss.

HIV contains its own reverse transcriptase, which is packaged within the viral capsid. This enzyme generates frequent errors in replication, resulting in the opportunity for rapid viral evolution and diversification. The clinical consequence is that HIV can mutate readily and escape both immunologic and pharmacologic control. The former occurs by changes in viral epitopes recognized by HLA molecules; the latter by changes at drug binding sites. Once HIV enters the cell, reverse transcription produces a DNA copy from the viral RNA template.

At this point, HIV can either undergo active viral replication or become integrated into the host genome as "proviral DNA" and enter a latent stage, which can persist indefinitely. When activation occurs, the proviral DNA transcribes genomic and messenger RNA. After viral proteins are synthesized in the replication pathway, new virions are assembled and bud from the infected cell. For budding virions to become functional, processing by a viral protease is required. Once accomplished, the virions circulate until they identify new target cells. Pharmacologic targets for almost all stages of cellular infection have been identified or are under active investigation (Figure 1-2). Left untreated, HIV infection leads to a gradual diminution of immune function in the vast majority of patients. The culmination of this immunologic

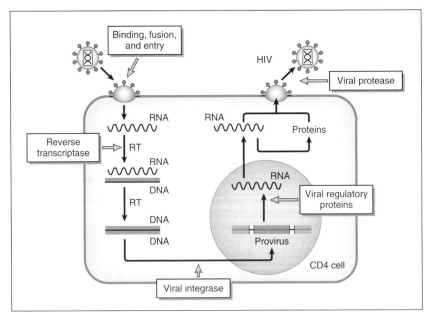

Figure 1-2.   Pharmacologic target sites of HIV/CD4 cell interaction.

deterioration is AIDS, which is characterized by the susceptibility to opportunistic infections and malignancies.

Disease Progression

Several viral and host factors affect the rate of HIV disease progression (Box 1-3).

Viral Factors

Disease progression varies based on degree of viral virulence, which is related to the following:

Syncytium Formation

Utilization of the CXCR4 coreceptor is associated with capacity for syncytium formation and more rapid disease progression. Most patients are infected with a wild-type R5 nonsyncytium-inducing (NSI) strain of HIV that does not lead to the formation of multinucleated giant cells (syncytia) in cell culture. NSI strains can mutate to syncytium-inducing (SI) strains over time and gain this capacity by switching to X4 tropic strains later in the disease course. Primary infection with an SI strain occurs in a minority of patients and has been associated with a more rapid decline in CD4 count and progression to AIDS.

Box 1-3.   Factors Affecting the Rate of HIV Disease Progression

Viral
- Syncytium formation
- Resistance
- Replication capacity

Host Genetic
- Co-receptor polymorphisms (CCR5Δ32 mutation)
- HLA type

Host Immune
- Cytotoxic T lymphocyte responses
- CD4+ proliferative responses
- Neutralizing antibodies
- Natural killer cells

Host Cellular
- APOBEC
- TRIM 5-alpha

Resistance

Resistance to antiretroviral therapy is mediated by mutations in viral genes. Most current drugs bind to and interfere with either reverse transcriptase or protease, two viral enzymes required for replication. Mutations of viral genes that code for these proteins can diminish the activity of antiretroviral drugs, usually by interfering with their ability to bind. The number of mutations required to diminish drug activity can vary considerably between classes, with only one mutation needed to develop high-level resistance to non-nucleoside reverse-transcriptase inhibitors (NNRTIs). In contrast, multiple mutations may be necessary to achieve the same effect with protease inhibitors (PIs) and with some nucleoside reverse-transcriptase inhibitors (NRTIs).

Viral resistance to antiretroviral drugs occurs in two forms: primary and acquired. Primary resistance refers to those mutations that are present at the time of acute HIV infection. The prevalence of primary resistance varies geographically, but one study showed that approximately 20% of isolates were found to harbor resistance to at least one class of antiretroviral drugs at the time of transmission, and 10% had multidrug resistance. Acquired resistance, in contrast, occurs over time in response to the selective pressure of medications. The high rate of viral replication that characterizes HIV infection, in conjunction with a relatively high reverse-transcriptase error rate, can lead to multiple mutations. In both primary and acquired resistance, genotypic mutations can compromise the effectiveness of antiretroviral drugs and result in ineffective suppression of viral replication. Antiretroviral therapy that only partially suppresses viral replication will result in the accumulation of additional mutations. Over time, resistance will develop and viral replication may increase substantially.

Replicative Capacity

Replicative capacity (RC) is a measurement of a particular viral strain's ability to generate new viral particles compared with a wild-type reference strain. It is reported as a percent (compared to wild type) on genotype testing. The factors contributing to RC are not completely understood, but the accumulation of genetic mutations generally decreases RC. Exceptions to this rule include the K103N mutation (causing decreased susceptibility to NNRTIs), which does not diminish fitness. Recently, the case of a man with primary resistance to three drug classes and rapid progression to AIDS was reported. The case generated significant publicity and concern because it represented the rare combination of multidrug-resistant virus without a decrement in viral fitness.

Host Genetic Factors

HLA Type

HLA class I haplotypes HLA-B27 and B57 have been associated with slower progression of HIV disease, whereas HLA-B35 alleles have been associated with more rapid development of AIDS in Caucasians.

CCR5Δ32 Mutation

Coreceptor polymorphisms can affect susceptibility to HIV infection. Persons who are homozygous for a 32-base-pair deletion in CCR5 are more resistant to infection with R5 strains. Persons who are heterozygous for the 32bp deletion may have a decreased risk of HIV disease progression and possibly a decreased risk of becoming infected. Among people of Western European descent, approximately 18% are heterozygous and 1% homozygous for the mutant CCR5Δ32 allele.

Host Immune Factors

The relative strength and breadth of the immune response can affect HIV disease progression. Initial control of viremia is temporally correlated with the appearance of HIV-specific cytotoxic T-lymphocyte (CTL) responses. HIV-specific CTL cells can be detected as early as 3 weeks after the onset of symptoms of primary infection and weeks before the development of neutralizing antibodies. HIV-specific CD4+ proliferative responses also play a role in disease control and have been found to be preserved in some long-term nonprogressors. Neutralizing antibodies probably contribute to viral suppression but generally appear later in the course of infection (average 4 to 6 months). The role of natural killer (NK) cells is also under investigation. HIV antibodies typically appear by 3 to 12 weeks following infection but can take up to 6 to 12 months to be detectable. Early treatment of acute HIV infection has been associated with lack of evolution or seroreversion of HIV antibodies in some instances. The clinical significance of these observations is unknown.

Host Cellular Factors

Several host cellular cofactors of viral replication have been identified that can promote infection. These include factors that aid virus entry (receptors and coreceptors), regulate viral gene expression (Tat, cyclin, Rev, Crm-1), and facilitate viral budding. Other host cofactors confer protection against viral infection, presumptively originating as innate cellular defenses to primate lentivirus replication.

APOBEC

The first such cellular defense to be identified is the APOBEC enzyme family. The mechanism by which APOBEC proteins block HIV infection remains to be fully characterized but is thought to be through catastrophic mutations in viral cDNA during reverse transcription, resulting in nonfunctional cDNA or cDNA that is targeted for destruction. HIV has a direct interaction with APOBEC; the viral accessory protein Vif depletes the infected cell of APOBEC. The Vif-APOBEC interaction has become an attractive target for therapeutic intervention.

TRIM 5-alpha

A second cellular restriction factor named TRIM 5-alpha was recently identified and is thought to interfere with viral uncoating upon cell entry.

Viral Dynamics

It is estimated that 10 billion viral particles are produced each day in the untreated HIV-infected patient. The cytopathic effect of viral replication is the postulated cause of CD4+ lymphocyte depletion and progressive immune deterioration. Plasma viremia reflects the net result of two opposing forces: viral production and viral clearance. During primary HIV infection, when activated CD4 lymphocytes are plentiful and the host HIV-specific immune response is minimal or absent, the plasma viral load often exceeds one million copies/mL. With the development of HIV-specific CD4 lymphocyte and CTL responses, the concentration of HIV-RNA declines precipitously and after a period of 6 to 12 months stabilizes at a set point (Figure 1-3). The viral and host factors discussed above may play a role in determining this value.

The development of effective drugs to slow HIV replication has led to an improved understanding of viral dynamics in the infected host. Measuring the slope of the initial fall in viremia after initiating antiretroviral therapy has permitted estimation of the plasma half-life of HIV virions to be 6 hours, implying a dynamic process of viral production and clearance.

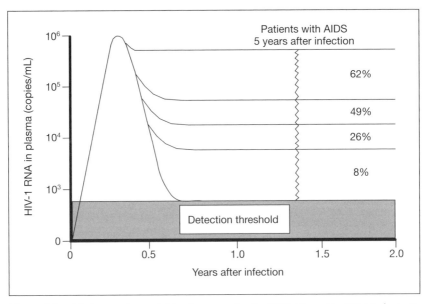

Figure 1-3. Viral set point and risk of progression to AIDS. (From Ho DD. Viral counts count in HIV infection. Science. 1996;272:1124-5; with permission. © 1996 by AAAS.)

The decline of plasma HIV RNA in response to treatment occurs in two phases. An initial rapid decline, which is characterized by a 1- to 2-log drop in viral load, occurs over approximately 2 weeks. This is believed to represent the rapid clearance of productively infected CD4 lymphocytes. A second, slower-decay phase may represent a virus produced by longer-living, chronically infected cells or by latently infected cells that have been activated to produce virus. The demonstration by model analyses that over 60 years of antiretroviral therapy would be required to eradicate infection from reservoir sites has shifted the treatment paradigm from "cure" to "control." Viral replication still occurs at low levels in patients receiving suppressive antiretroviral therapy and may contribute to the formation of genetic mutations and escape from pharmacologic and immunologic control.

The level of HIV RNA (viral load) in the plasma is a useful clinical marker of disease progression. The plasma viral load generally correlates with viral replication in other tissue compartments, but this association is not necessarily linear or consistent. For example, presence of an STD can increase local HIV replication in the genital compartment.

Reservoirs and Compartments

Cellular reservoirs for HIV infection are established early in infection. Because these "resting" cells are not actively multiplying, HIV antigens are not expressed and the virus cannot be targeted by antiretroviral drugs. HIV may also reside in "immunologic" havens, where it is not as readily identified, or in anatomic compartments (e.g., central nervous system [CNS]), where therapeutic antiretroviral drug levels may not be readily available. The relative differences in drug penetration result in distinct viral dynamics and evolution in these compartments. For example, different resistance patterns in a virus isolated from a patient's plasma and CNS have been demonstrated.

Immune Reconstitution

The institution of antiretroviral therapy can dramatically reduce the plasma viral load and increase the CD4 cell count, resulting in enhanced responses to antigen stimulation and a decrease in opportunistic infections. To date, however, experience suggests that immune function improvement may be incomplete in some patients. A broad disruption of CD4 lymphocyte function occurs as a consequence of HIV infection, and subpopulations of these cells may be irrecoverable despite treatment. The large increase in CD4 lymphocytes that is observed in some patients on antiretroviral therapy may represent an expansion of a limited number of CD4 cell clones, resulting in only partial reconstitution of the host immune system. In some instances, immune reconstitution may be associated with a clinical syndrome manifesting as a "flare" in underlying opportunistic infections caused by cytomegalovirus

(CMV), *Mycobacterium tuberculosis, Mycobacterium avium* complex (MAC), *Cryptococcus neoformans*, JC virus (progressive multifocal leukoencephalopathy), and other pathogens. These immune reconstitution syndromes are generally inflammatory in nature and can be managed with treatment of the opportunistic infection and the use of antiinflammatory drugs (see Chapter 9).

KEY POINTS

- HIV infection is established by viral entry into cells bearing the CD4+ cell surface receptor and associated coreceptor molecules.
- The deterioration of immune function that is characteristic of HIV infection occurs through CD4 lymphocyte depletion, which is caused primarily by viral replication.
- The gut has been recognized as an important site for early CD4 cell depletion and likely plays a key role in acute HIV infection.
- The rate of HIV disease progression can be affected by a number of different host and viral factors including coreceptor polymorphisms (CCR5Δ32 mutation), HLA type, viral replication capacity, breadth and strength of the immune response, and innate host cellular factors.
- Cellular reservoirs of latent HIV are established early in infection and have changed the treatment paradigm from "cure" to "control." The relative differences of drug penetration into different anatomic compartments can result in independent viral dynamics, evolution, and resistance patterns.
- HIV replicates rapidly in untreated patients, with estimates of up to 10 billion viral particles produced each day. Random-point mutations are common because of its error-prone reverse transcriptase.
- High-level viral resistance may develop over time in patients receiving antiretroviral therapy from mutations that confer drug resistance.

SUGGESTED READINGS

Boden D, Hurley A, Zhang L, et al. HIV-1 drug resistance in newly infected individuals. JAMA. 1999;282:1135-41.

Finzi D, Blankson J, Siliciano JD, et al. Latent infection of CD4+ T cells provides a mechanism for lifelong persistence of HIV-1, even in patients on effective combination therapy. Nat Med. 1999;5:512-7.

Geijtenbeek T, van Kooyk Y. DC-SIGN: a novel HIV receptor on DCs that mediates HIV-1 transmission [Review]. Curr Top Microbiol Immunol 2003;276:31-54.

Koup RA, Safrit JT, Cao Y, et al. Temporal association of cellular immune responses with the initial control of viremia in primary human immunodeficiency virus type 1 syndrome. J Virol. 1994;68:4650-5.

Little SJ, Daar ES, D'Aquila RT, et al. Reduced antiretroviral drug susceptibility among patients with primary HIV infection. JAMA. 1999;282:1142-9.

Little SJ, Holte S, Routy JP, et al. Antiretroviral-drug resistance among patients recently infected with HIV. N Engl J Med. 2002;347:385-94.

Markowitz M, Mohri H, Mehandru S, et al. Infection with multidrug resistant, dual-tropic HIV-1 and rapid progression to AIDS: a case report. Lancet. 2005;365:1031-8.

Michael NL, Chang G, Louie LG, et al. The role of viral phenotype and CCR-5 gene defects in HIV-1 transmission and disease progression. Nat Med. 1997;3:338-40.

Montefiori DC, Hill TS, Vo HT, et al. Neutralizing antibodies associated with viremia control in a subset of individuals after treatment of acute human immunodeficiency virus type 1 infection. J Virol. 2001;75:10200-7.

Moore JP, Kitchen SG, Pugach P, Zack JA. The CCR5 and CXCR4 coreceptors—central to understanding the transmission and pathogenesis of human immunodeficiency virus type 1 infection. AIDS Res Hum Retroviruses. 2004;20:111-26.

Musey L, Hughes J, Schacker T, et al. Cytotoxioc T-cell responses, viral load, and disease progression in early human immunodeficiency virus type 1 infection. N Engl J Med. 1997;337:1267-74.

Niu MT, Jermano JA, Reichelderfer P, Schnittman SM. Summary of the National Institutes of Health workshop on primary human immunodeficiency virus type 1 infection. AIDS Res Hum Retroviruses. 1993;9:913-24.

Samson M, Libert F, Doranz BJ, et al. Resistance to HIV-1 infection in Caucasian individuals bearing mutant alleles of the CCR-5 chemokine-receptor gene. Nature. 1996;382:722-5.

Tang J, Shelton B, Makhatadze N, et al. Distribution of chemokine receptor CCR2 and CCR5 genotypes and their relative contribution to human immunodeficiency type 1 (HIV-1) seroconversion, early HIV-1 RNA concentration in plasma, and later disease progression. J Virol. 2002;76:662-72.

Troyer RM, Collins KR, Abraha A, et al. Changes in human immunodeficiency virus type 1 fitness and genetic diversity during disease progression. J Virol. 2005;79:9006-18.]

Zhang L, Ramratnam B, Tenner-Racz K, et al. Quantifying residual HIV-1 replication in patients receiving combination antiretroviral therapy. N Engl J Med. 1994;340:1605-13.

III. Natural History
SIGALL K. BELL

Acute HIV Infection

Acute HIV infection, also called primary HIV infection, is defined as the time from initial HIV infection until HIV antibody seroconversion. Acute retroviral syndrome (ARS) refers to the clinical manifestations associated with it. The formation of HIV-specific antibodies marks the completion of seroconversion; antibodies are often detectable within 3 to 12 weeks of infection but may take up to 6 to 12 months in some patients. Early HIV infection is less clearly defined but generally refers to the first 6 to 12 months of infection, after antibody has been formed. This stage is clinically important because of the establishment of the viral "set point," the magnitude of which correlates with the rate of HIV disease progression.

Infection with HIV typically occurs across mucosal surfaces or by percutaneous inoculation. The virus first encounters dendritic cells and is transported to regional lymph nodes. HIV resides and replicates in lymphoid tissue for days to weeks. Once HIV infects a cell, the virus either can begin replicating immediately or can integrate into host genome resulting in latent infection. The establishment of such latently infected cellular reservoirs has been shown to occur early in infection. Rapid replication in actively infected cells results in widespread dissemination. Estimated time to viremia has been reported as early as 4 to 11 days after exposure. The average incubation period from infection to onset of ARS is 2 weeks, which typically coincides with high-level viremia and the host's initial immunologic responses. Both viral cytopathic effect and immune-mediated toxicity including cytokine elaboration likely contribute to the clinical manifestations of ARS.

Peak viremia during acute HIV infection can reach several million copies/mL, which is higher than at any other disease stage. Several studies have now correlated an increased risk of transmission during acute HIV infection. Wawer and colleagues demonstrated that transmission during early infection was 10 to 12 times higher than in chronic infection, raising public health issues related to recognition of early infection to prevent "unknowing transmission."

Acute Retroviral Syndrome

An estimated 40% to 90% of patients with acute HIV infection experience ARS. Its severity varies from a subclinical presentation to manifestations requiring hospitalization. Symptoms typically occur 2 to 6 weeks from exposure and include fever, night sweats, fatigue, weight loss, pharyngitis (often severe), rash, lymphadenopathy, myalgias, headache, nausea, vomiting, and diarrhea (Table 1-5).

The rash of ARS is a diffuse, erythematous, maculopapular eruption that can involve the trunk and extremities and occasionally the face, palms, and soles. A vesicular, pustular exanthem also has been reported, as have urticaria and genital and anal ulcers. HIV-associated oral ulcers are similar in appearance to aphthous ulcers but have a surrounding zone of erythema. They may involve the lips, tongue, floor of the mouth, palate, tonsils, and uvula.

Neurologic manifestations include aseptic meningitis (present in 24% of patients in one series), cranial nerve VII palsy, and radiculopathy. Other unusual presentations of ARS include acute renal failure, rhabdomyolysis, myopericarditis, pulmonary alveolitis, and Guillain-Barré syndrome. Patients may occasionally present with opportunistic infections, including *Pneumocystis jiroveci* (previously *Pneumocystis carinii* pneumonia [PCP]), esophageal candidiasis, or CMV infection, related to a transient acute decrease in the CD4 cell count. Frequently associated laboratory findings include leukopenia, thrombocytopenia, and mildly increased serum transaminase levels.

Table 1-5.   Symptoms, Signs, and Laboratory Abnormalities Associated with Acute Retroviral Syndrome

Fever	>80-90%
Fatigue	>70-90%
Rash	50-60%
Myalgia/arthralgia	50-70%
Pharyngitis	50-70%
Night sweats	50%
Nausea/vomiting/diarrhea	30-60%
Leukopenia/thrombocytopenia	40-45%
Weight loss	25%
Aseptic meningitis	24%
Anorexia	21%
Increased serum transaminases	20%
Oral ulcers	10-20%
Genital ulcers	5-15%

Adapted from Kahn JO, Walker BD. Acute human immunodeficiency virus type 1 infection. N Engl J Med. 1998;339:33-9.

Symptoms of ARS typically last 2 to 4 weeks but can continue for as long as 10 or more weeks. Some studies have suggested that increased intensity or duration of ARS symptoms is correlated with more rapid disease progression. Initiation of antiretroviral therapy for acute infection can expedite resolution of ARS.

Diagnosis

The protean clinical manifestations of acute HIV infection give rise to a broad differential diagnosis, including both infectious and noninfectious etiologies (Box 1-4). Mild or subclinical presentations with a "flu-like" illness also make the diagnosis particularly challenging and result in significant underdiagnosis of this condition. ARS is accurately diagnosed in only 19% to 26% of patients presenting at primary care facilities, urgent care centers, and emergency departments.

One study of unselected visits to an inner city hospital emergency department showed that 0.3% of patients had ARS regardless of the presenting complaint. In another study, 1% of all patients with a "viral-like" illness were diagnosed with ARS in an urban urgent care clinic. Similarly, 1% of patients presenting with a mononucleosis-like illness with a negative heterophile antibody assay (monospot) were found to have ARS.

Making the diagnosis of acute HIV infection requires maintaining a high clinical index of suspicion and incorporating history-taking and careful examination skills. It should be considered in the differential diagnosis in

---

Box 1-4.   Differential Diagnosis of Acute Retroviral Syndrome

Viral
- Epstein-Barr virus
- Cytomegalovirus
- Primary HSV
- Influenza
- Viral hepatitis
- Parvovirus B19
- Rubella

Bacterial
- Streptococcal disease
- Secondary syphilis
- Lyme disease
- Rickettsial disease
- Disseminated gonococcal infection

Non-infectious
- Adult Still's disease
- Systemic lupus erythematosus
- Systemic vasculitides

Adapted from Kassutto S, Rosenberg ES. Primary HIV-1 infection. Clin Infect Dis. 2004;38:1447-53.

---

patients with an atypical or prolonged viral illness or with a heterophile-negative mononucleosis-like syndrome.

If the diagnosis of acute HIV infection is being considered, an HIV antibody test along with a plasma viral load should be obtained. A typical result pattern includes a positive viral load at a very high level (millions of copies/mL), a negative or (weakly) positive HIV antibody ELISA (screening test), and a negative or indeterminate HIV antibody Western blot (confirmatory test). The latter finding usually represents HIV antibody evolution, and repeat HIV antibody testing after 6 weeks typically shows a positive result. Also, p24 (core) antigen has been used as a supplemental test in this setting, but its sensitivity wanes over time.

Given the classically high magnitude of viremia during acute HIV infection, a low (<5000 copies/mL) level should prompt repeat testing to rule out a false-positive result. The presence of an indeterminate Western blot with a negative viral load should prompt consideration of HIV-2 in epidemiologically appropriate settings (e.g., patients from or having sexual partners from West Africa). In patients with a positive HIV antibody test and a recent history of ARS or high-risk exposure, a "detuned" ELISA can be used to identify patients with early infection. This less-sensitive assay turns positive on average 129 days after infection. A positive HIV antibody test and a nonreactive detuned ELISA indicate recent acquisition of HIV infection. The detuned ELISA is not currently commercially available and is best pursued in the context of an acute HIV referral center. The use and interpretation of these diagnostic tests are presented in Figure 1-4.

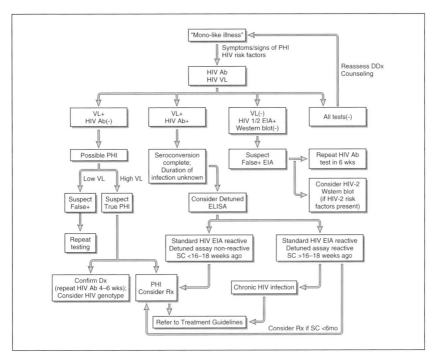

Figure 1-4. Testing algorithm for diagnosis of primary HIV infection (PHI). Ab = antibody; DDx = differential diagnosis; Rx = treatment; SC = seroconversion; VL = viral load.

Management

Enthusiasm for the "hit early, hit hard" approach to HIV management was supported by early data showing that treatment of acute infection can preserve HIV-specific CD4+ T lymphocyte responses. In addition, initial reports of successful structured treatment interruption (STI) piqued interest in early treatment as a means of gaining control of HIV infection without the need for chronic antiretroviral therapy. The first such reported case was that of the "Berlin patient," who started therapy during acute infection and then stopped it briefly at day 15 because of an episode of epididymitis, with associated rebound in HIV viral load. He resumed treatment but then stopped again on day 121 because of hepatitis A infection. This time there was no rebound viremia. He then resumed treatment a third time until self-discontinuing medications on day 176, with sustained control of viremia for several years thereafter.

The theory behind STI is that periods of permissive viremia act as "autologous vaccination," allowing the host to respond to HIV antigenemia exposure by producing HIV-specific immune responses in repetitive cycles with serially increased amplitude of immune competency (and subsequently decreased levels of viremia) until the immune system can control HIV without medication.

Unfortunately, STI in the clinical realm has been met with less success. A small study showed that sustained control was not achievable in the majority of patients treated during acute infection and that no identifiable variables could predict which individuals would maintain virologic control. More recent studies of STI in chronic HIV infection have raised significant concerns about this treatment strategy. Patients undergoing CD4-driven STI in the large multicenter SMART study showed worse outcomes with respect to both disease progression and adverse events compared with those on continuous therapy. One potential explanation for these surprising results is that interrupted therapy and rebound viremia result in a proinflammatory state that may induce disease progression and end-organ damage.

Currently, initiation of antiretroviral therapy should be viewed as a lifelong commitment. The advantages and disadvantages of early versus delayed antiretroviral therapy are described in Table 4-2. Treatment of acute HIV infection may confer immunologic, virologic, and public health benefits, but to date no survival advantage has been proven.

The decision of whether or not to initiate therapy for acute HIV infection remains controversial and is best accomplished in the setting of a clinical trial. One approach is to consider therapy for patients who are committed to it and to stop if toxicities develop or if resistance emerges. This strategy gives the patient the greatest chance of responding to future therapies by "freeze-framing" the immune system in its most preserved state.

If early treatment is chosen, the importance of medication adherence should be emphasized, especially given the presence of high-grade viremia. The preferred antiretroviral drug combinations are the same as those for the treatment of chronic HIV infection. A genotype test should be obtained at the time of initiation of therapy to look for evidence of primary resistance, with adjustment of the regimen as warranted based upon the results.

Analysis of over 100 subjects with acute and early HIV infection showed that average time to virologic suppression was 11 weeks. Patients on therapy showed an average CD4 count increase of 217 cells/mm^3 over the first year of therapy, and additional incremental gains persisted over the ensuing 4 years in those remaining on it. Over 90% of patients maintained an undetectable viral load after 12 months of treatment.

Progression to Symptomatic HIV Infection and AIDS

HIV viral load and CD4 cell count are the two most useful clinical markers to assess disease progression (Figure 1-5). After the high viral level associated with acute HIV infection is suppressed by the initial immunologic response, an asymptomatic period ranging from several months to more than 10 years ensues. Although symptoms are not present during this period of

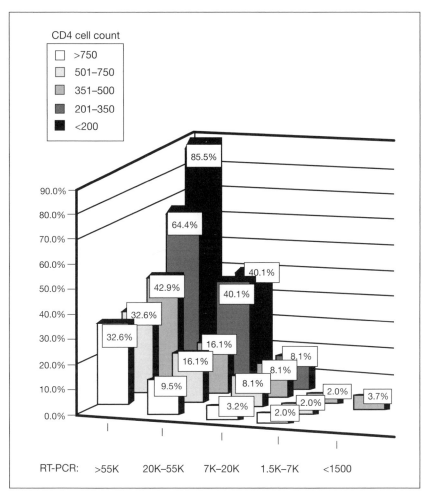

Figure 1-5. Risk of developing AIDS within three years based on CD4 cell count and viral load. RT-PCR = reverse transcriptase-polymerase chain reaction. (Adapted from Centers for Disease Control and Prevention. Report of the NIH panel to define principles of therapy of HIV infection and guidelines for the use of antiretroviral agents in HIV-infected adults and adolescents. MMWR. 1998;47:1-82.)

clinical latency, viral replication is ongoing, leading to a CD4 count decline of approximately 10% (or 100/mm³) per year in most patients.

The clinical progression to AIDS, as defined by a CD4 count of less than 200 cells/mm³ or an indicator disease (see Box 1-1), typically occurs an average of 8 to 12 years from the time of infection. The CD4 cell count at any given time correlates with the risk for particular opportunistic diseases (Figure 1-6).

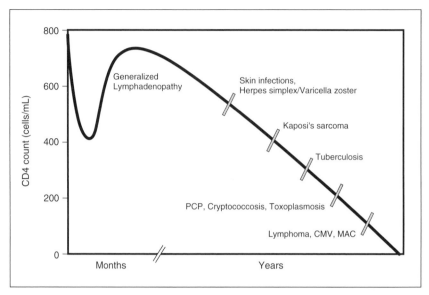

Figure 1-6. Opportunistic disease thresholds with declining CD4 counts.

Minor infections may develop as the CD4 count drops to less than 500 cells/mm³, with relapsing and increasingly severe manifestations associated with lower counts. Initial presentations may include bacterial cellulitis, HSV and varicella-zoster infections, and candidal infections of the mouth and vagina. If the count drops to less than 200 cells/mm³, more serious infections such as PCP, cerebral toxoplasmosis, and cryptococcal meningitis may occur. If the CD4 count drops to less than 50 cells/mm³, systemic infection with CMV and MAC may develop.

In addition to opportunistic infections, malignancies such as Kaposi's sarcoma and lymphoma may occur with progressive immunologic dysfunction. HIV-infected patients with advanced disease also may experience fever and night sweats, chronic diarrhea, wasting syndrome, and significant neurocognitive dysfunction.

Long-Term Nonprogression

A small percentage of HIV-infected persons will remain asymptomatic for 10 or more years in the absence of antiretroviral therapy. Many have CD4 counts in the normal range and have low viral loads. These patients are immunologically and epidemiologically diverse, and active research of such individuals may help further our understanding of HIV pathogenesis and control.

KEY POINTS

- Acute HIV infection is characterized by nonspecific symptoms and signs, and maintaining a high clinical index of suspicion is necessary to establish the diagnosis. Characteristic laboratory findings include a negative HIV antibody test (or positive ELISA with a negative or indeterminate Western blot) and a very high plasma viral load.

- Early treatment may offer the opportunity for immunologic preservation and long-term disease control, but a survival advantage has not been demonstrated.

- HIV transmission occurs 10 to 12 times more frequently during early infection than in chronic infection. There is a public health benefit in identifying newly acquired cases and preventing "unknowing transmission."

- Acute HIV infection is followed by an asymptomatic period ranging from several months to 10 years or more. During this time, viral replication continues and the CD4 cell count declines. Symptomatic disease and ultimately AIDS develop in the vast majority of untreated patients.

- Long-term nonprogression of HIV disease has been described in a small percentage of patients, and the factors responsible for it appear to be diverse.

SUGGESTED READINGS

Blankson JN. Primary HIV-1 infection: to treat or not to treat? AIDS Read. 2005;15:245-6, 249-51.

Hecht FM, Busch MP, Rawal BD, et al. Use of laboratory tests and clinical symptoms for identification of primary HIV infections. AIDS. 2002;16:1119-29.

Kahn JO, Walker BD. Acute human immunodeficiency virus type 1 infection. N Engl J Med. 1998;339:33-9.

Kassutto S, Maghsoudi K, Johnston MN, et al. Longitudinal analysis of clinical markers following antiretroviral therapy initiated during acute or early HIV type 1 infection. Clin Infect Dis. 2006;42:1024-31.

Kassutto S, Rosenberg ES. Primary HIV-1 infection. Clin Infect Dis. 2004;38:1447-53.

Kaufmann DE, Lichterfield M, Altfeld M, et al. Limited durability of viral control following treated acute HIV infection. PLOS Med. 2004;1:e36.

Lisziewicz J, Rosenberg E, Lieberman J, et al. Control of HIV despite the discontinuation of antiretroviral therapy. N Engl J Med. 1999;340:1683-4.

Lyles RH, Munoz A, Yamashita TE, et al. Natural history of human immunodeficiency virus type 1 Viremia after seroconversion and proximal to AIDS in a large cohort of homosexual men. J Infect Dis. 2000;181:872-80.

Pantaleo G, Demarest JF, Schacker T, et al. The qualitative nature of the primary immune response to HIV infection is a prognosticator of disease progression independent of the initial level of plasma viremia. Proc Natl Acad Sci USA. 1997;94:254-8.

Pilcher CD, Fiscus SA, Nguyen TQ, et al. Detection of acute infections during HIV testing in North Carolina. N Engl J Med. 2005;352:1873-83.

Pincus JM, Crosby SS, Losina E, et al. Acute human immunodeficiency virus infection in patients presenting to an urban urgent care center. Clin Infect Dis. 2003;37:1699-704.

Rosenberg ES, Altfeld M, Poon SH, et al. Immune control of HIV-1 after early treatment of acute infection. Nature. 2000;407:523-6.

Rosenberg ES, Billingsley JM, Caliendo AM, et al. Vigorous HIV-1-specific CD4+ T cell responses associated with control of viremia. Science. 1997;278:1447-50.

Rosenberg ES, Caliendo AM, Walker BD. Acute HIV infection among patients tested for mononucleosis. N Engl J Med. 1999;340:969.

Schacker T, Collier AC, Hughes J, et al. Clinical and epidemiologic features of primary HIV infection. Ann Intern Med. 1996;125:257-64. Erratum in: Ann Intern Med. 1997;126:174.

Smith DE, Walker BD, Cooper DA, et al. Is antiretroviral treatment of primary HIV-1 infection clinically justified on the basis of current evidence? AIDS. 2004;18:709-18.

Strain MC, Little SJ, Daar ES, et al. Effect of treatment, during primary infection, on establishment and clearance of cellular reservoirs of HIV-1. J Infect Dis 2005;191:1410-8.

Wawer MJ, Gray RH, Sewankambo NK, et al. Rates of HIV-1 transmission per coital act, by stage of HIV-1 infection, in Rakai, Uganda. J Infect Dis. 2005;191:1403-9.

Weintrob AC, Giner J, Menezes P, et al. Infrequent diagnosis of primary human immunodeficiency virus infection: missed opportunities in acute care settings. Arch Intern Med. 2003;163:2097-2100.

Chapter 2

Prevention of HIV Infection

HARVEY J. MAKADON, MD
STEVEN A. SAFREN, PhD

Although significant advances in the management of HIV disease have occurred during the past two decades, a cure or preventive vaccine remains elusive. The Centers for Disease Control and Prevention (CDC) estimates that 1,039,000 to 1,185,000 people in the United States were living with HIV infection at the end of 2003, with 24% to 27% undiagnosed and unaware of their serostatus. Over 38,000 new HIV cases were diagnosed in 2005, 74% of which were in men and 26% of which were in women. While most of the prevention literature has focused on public health efforts to prevent HIV infection in high-risk persons, it is clear that primary care providers also play an important role in this area. Since the advent of effective combination antiretroviral therapy, there are more people living with HIV infection, all of whom need to engage in consistent behavioral changes to reduce the chance of infecting others or putting themselves at risk for additional sexually transmitted diseases (STDs).

Barriers to Providing HIV Prevention Information

Traditionally, our health care system has placed a higher priority on acute care needs than on disease prevention, and time constraints in clinical practice have accentuated this pattern. A clinician's potential to influence patients' attitudes and behaviors has gone largely unrealized. Physicians are cited regularly by the public as the most trusted source of health information, and patients often heed their counsel. As such, primary care providers have the potential to play a key role in HIV prevention efforts.

While physicians are considered valuable sources of information about health issues, one national survey showed that counseling and advice about HIV transmission were given in less than 1% of primary care visits. The CDC now recommends that HIV antibody testing be included as part of the routine care of healthy adults, adolescents, and pregnant women. The aim is to identify the estimated 250,000 HIV-infected Americans who are unaware of their serostatus. It is hoped that, through this process, they will be provided earlier access to treatment and prevention counseling.

Four major barriers have been identified to communicating information about HIV prevention in clinical settings:

1) A narrow conception of health care and the physician's role in prevention efforts
2) Physicians' attitudes toward HIV-infected people, including the stigma associated with the disease and discomfort discussing sexual and drug-use behaviors
3) Practical constraints of time and resources
4) Ambiguities in the HIV prevention message, including imprecise information about sexual risk transmission rates associated with various behaviors

In 1992, the CDC and the Health Resources and Services Administration commissioned a survey of primary care physicians to learn more about practices in the prevention of HIV infection. Although most physicians indicated that they "usually" or "always" asked new adult patients about cigarette smoking, inquiries about STDs, condom use, sexual orientation, and number of sexual partners were far less frequent. One-quarter of physicians surveyed believed that their patients would be offended by questions about their sexual behavior, whereas a corresponding survey of patients indicated that nearly all would not object to discussing AIDS. These results highlight missed opportunities for HIV prevention counseling during patient encounters and indicate an increased need for focused skills-based training of clinicians in areas such as sexual history-taking and HIV risk assessment.

What is HIV Prevention?

The American Medical Association has recommended that a discussion about HIV infection and prevention be part of routine health care maintenance for all patients. Clinicians see patients in a variety of settings, and these often dictate the nature and scope of issues that can be addressed. Primary care practitioners may not be able to identify easily which patients are at high risk for HIV infection, and therefore adding regular conversations about sexual and drug-use safety may be a way to assist with these important self-care behaviors. The clinician should inquire about high-risk behaviors in a manner that is sensitive and comprehensive (Box 2-1).

While some primary care providers may feel uncomfortable asking about these topics, one successful approach was recently described. In it, providers introduce the topic with all patients, using language such as "One topic we are making sure to discuss with our patients is the issue of sexual safety." Once a patient's risk has been assessed, clinical prevention activities are guided by the three components of behavioral change: 1) information, 2) motivation, and 3) skills. Each of these is thought to be critical to sexual and other health behavior change.

Box 2-1.   Sample HIV Risk-Assessment Questions

- Did you receive a transfusion of blood or blood products between 1978 and 1985?
- Have you ever, even once, used any kind of injected drug?
- Have you ever had a disease that you contracted sexually?
- Are you sexually active with men, women, or both?
- How many sexual partners have you had during your life?
- Have you ever, even once, had sex with a prostitute (ask of male patients), bisexual man (ask of female patients), or someone who has used injected drugs?
- Do you have any other reason to suspect you might be at risk for HIV or AIDS?

Adapted from Libman H, Witzburg RA, eds. HIV Infection: A Primary Care Manual. Boston: Little, Brown; 1996.

Conducting HIV prevention in the context of a clinical visit should be done in a nonjudgmental way, using language that normalizes the range of potential patient experiences. Prevention information includes providing patients with basic facts regarding HIV transmission and prevention and answering their questions. One way to employ a nonjudgmental approach is to use open-ended questions such as, "What questions do you have about what I just said?" This approach can be more effective than using closed-ended questions, such as "Do you have any questions?" In the latter scenario, the reply may more likely be "No."

Information alone, however, does not necessarily lead to change. Illustrations include persons with a history of lung cancer who continue to smoke and people with chronic liver disease who drink alcohol. Motivation and skills are essential to modifying behavior. Additionally, behavioral research suggests that individuals may be ready at different times to make a change. This transtheoretical model describes five stages of change, including: 1) precontemplation, when a person has no intention of changing; 2) contemplation, when a person intends to take action at some point; 3) preparation, when a person has taken some initial steps towards changing; 4) action, when a person has made behavioral changes in the short term; and 5) maintenance, when a person has changed his or her behavior for a substantial period of time.

The most effective health-related counseling is individualized based on where a patient is on this spectrum of readiness to change. Patients who are further away from action tend to benefit most from counseling that increases one's motivation to change. This might entail asking the patient about the pros and cons of making changes and following up with questions about what would need to be different to have the pros outweigh the cons. Providers should realize that for many individuals there are significant and meaningful advantages of not modifying behavior and many barriers to making changes. Hence, inquiring about these advantages and disadvantages may stimulate dialogue about the patient's ambivalence and facilitate the process of moving to the next level in the model.

Patients who are further along in terms of their readiness to change may benefit most from counseling geared toward maintaining motivation and increasing behavioral skills. Individuals may have adequate information about the need to make a change and excellent motivation but not have the necessary skills to do so. Skills-based training, including activities such as having a model to demonstrate how condoms are used, practicing role-playing assertiveness, and providing a referral for psychotherapy when needed, may be useful in this setting.

When counseling about HIV risk behaviors, clinicians need to be aware that permanent behavioral change is difficult to achieve and that no single intervention strategy will be completely effective. Successful prevention efforts involve the primary care provider and patient as part of a system of care that includes community-based services and public health interventions.

Reducing HIV transmission also requires institution of prevention efforts in HIV-infected persons. These include: 1) screening for risk behaviors; 2) communicating prevention messages; 3) referring patients for services such as substance abuse and mental health care, as needed; 4) facilitating partner notification, counseling, and testing; and 5) identifying and treating other STDs.

Prevention of Sexual Transmission

High-Risk Sexual Activities

Clinicians should communicate information about the relative risk of sexual behaviors when educating patients about options for decreasing HIV transmission (see Box 2-1). However, simply advising abstinence may be an unrealistic foundation on which to build an effective HIV prevention strategy, particularly among adolescents and young adults. Sexual activity is a normal part of human development, and it is often initiated during adolescence. Most people will choose to have sex, and they should be provided with instructions on safer sexual behaviors. Sexually active people can be reached more effectively with nonjudgmental messages that emphasize the importance of having satisfying intimate experiences, improving interpersonal communication, maintaining control over their sexual behavior, and protecting themselves from HIV and other STDs (Box 2-2).

Over the years, safer sex guidelines have emphasized the importance of limiting the number of sexual partners and avoiding contact with persons who are at risk for HIV. This message also should include using condoms consistently and limiting oneself to lower-risk sexual activities. Patients should be encouraged to discuss openly their serostatus before engaging in sexual activity because evidence suggests that high-risk behaviors (e.g., unprotected anal intercourse between homosexual men) are more

---

Box 2-2.   Sexual Risk Reduction Topics for Discussion with Patients

- Importance of taking care of oneself and others by reducing the risk for HIV transmission
- Role of "safer sex" in the patient's life with all partners—whether regular, occasional, and/or paid
- Importance of limiting the number of sexual partners
- Importance of knowing the HIV serostatus of sexual partners and frankly discussing risk behaviors with them
- Risk of unplanned or unprotected sexual contact when using drugs or alcohol
- Use of condoms in male–female and male–male sexual activity, and the identification of obstacles and appropriate strategies for overcoming them

---

Adapted from Libman H, Witzburg RA, eds. HIV Infection: A Primary Care Manual. Boston: Little, Brown; 1996.

---

likely to occur within the context of an ongoing relationship than in anonymous sexual encounters. Among HIV-infected patients, clinicians must recognize that sexual activity is an important quality-of-life indicator.

There are many complicated issues regarding the transmissibility of HIV. For example, there are data to suggest that HIV-infected patients with a lower plasma viral load may be less infectious to others. However, this observation does not mean that such an individual cannot transmit HIV infection. Viral load measurements in semen and vaginal secretions may not correlate closely with plasma viral loads, and it is important that patients be aware of this information.

HIV-infected sexual partners, especially if they are mutually monogamous, may be inclined to forgo regular condom use as a demonstration of their intimacy and trust. However, concerns about HIV superinfection—that is, becoming infected with a second, perhaps more virulent and/or resistant viral strain—should be considered in making such a decision.

Treatment of Sexually Transmitted Diseases

Among people who are sexually active, a compelling body of evidence has shown that STD prevention and treatment are important components of a successful HIV prevention strategy (see Chapter 1). Treatment of STDs has been associated with decreased acquisition and transmission of HIV. Unfortunately, comprehensive STD care is not readily available in all parts of the United States, and many local public health departments do not provide such services. Expanding STD surveillance programs and improving detection and treatment services for people who have or are at risk for STDs should be part of any comprehensive HIV prevention strategy.

Appropriate Use of Condoms

In addition to STD management, consistent use of latex condoms during sexual activity is essential to HIV prevention efforts. Physicians must be able to provide patients with specific instructions about the appropriate use of condoms because improper use can lead to slippage, breakage, and unnecessary HIV exposure. This type of counseling is consistent with the provision of behavioral skills as one component of effective health counseling discussed above.

Instructions for correct latex condom use include:

1) Using a new condom for each act of intercourse
2) Checking the expiration date on the package
3) Carefully handling the condom to avoid damaging it with sharp objects (e.g., do not use teeth to open the package)
4) Ensuring that the condom is placed on an erect penis before any genital contact with a partner
5) Ensuring that no air is trapped in the tip of the condom
6) Ensuring adequate lubrication during intercourse with water-based (not oil-based) products
7) Holding the condom at the base of the erect penis during withdrawal to prevent slippage

Persons who are allergic to latex should use a polyurethane condom, although its effectiveness in HIV prevention has not been demonstrated. The female condom was introduced as a method that women can control for preventing pregnancy and STDs. Although the female condom is impenetrable to HIV, its efficacy in preventing infection has also not been established. Dental dams (small squares of latex) or, alternatively, nonmicrowaveable plastic wrap is recommended as a barrier during cunnilingus and analingus. Data on the safety and effectiveness of topical microbicides are lacking, but research is ongoing in this important area.

Prevention of Transmission by Injection-Drug Use

Approximately one-third of AIDS cases in the United States have been associated with injection-drug use (see Chapter 11). These statistics do not include patients who contracted HIV through high-risk sexual behaviors associated with the use of noninjection drugs, such as alcohol, cocaine, and methamphetamine. Data from a CDC study of young adults aged 18 to 29 years showed a high prevalence of HIV infection among women who recently had unprotected sex in exchange for crack cocaine or money. In fact, these women were as likely to be HIV-infected as men who had sex with men. Therefore, in addition to sharing needles, engaging in high-risk sexual activity while under the influence of drugs (either injection or non-injection) and exchanging sex for drugs or money can contribute significantly to HIV transmission in the substance-using population.

Needles and syringes are the primary equipment involved in transferring HIV-infected blood between injection-drug users. Hepatitis C, which results in chronic infection in most patients, is also effectively transmitted in this manner. Providing nonjudgmental counseling and medical care are the initial components of an HIV prevention strategy in a substance-using patient (Box 2-3).

Establishing trust with the individual is critical to the goals of referral to drug treatment programs and abstinence from drug use. Unfortunately, these are not always attainable because patients may be unwilling to accept treatment, and access to treatment programs may be limited. In this scenario, the clinician needs to set more realistic goals, emphasizing harm reduction rather than absolute risk elimination. A harm-reduction model accepts that drug use exists but attempts to minimize the adverse consequences of the behavior. For the active injection-drug user, clinicians can advise that the most effective way to reduce HIV transmission risk is to not share needles and to use sterile needles for each injection. Users who share needles should disinfect their injection equipment with bleach, although this practice is not as safe as always using a sterile needle and syringe. In order to eradicate HIV, drug apparatus must first be flushed with clean water and then soaked in full-strength bleach for at least one minute, followed by another thorough rinse with clean water.

As rates of HIV infection related to drug use continue to rise, there is growing pressure to identify effective prevention strategies. In some localities in the United States, physicians can refer injection-drug users to needle exchange programs (NEPs). Proponents of needle exchange cite an emerging body of scientific evidence supporting its efficacy in reducing HIV transmission among injection-drug users. In contrast, opponents fear that NEPs may serve as a deterrent for patients to seek drug treatment and that they send the "wrong message" to young people. However, studies

---

Box 2-3.   Drug-Use Risk Reduction Topics for Discussion with Patients

- Importance of using bleach to clean drug paraphernalia
- Avoidance of "shooting galleries" or trading sex for drugs
- Importance of drug treatment and rehabilitation
- Opportunity to discuss harm reduction topics and/or offer referral to community-based educational services

Adapted from Libman H, Witzburg RA, eds. HIV Infection: A Primary Care Manual. Boston: Little, Brown; 1996.

have shown consistently that needle exchange is not associated with an increase in injection- or noninjection-drug use. Some data even suggest that needle exchange actually may serve as a vehicle for patients to seek ongoing treatment for substance use. Along with continued counseling, support, and education aimed at decreasing rates of high-risk behaviors, NEPs appear to be an important HIV preventive intervention in this complex patient population.

Prevention of Perinatal Transmission

Transmission of HIV from mother to infant accounts for the majority of pediatric AIDS cases. The number of infected infants has decreased significantly over the past decade. It is now clear that most cases of perinatal HIV transmission can be prevented by appropriate evaluation and treatment of pregnant women and their newborns (see Chapter 11). Important interventions include: 1) using antiretroviral therapy in the mother during the second and third trimesters and peripartum and in the infant postpartum, 2) minimizing trauma at the time of delivery and considering elective cesarean section, and 3) avoiding breastfeeding postpartum when suitable alternatives exist.

HIV Postexposure Prophylaxis

A retrospective study of health care workers found that treatment with zidovudine (ZDV) after needle-stick exposure to HIV-infected blood reduced the odds of HIV infection by approximately 80%. Although this observation has not been confirmed in a randomized controlled trial, these findings and other data led the CDC to recommend postexposure prophylaxis (PEP) for health care workers who were exposed accidentally to HIV-infected body fluids.

The CDC has also published PEP recommendations for sexual and injection-drug use exposures. Deciding whether PEP is appropriate for an individual is often difficult and requires a careful assessment of the following issues:

1) *Type of Sexual Exposure*—Data suggest that the probability of transmission through a single episode of unprotected rectal or vaginal intercourse with someone known to be infected with HIV is similar in magnitude to that associated with occupational needle punctures (see Box 1-2). The probability is highest for unprotected receptive anal intercourse. Unprotected receptive vaginal intercourse seems to be of higher risk than unprotected insertive anal or vaginal intercourse. The per-episode risk of re-

ceptive oral sex with ejaculation is uncertain, but this behavior
has been shown to transmit HIV.

2) *HIV Status of the Patient and Sexual Partner*—PEP is given with
the assumption that a patient is not already infected with HIV. As
such, baseline HIV antibody testing should be performed. For
patients who report multiple exposures in the recent past, an
HIV viral load should also be done to detect primary HIV infection. The HIV status of the sexual partner may or may not be
known. If the partner is known to be infected with HIV, additional information (e.g., stage of disease, recent viral load) may
affect treatment decisions. If the partner's HIV status is unknown
and he or she is willing to be tested, treatment can be started
and then stopped if the partner tests negative. If the partner is
unavailable or unwilling to be tested, the decision to initiate PEP
is based on the type of exposure and knowledge of the patient's
risk behaviors. *In cases of rape in which the perpetrator is unknown, PEP always should be considered.*

3) *Patient's Attitude Toward Safer Sex*—Some patients diligently
practice safer sex but are exposed accidentally to HIV when a
condom breaks. Others have isolated episodes of unsafe sex
while under the influence of alcohol or drugs. Still others have
many unsafe sexual exposures with a variety of partners of unknown HIV status. PEP may not be appropriate for people who
intend to continue high-risk behaviors because it is unlikely to
be effective in the long term and may contribute to the development of viral resistance in the community. However, in am-
biguous cases, clinicians may choose to offer PEP and to
emphasize the importance of condom use and safer sexual practices in the future.

4) *Length of Time Since Exposure*—The timing of the risk behavior
is an important component of the PEP evaluation. Few data exist on which to base a precise cutoff time after exposure, but animal models suggest that delaying therapy more than 24 to 36
hours dramatically decreases its likelihood of effectiveness.
Although immediate treatment is optimal, PEP can be initiated
up to 72 hours after exposure.

Consideration of PEP after sexual encounters or injection-drug use provides physicians in primary care practice, emergency departments, and STD
clinics a valuable opportunity to reach patients at high risk for HIV and to
provide them with evaluation, treatment, and counseling. However, we
must be careful not to undermine existing prevention efforts and make sure
patients know that PEP may not be effective in all instances. Condom use,
safer sexual practices, and avoidance of high-risk behaviors remain the
most important components of HIV prevention. Detailed information about

nonoccupational PEP, including recommended drug regimens, can be found in Chapter 12.

KEY POINTS

- Primary care physicians have the opportunity to play an important role in HIV prevention. Clinical prevention of HIV infection requires assessing patient risk and providing health education tailored to help modify high-risk behaviors.
- The CDC now recommends that HIV antibody testing be included as part of the routine care of healthy adults, adolescents, and pregnant women.
- Discussion of HIV prevention with patients should include providing information, increasing motivation, and increasing behavioral skills. Clinicians should be aware that patients are at different stages of "readiness" to change and should work with them over time to reach the next level.
- Clinicians should emphasize the importance of safer sexual behaviors, particularly the consistent and appropriate use of condoms. Sexual behaviors can be stratified by their relative risk.
- Because STDs are associated with an increased risk of HIV acquisition and transmission, the prevention and treatment of these infections are essential in HIV prevention.
- Primary care physicians should advise injection-drug users to avoid sharing paraphernalia. Despite political controversies, needle exchange programs appear to be effective at reducing the risk of HIV transmission.
- Perinatal transmission of HIV infection has been greatly reduced over the past decade through the use of antiretroviral therapy, minimizing trauma at the time of delivery, and avoidance of breastfeeding if possible.
- Postexposure antiretroviral therapy prophylaxis should be considered in appropriate persons presenting within 72 hours of HIV exposure through sexual contact or injection-drug use.

SUGGESTED READINGS

Centers for Disease Control and Prevention. HIV prevention practices of primary care physicians: United States. MMWR. 1994;42:988-92.

Centers for Disease Control and Prevention. Antiretroviral postexposure prophylaxis after sexual, injection-drug use, or other nonoccupational exposure to HIV in the United States: recommendations from the U.S. Department of Health and Human Services. MMWR. 2005; 54(RR-2):1-19.

Centers for Disease Control and Prevention. Revised recommendations for HIV testing of adults, adolescents and pregnant women in health care settings. MMWR. 2006; 55(RR-14); 1-17.

DeGruttola V, Seage GR 3rd, Mayer KH, Horsburgh CR Jr. Infectiousness of HIV between male homosexual partners. J Clin Epidemiol. 1989;42:849-56.

Fisher JD, Fisher WA, Cornman DH, Amico RK, Bryan A, Friedland GH. Clinician-delivered intervention during routine clinical care reduces unprotected sexual behavior among HIV-infected patients. J Acquir Immune Defic Syndr. 2006;41:44-52.

Gerberding JL. Prophylaxis of occupational exposure to HIV. Ann Intern Med. 1996;25: 497-501.

Hurley SF, Jolley DJ, Kaldor JM. Effectiveness of needle-exchange programmes for prevention of HIV infection. Lancet. 1997;349:1797-800.

Makadon HJ, Silin JG. Prevention of HIV infection in primary care: current practices, future possibilities. Ann Intern Med. 1995;123:715-9.

Mayer KH, Safren SA, Gordon CM. HIV care providers and prevention: opportunities and challenges. J Acquir Immune Defic Syndr. 2004;37 (Suppl 2):S130-2.

Prochaska JO, DiClementne CC. The Transtheoretical Approach: Crossing Traditional Boundaries of Change. Homewood, IL: Dow Jones/Irwin; 1984.

Quinn TC, Wawer MJ, Sewankambo N, et al. Viral load and heterosexual transmission of human immunodeficiency virus type 1. Rakai Project Study Group. N Engl J Med. 2000;342; 921-9.

Chapter 3

Primary Care of HIV Infection

HOWARD LIBMAN, MD
JON D. FULLER, MD

The management of HIV-infected patients has undergone dramatic changes since the advent of combination antiretroviral therapy and the introduction of viral plasma load and resistance testing in clinical practice. As a result, patients in care are being diagnosed less frequently with opportunistic infections and are living longer. However, with this encouraging news have come important challenges. For patients, they include difficulties in adhering to a medical regimen, drug toxicities, and quality of life issues. For primary care clinicians, they include keeping up with a rapidly changing knowledge base and addressing the needs of complicated outpatients within time constraints.

Competence in HIV care requires clinical experience and continuing education in the field rather than specific subspecialty training. Also essential are nursing support, social services, subspecialty consultations, mental health and pharmacy expertise, and, where possible, linkage to clinical trials and to expanded access programs for drugs in development. Experience has shown that a multidisciplinary approach is optimal for both patients and clinicians.

This chapter reviews the major issues related to outpatient HIV care, including antibody testing, clinical assessment, laboratory testing, antiretroviral therapy, opportunistic infection prophylaxis, and health care maintenance issues. HIV prevention, which is also important in primary care practice, is addressed in Chapter 2.

HIV Antibody Testing

HIV antibody testing has traditionally been recommended to patients at historical risk for HIV infection and to those with suggestive clinical findings (Box 3-1). However, the Centers for Disease Control and Prevention (CDC) recently advised performing such testing as part of the routine health care of adults, adolescents, and pregnant women. Primary care physicians can order the test in an office setting. In addition, both confidential and anonymous testing sites exist in most urban centers, and a home testing kit is available.

Box 3-1.   Traditional Indications for HIV Antibody Testing

Historical
- Men who have sex with men
- People with multiple sexual partners
- Current or past injection-drug users
- Recipients of blood products between 1978 and 1985
- People with current or past sexually transmitted diseases
- Commercial sex workers and their sexual contacts
- Pregnant women and those of childbearing age
- Children born to HIV-infected mothers
- Sexual partners of those at risk for HIV infection
- Persons who consider themselves at risk or who request testing

Clinical
- Tuberculosis
- Syphilis
- Recurrent shingles
- Unexplained chronic constitutional symptoms
- Unexplained generalized adenopathy
- Unexplained chronic diarrhea or wasting
- Unexplained encephalopathy
- Unexplained thrombocytopenia
- Thrush or chronic/recurrent vaginal candidiasis
- HIV-associated opportunistic diseases (e.g., *Pneumocystis jiroveci [carinii]* pneumonia, Kaposi's sarcoma)
- Suspected acute retroviral syndrome (to rule out prior infection)

Knowledge of HIV serostatus has many potential individual health benefits, including initiation of HIV primary care, provision of antiretroviral therapy and prophylaxis for opportunistic infections where indicated, screening and prophylaxis for tuberculosis (TB), screening for and treatment of sexually transmitted diseases (STDs), administration of appropriate vaccinations, and institution of other health care maintenance measures. Public health benefits of HIV testing include the adoption of safer sex and drug use practices to avoid secondary transmission (see Boxes 2-2 and 2-3 in Chapter 2), tracking of the epidemic, and, where appropriate, the institution of antiretroviral therapy. This last intervention has the potential to reduce HIV transmission by lowering the concentration of virus in body fluids.

Potential risks of HIV antibody testing include receiving a false-positive test result, receiving a false-negative test result, adverse psychological reactions, breach of confidentiality, and discrimination when applying for life insurance, health insurance, employment, and housing. Patients who undergo HIV antibody testing would ideally have an understanding of its ramifications through pre-test and post-test counseling, although it is not required in the new CDC recommendations (Box 3-2). Antibody testing is contraindicated in patients who cannot provide informed consent, are unable to understand the implications of test results, are psychotic or suicidal, or lack adequate personal support systems to cope with the stress of receiving a positive test result.

Box 3-2.   Features of Pre-Test and Post-Test Counseling

Pre-Test Counseling
- Distinguish between anonymous and confidential testing and discuss the availability of home-testing kit
- Review natural history of HIV infection
- Review reasons for testing and expectations
- Review individual risk behaviors and risk-reduction measures
- Discuss meaning of positive and negative results
- Assess personal and social supports

Post-Test Counseling
- Review meaning of test results and implications
- If test result is positive:
  - Assess patient's reaction and ability to cope
  - Anticipate need for immediate support and plan for medical evaluation
- If test result is negative:
  - Restate possibility of seroconversion if patient is involved in high-risk activities
  - Dispel any false beliefs regarding invulnerability or immunity to HIV infection

---

Characteristics of Testing

HIV antibody testing is performed in a two-step fashion, the first of which is a highly sensitive enzyme-linked immunosorbent assay (ELISA). HIV seroconversion, or the development of detectable anti-HIV antibodies, generally occurs 6 to 8 weeks after infection. If the ELISA is negative, the HIV antibody test is reported as being negative; if it is positive, the test is repeated. If the repeat ELISA is positive, a Western blot (WB) assay, which is more specific, is performed for confirmation. If the WB assay result is positive, the HIV antibody test is reported as being positive. These sequential testing modalities are 99.5% sensitive and over 99% specific. WB results occasionally are reported as being indeterminate. In these instances, repeat or supplemental testing, such as an HIV viral load, may be recommended. Indeterminate WB results may indicate recently acquired HIV infection.

It is important to note that the "window period," the time between infection and first detectable sign of antibody positivity, may last from 3 to 6 months after a high-risk behavior. In people with suspected acute HIV syndrome, an HIV antibody test should be obtained at baseline (result should be negative or indeterminate), and an HIV viral load (often >1,000,000 copies/mL) is also necessary to establish the diagnosis. Low-titer false-positive HIV viral load assays (<5000 copies/mL) have been reported in patients with acute non–HIV-related illness, so expert consultation is advised in their interpretation.

Rapid tests to detect HIV antibody within 20 minutes also have been developed. These enable clinicians to provide definitive negative and preliminary positive results immediately and are especially useful in settings in which patients are less likely to return for their test results (e.g., anonymous test sites, STD clinics). Positive rapid HIV tests must be confirmed with the ELISA/WB sequence to identify potential false-positive results.

A low CD4 cell count is not in itself diagnostic of HIV disease and should never be used as a surrogate for HIV antibody testing. Some HIV antibody tests do not reliably detect HIV-2, which is common in West Africa. If this virus is suspected by history, a specific ELISA and WB can be requested.

Clinical Assessment

The clinical evaluation of HIV-infected patients should include a careful history, review of systems, physical examination, and attention to psychosocial and educational concerns. In newly diagnosed patients, understanding the patient's emotional state and knowledge of HIV disease should be the first priority. Denial, anxiety, isolation, depression and increased substance use or high-risk sexual activity may be seen in this setting. Mental health concerns should be addressed before dealing with nonurgent medical issues. Patients show great variability in their knowledge of HIV disease despite the widespread availability of information in the press and on the Internet. Comprehension of the natural history of HIV infection, how HIV is spread, and when and how it should be treated is essential. Information should be provided in the patient's primary language and should be appropriate to his or her level of education.

History

Taking a history from an HIV-infected patient allows the clinician to establish rapport and to gather important data. The first visit often provides insight into the patient's understanding of HIV disease. It also serves as an opportunity to discuss psychological factors, social supports, and financial resources, which likely will prove critical for adherence to recommended therapies. Exploration of possible modes by which the patient acquired HIV infection directs the clinician to specific interventions for prevention of secondary transmission (see Boxes 2-2 and 2-3 in Chapter 2).

The initial medical history should include the items listed in Box 3-3. The patient should be asked about any history of opportunistic diseases and about antiretroviral drugs received in the past. If the patient was previously treated, it is important to know the first, lowest, and most recent CD4 cell counts; the first, highest, and most recent viral loads; and whether there has been evidence of HIV drug resistance or toxicity.

It is also important to ask about a history of syphilis because atypical manifestations and responses to treatment have been described in some patients. A history of genital or anal warts or abnormal Pap smears also should be sought because of the association of advanced immunodeficiency with

---

Box 3-3.   History Taking in an HIV-Infected Patient

Medical History
- Opportunistic diseases
- CD4 cell count results (first, lowest, and most recent) and viral load results (first, highest, and most recent)
- Previous use of antiretroviral drugs
- Previous results of HIV resistance testing
- Exposure to tuberculosis, viral hepatitis, syphilis, and other sexually transmitted diseases
- Previous medical, surgical, and psychiatric care
- Gynecologic and obstetric history
- Alcohol or drug use
- Travel history
- Immunizations
- Current medications
- Drug allergies

Psychosocial History
- HIV risk behaviors
- Knowledge of HIV disease
- Emotional response
- Family/social situation
- Employment/insurance status

---

cervical and anal dysplasia/carcinoma in patients coinfected with human papillomavirus (HPV).

Inquiry should be made into any history of viral hepatitis. Hepatitis A exposure is common in men who have sex with men (MSM), hepatitis B is frequent in both MSM and injection-drug users, and hepatitis C often occurs in injection-drug users but has also been described in MSM. A history of TB exposure or positive reaction to purified protein derivative (PPD) in HIV-infected patients indicates a significantly increased risk of developing active disease in the absence of antimicrobial prophylaxis.

Review of medications should include all forms of treatment, since the use of over-the-counter drugs and complementary therapies is common in this patient population. An HIV medication poster or chart often is helpful to review timing and doses of specific medications by sight rather than relying on names. There should also be discussion of the nature and severity of any medication side effects.

Mental health issues are important at all stages of HIV disease. Psychological trauma is common, and some patients face rejection and discrimination by family and friends. Disclosure of HIV serostatus to sexual partners is a matter of personal responsibility (although some state health departments now have partner-notification programs to assist in this process). Many HIV-infected people have concerns related to insurance and housing at some time in the course of their disease. These may require the expertise of case managers or social workers familiar with community resources.

Finally, each visit should include a discussion of current health habits. It is important to ask explicitly about new sexual partners and practices. This allows the health care provider the opportunity to counsel patients about protecting themselves and their partners. Patients need to understand that they should still practice safer sex even with other HIV-infected persons because of possible superinfection and viral recombination, both of which may have deleterious clinical consequences. A discussion of any ongoing substance abuse is also critical. For patients who continue to inject drugs, harm-reduction techniques may be helpful in self-protection and in assessing their readiness to enter drug treatment programs. Heavy alcohol use may contribute to sexual risk-taking and has its own adverse health effects. Both cocaine and crystal methamphetamine use have been associated with increased risk of HIV transmission.

Physical Examination

Because HIV infection and its complications may involve nearly every organ system, a comprehensive review of systems and physical examination should be performed, with special focus on the skin, mouth, anogenital region, and central nervous system (Box 3-4).

Weight loss often suggests undiagnosed opportunistic infections, progressive HIV disease, depression, or substance abuse. As one of the earliest and most meaningful signs of deteriorating clinical status, the patient's weight should be measured at each visit.

The skin may also be involved early in the course of HIV disease. HIV-infected patients are at increased risk for a variety of infectious and inflammatory skin conditions. Bacterial agents may cause folliculitis, cellulitis, and bacillary angiomatosis. People actively injecting drugs may have infected or inflamed "tracks" or skin abscesses. Methicillin-resistant *Staphylo-*

Box 3-4.   Review of Systems and Physical Examination

- *Constitutional symptoms:* fever, chills, night sweats, weight loss
- *Integument:* seborrhea, psoriasis, onychomycosis, molluscum contagiosum, petechiae, herpes simplex virus, varicella-zoster virus, Kaposi's sarcoma, generalized adenopathy
- *HEENT:* altered vision, dysphagia, cytomegalovirus retinitis, thrush, oral hairy leukoplakia, periodontal disease
- *Pulmonary:* cough, dyspnea, evidence of pneumonia
- *Gastrointestinal:* odynophagia, diarrhea, organomegaly, perianal pathology
- *Genitourinary:* vaginitis, pelvic inflammatory disease, human papillomavirus, cervical and anal dysplasia/carcinoma
- *Neurological:* headache, problems with memory, change in behavior or personality, focal findings

coccus aureus (MRSA) infection has been reported in HIV-infected patients (especially MSM) presenting as severe or recurrent cellulitis or furunculitis. Superficial fungal infections and warts are common. Molluscum contagiosum, which are centrally umbilicated, pearly papules most often on the genitalia and face, also may be seen. Herpes simplex virus (HSV) or varicella-zoster virus (VZV) infection may be the initial presentation of HIV disease and can be severe and recurrent. Inflammatory disorders, such as seborrheic dermatitis, eosinophilic folliculitis, and psoriasis, may be difficult to treat. Kaposi's sarcoma (KS) presents as purplish nodules and plaques, usually on the trunk, legs, or oral mucosa (see Chapter 10).

Most HIV-infected people have palpable lymph nodes at some point during the course of their disease. Such nodes, which may involve multiple sites, do not predict disease progression but often cause discomfort and distress. Patients should be reassured that enlarged nodes are common and often spontaneously change in size. To exclude an opportunistic disease, lymph node biopsy should be considered if gland enlargement is rapid or asymmetric, if nodes are fixed or bulky, or if lymphadenopathy is associated with constitutional symptoms or cytopenias.

Direct ophthalmoscopy with dilatation of the pupils should be performed regularly even in asymptomatic patients with a CD4 count of less than 100 cells/mm^3. Cytomegalovirus (CMV) retinitis presents with hemorrhagic exudates and can progress quickly to blindness by affecting the macula or by leading to retinal detachment (see Chapter 9).

Mouth lesions may cause discomfort and adversely affect nutrition. Oral candidiasis manifests as white plaques (pseudomembranous form or "thrush") or as painful erythematous lesions (atrophic form) (see Chapter 9). Without treatment, oral candidiasis may spread throughout the mouth; in patients with advanced HIV disease, it can involve the esophagus, which leads to severe odynophagia. Angular cheilitis, which is fissuring of the corners of the mouth, may be from candida or HSV infection. Oral hairy leukoplakia (OHL), which is caused by Epstein-Barr virus, presents as a corrugated, vertical white plaque on the side of the tongue. It is usually asymptomatic and often regresses spontaneously. Ulcerations also are frequent in HIV-infected patients. Lesions appearing on keratinized epithelium, the lips, tongue, and hard palate are likely herpetic, whereas those on the buccal mucosa are often aphthous. Periodontal disease can be severe and, if untreated, lead to necrotizing gingivitis and tooth loss.

Patients with HIV disease are at risk for other STDs, including syphilis, chlamydia, gonorrhea, HSV and HPV infections, chancroid, and lymphogranuloma venereum. HIV-infected women with HPV infection are at increased risk for cervical dysplasia and cancer. A cervical Pap smear should be performed initially every 6 months. If two sequential tests are normal, further testing may be done annually (see below).

Bacterial vaginosis, candidal vaginitis, and trichomoniasis are also common. These infections often are recurrent and sometimes are difficult to manage. Patients with a history of receptive anal intercourse or anogenital warts are at increased risk for HPV-related anal squamous cell dysplasia and cancer. Consideration should be given to performing an anal Pap smear on a regular basis in those at risk, although formal recommendations are lacking (see below). Anal warts, herpetic ulcers, hemorrhoids, fissures, and traumatic tears are common in MSM.

Clinicians should screen for affective disorders and alcohol or drug use when evaluating complaints of memory difficulty. The other essential part of the neurologic exam involves looking for evidence of peripheral neuropathy, which may be a manifestation of HIV disease or drug toxicity.

Laboratory Testing

Baseline laboratory evaluation of the HIV-infected patient is important to screen for occult systemic disease, to identify latent infections that may reactivate, and to monitor for drug toxicity (Box 3-5).

Confirmation of HIV antibody status is recommended if documentation is not available. A complete blood count with differential should be performed on all patients, as cytopenias may occur without symptoms and should prompt appropriate evaluation. Anemia, leukopenia, and/or thrombocytopenia may result from HIV-induced bone marrow suppression, from toxicity related to antiviral therapy, or from infiltration of the bone marrow by infection or tumor; leukopenia and thrombocytopenia also may be mediated by autoantibody production. Fasting glucose and lipid profile are important for health care maintenance and for establishment of a baseline, especially given the metabolic complications associated with combination antiretroviral therapy (see Chapter 6). Given the incidence of resistance to antiretroviral drugs in newly infected patients (ranging from 8% to 16%), baseline genotypic resistance testing has been recommended for all those being considered for initiation of antiretroviral therapy.

Box 3-5.   Baseline Laboratory Studies

- Complete blood and differential counts
- BUN/creatinine, liver function tests, glucose, lipid profile
- CD4 cell count
- HIV viral load
- HIV genotype test (see Chapter 5)
- RPR or VDRL
- Anti-HAV
- Anti-HCV

- HBsAg, HBcAb (HBsAb if prior immunization)
- Toxoplasmosis (IgG) serology
- PPD testing
- *Chlamydia* and GC assays in persons at risk
- Pap smear in women
- Consider anal Pap smear in persons at risk

As hepatitis A, B, and C are known to occur with increased frequency among some patients with HIV infection, liver function tests and serologic tests for these viruses are recommended as part of the initial evaluation (see Chapter 8). These studies help to identify people who would benefit from hepatitis A and B immunizations and to alert clinicians to the possible presence of chronic hepatitis B or C virus infections. An isolated increased serum alkaline phosphatase level may prompt evaluation for infiltrative diseases of the liver.

Syphilis may progress more rapidly and may be more resistant to standard therapies, more prone to reactivation, and more difficult to detect by serologic tests in HIV-infected patients (see Chapter 9). Baseline screening for syphilis and periodic retesting in those at continued risk are warranted.

HIV is one of the most potent known activators of latent TB infection, and baseline and follow-up skin testing is important in identifying patients in whom antimicrobial prophylaxis is indicated (see Chapter 7). Because skin testing depends on intact cell-mediated immunity, lack of reactivity to antigens is more common with advanced immunodeficiency, which may lead to a false-negative result. A positive PPD (defined as 5 mm of induration in the context of HIV infection) is an indication for prophylactic antimicrobial therapy in the previously untreated patient, regardless of his or her age, timing of PPD conversion, and whether BCG was received during childhood.

A toxoplasma antibody titer should be obtained as part of the baseline evaluation. This information may have value in selecting patients for antimicrobial prophylaxis and in identifying those at risk for developing active disease (see Chapter 7). Some clinicians have advocated CMV serology as a screening test to determine which patients with advanced HIV disease are at increased risk for developing symptomatic infection. It also may be useful in patients who require a blood transfusion to identify CMV-seronegative patients who should be given white blood cell–poor products, which carry a lowered risk of CMV transmission. Serum cryptococcal antigen testing of asymptomatic patients has little clinical utility.

CD4 Cell Count

The CD4 cell count correlates highly with the progression of HIV disease and is the main surrogate marker for immunologic function (see Figure 1-5 in Chapter 1). Its clinical uses are to determine the need for and response to antiretroviral therapy; to determine the risk of opportunistic diseases and need for antimicrobial prophylaxis; and to assess prognosis. In the absence of effective antiretroviral therapy, the average decline per year in CD4 count is 75 to 100 cells/mm^3, but there is a great deal of variability among patients and in a given patient over time. A normal CD4 count is generally greater than 500 cells/mm^3 in healthy people, but it may be as low as 350 cells/mm^3.

Opportunistic infections usually do not occur with CD4 counts of greater than 500 cells/mm³; therefore, conventional bacterial infection, HSV and VZV infections, thrush, TB, KS, generalized lymphadenopathy, and chronic skin conditions may be seen as the count declines (see Figure 1-6 in Chapter 1). A CD4 count of less than 200 cells/mm³ indicates significant immunodeficiency with increased risk for serious opportunistic infections, such as *Pneumocystis jiroveci* pneumonia (formerly *Pneumocystis carinii* pneumonia [PCP]), toxoplasmosis, and cryptococcal meningitis. Patients with a count of less than 50 cells/mm³ are also at risk for CMV and *Mycobacterium avium* complex (MAC) infections and for lymphoma. The highest risk for death in HIV-infected patients occurs with a CD4 count less than 50 cells/mm³.

Because CD4 cell count results have a diurnal variation, samples should be obtained at the same time of day if possible. Intercurrent illnesses, especially herpesvirus infections, may cause transient CD4 count decline. Due to inter- and intra-laboratory variation in test results, it is wise to confirm the initial CD4 count and any subsequent values that are grossly different from the preceding one. Spurious results could lead to unwarranted therapeutic interventions.

Some investigators have suggested that the ratio of CD4 to total lymphocytes (CD4 percentage) may provide a more reliable indication of immune function than the absolute CD4 cell count, but use of this parameter has not gained widespread acceptance. Other proposed surrogate markers of immune function, such as beta-2-microglobulin and neopterin levels, are not used routinely.

Viral Load

The ability to measure HIV viral level in plasma has revolutionized disease management. Its clinical uses are to assess prognosis and to determine the need for and response to antiretroviral therapy. Measurement of HIV viral RNA in blood is performed using polymerase chain reaction (PCR) or branched-chain DNA (bDNA) techniques. The lower threshold for detection of newer assays is between 75 and 20 copies/mL. Viral load results provide complementary information to the CD4 cell count. They directly correlate with clinical disease progression and inversely correlate with CD4 count decline (see Figures 1-3 and 1-5 in Chapter 1). In general, the level of HIV in plasma reflects tissue levels, but virus may still be detectable in semen and vaginal secretions in patients with a suppressed plasma viral load. Importantly, there is a 0.3 log (three-fold to five-fold) variability in the viral load assay, meaning that differences between sequential values must exceed this threshold to be considered significant. Because intercurrent illnesses and immunizations may affect results transiently, the use of the assay in this context is not recommended.

Management

General Approach

Specific management issues in HIV-infected patients include initiation and maintenance of antiretroviral therapy where indicated, prophylaxis against PCP and other opportunistic infections where indicated, and health care maintenance issues. Patients are stratified based on their CD4 cell count (Box 3-6).

Box 3-6.   Management of HIV Disease Stratified by CD4 Cell Count

CD4 Cell Count > 350/mm³
- Initiate antiretroviral therapy if patient is symptomatic or pregnant after addressing factors that could negatively affect adherence
- Consider initiation of antiretroviral therapy if patient is asymptomatic with a high (>100,000 copies/mL) viral load
- If above criteria are not met, monitor patient off antiretroviral therapy
- Initiate TB prophylaxis in patient with positive PPD
- Address immunizations and other health care maintenance

CD4 Cell Count 350-200/mm³
- Initiate antiretroviral therapy if patient is symptomatic or pregnant after addressing factors that could negatively affect adherence
- Offer initiation of antiretroviral therapy if patient is asymptomatic
- Maintain antiretroviral therapy in patient who is already receiving it with modification of regimen as necessary based upon effectiveness and tolerability
- Initiate TB prophylaxis in patient with positive PPD
- Address immunizations and other health care maintenance

CD4 Cell Count 200-50/mm³
- Initiate antiretroviral therapy in all patients after addressing factors that could negatively affect adherence
- Maintain antiretroviral therapy in patient who is already receiving it with modification of regimen as necessary based upon effectiveness and tolerability
- Initiate PCP prophylaxis*
- Initiate TB prophylaxis in patient with positive PPD
- Address immunizations and other health care maintenance

CD4 Cell Count < 50/mm³
- Initiate antiretroviral therapy in all patients after addressing factors that could negatively affect adherence
- Maintain antiretroviral therapy in patient who is already receiving it with modification of regimen as necessary based upon effectiveness and tolerability
- Initiate or maintain PCP prophylaxis*
- Initiate prophylaxis for MAC infection
- Initiate TB prophylaxis in patient with positive PPD
- Address immunizations and other health care maintenance

PCP = *Pneumocystis jiroveci (carinii)* pneumonia; MAC = *Mycobacterium avium* complex.
* Alternative prophylaxis for toxoplasmosis should be initiated in the patient with CD4 count < 100/mm³ and positive toxoplasmosis serology who is not receiving TMP-SMX for PCP prophylaxis.

In general, antiretroviral therapy is recommended if the patient is symptomatic, has a CD4 count of less than 350 to 200/mm^3, or is pregnant. Antiretroviral therapy should also be considered if the patient is asymptomatic and has a CD4 count of greater than 350/mm^3 and a viral load of greater than 100,000 copies/mL. Prophylaxis against PCP is started in patients with a CD4 count of less than 200 cells/mm^3 and against toxoplasmosis if the CD4 count is less than 100 cells/mm^3. Preventive therapy against MAC is begun in patients with a CD4 count of less than 50 cells/mm^3.

Medical visits should be scheduled at appropriate intervals in order to monitor for disease progression and complications of therapy and to assess the efficacy of drug therapies. In general, patients with advanced HIV disease require more frequent visits than those at earlier stages.

The initial evaluation generally is completed in two appointments. At the first visit, a history and physical examination are performed, and baseline laboratory studies are obtained. At the second visit, results of the evaluation are reviewed, and the management plan is discussed. Before starting antiretroviral drugs, factors that could have a negative impact on medication adherence should be addressed (Box 3-7). Frequently missed doses will render a drug regimen ineffective by leading to the development of viral resistance. Every effort should be made to address substance abuse, alcoholism, an unstable housing situation, or significant psychological problems, all of which may interfere with a patient's ability to take medications reliably. Clear therapeutic goals should be established before starting antiretroviral therapy, and a plan should be in place to facilitate adherence and to monitor for drug toxicity.

If antiretroviral therapy is initiated, a follow-up visit is arranged in 2 to 4 weeks to assess the tolerability of the medical regimen and to repeat laboratory studies. Once a patient is on a stable regimen with an undetectable viral load, visits every 3 to 4 months are recommended unless active medical problems necessitate more frequent appointments. Follow-up laboratory studies should include complete blood and differential counts, glucose (every other visit), lipid profile (every other visit), renal and hepatic function tests, CD4 cell count, and viral load. In patients not on antiretroviral therapy, only a CD4 count and viral load are necessary.

Box 3-7.   Factors That Have a Negative Impact on Medication Adherence

- Lack of education about HIV disease
- Denial, anxiety, or depression
- Alcohol or drug use
- Poor social situation
- Inadequate health insurance
- Concerns about drug-related fat redistribution (e.g., facial lipoatrophy)

- Number of medications/pills
- Frequency of dosing
- Stringent dosing requirements
- Presence of side effects

When intercurrent medical conditions, gastrointestinal tract dysfunction, or interruption in the drug supply interferes with the ability of the patient to take medications, all antiretroviral drugs should be held temporarily. Viral resistance is more likely to occur if medications are continued but some doses are missed or not absorbed.

Antiretroviral Therapy

The following recommendations are based on our current understanding of the pathophysiology of HIV disease and the results of clinical trials. They reflect guidelines of U.S. Department of Health and Human Services and the International AIDS Society USA Panel (see Chapter 4). Because of the rapidly changing nature of management in this area, clinicians with limited experience should seek consultation when starting or changing antiretroviral drug regimens.

Viral replication occurs throughout the course of HIV infection at astonishing rates. It is estimated that 10 billion viral particles are produced each day. The patient's immune system keeps pace with this activity during the clinical latency period. However, in the absence of effective antiretroviral treatment, the immune system ultimately reaches a "point of exhaustion," at which viral replication exceeds its ability to produce CD4 cells. This leads to a decline in immunologic function and to the development of clinical disease manifestations, including opportunistic infections and neoplasms. The rate of viral replication is thought to stabilize after primary infection at a particular level or "set point." This level may be maintained within a 10-fold range over months and possibly years. The viral load is highly correlated with the rate of CD4 count decline, disease progression, and mortality.

The primary goal of antiretroviral therapy is to keep the viral load as low as possible for as long as possible. Maximal suppression of the virus makes it more difficult for resistance to develop. Lack of supression or partial suppression results in the homogeneous viral population diversifying through random errors in reverse transcription into numerous "quasispecies," some of which will contain mutations for drug resistance.

Approximately two-thirds of patients started on combination antiretroviral therapy will achieve virologic suppression. Patient adherence to medical therapy is key, with even 10% of doses missed being associated with decreased effectiveness of some regimens. Second and subsequent attempts at viral suppression are less often successful. Current antiretroviral drugs are not thought to be curative because of persistence of HIV in latently infected CD4 lymphocytes, which have a long life span, and in "sanctuary sites" (regions of the body such as the central nervous system and gonads) in which some drugs may not penetrate well.

Combination antiretroviral therapy with three active drugs is now considered the standard of care for HIV infection. Monotherapy and less potent combination regimens can lead to the development of viral resistance within weeks to months. To date, the Food and Drug Administration has approved 22 antiretroviral agents. They are classified by their mode of action against the virus into the following categories: 1) nucleoside and nucleotide reverse-transcriptase inhibitors (NRTIs), 2) nonnucleoside reverse-transcriptase inhibitors (NNRTIs), 3) protease inhibitors (PIs), and 4) entry inhibitors. Antiretroviral drugs vary considerably in dosing and frequency, in side effect profiles, in interactions with other drugs, and in how they should be administered in relation to food (see Chapter 4 tables).

When Should Antiretroviral Therapy Be Initiated?

Antiretroviral therapy is recommended in HIV-infected patients who meet any of the criteria listed in Box 3-8. Baseline laboratory testing, including CD4 cell count and viral load measurement, should be performed before starting therapy. Because of potential variability in test results, it may be prudent to obtain repeat baseline CD4 count and viral load over a 2- to 4-week period before initiation of therapy.

What Drugs Should Be Used?

Combination therapy using 3 drugs is recommended initially in most patients. They most commonly include two NRTIs given in conjunction with an NNRTI or a PI (often boosted with ritonavir). Three NRTIs are generally not recommended because of reports of failure of such combinations, especially in patients with viral loads of >100,000 copies/mL. The use of all monotherapies, d4T with ZDV (antagonistic thymidine analogues), indinavir with atazanavir (overlapping toxicity: hyperbilirubinemia), ddI and d4T (overlapping toxicities: peripheral neuropathy; acute pancreatitis; lactic acidosis), ddC with ddI or d4T (overlapping toxicity: peripheral neuropathy), and ddC with 3TC (inhibition of ddC phosphorylation) are not recommended. At least in treatment-naïve patients, the combination of tenofovir and ddI should be avoided because of suboptimal CD4 count responses. Specific combinations may necessitate dosage adjustments. NNRTIs and PIs have many potential drug interactions (see Chapter 4 tables). Medication lists should be reviewed carefully before starting these agents.

Box 3-8.   Indications for Antiretroviral Therapy

- Symptomatic HIV infection or AIDS regardless of CD4 cell count or HIV viral load
- CD4 cell count < 200/mm^3
- Pregnancy
- Offer in the asymptomatic patient with CD4 count 350-200/mm^3
- Consider in the asymptomatic patient with CD4 count > 350/mm^3 and a high (>100,000 copies/mL) viral load

How Should Antiretroviral Therapy Be Monitored?

Patients started on antiretroviral therapy should return in 2 to 4 weeks to assess the toxicity of the regimen and to repeat the CD4 cell count and viral load. If the drug regimen is well tolerated, the CD4 count is rising, and the viral load is decreasing, treatment is continued. Repeat laboratory parameters are obtained monthly until the viral load becomes undetectable. Viral loads can be expected to drop by approximately one log after one month on treatment but may take as long as 4 to 6 months to become undetectable in some individuals.

When Should an Antiretroviral Drug Regimen Be Modified?

Indications for modification of an antiretroviral regimen include the inability to tolerate drug(s), lack of suppression or rising viral load, declining CD4 cell count, or clinical disease progression. An unsuppressed or rising viral load necessitates inquiry into the patient's medication adherence and may indicate the emergence of viral resistance.

If a Modified Antiretroviral Regimen Is Necessary, How Should New Drugs Be Chosen?

If the drug regimen is being changed because of the development of viral resistance, an entirely new combination that does not share cross-resistance with drugs that the patient is currently taking is recommended. A careful history of previous antiretroviral drugs and an HIV resistance test (see Chapter 5) are useful in this setting. If the regimen is being modified because of toxicity to one drug, a single agent may be substituted.

HIV resistance tests assess the genotype or phenotype of the virus. The genotype test provides a genetic "blueprint" of the predominant viral strain and determines if specific mutations are present in the HIV genome that correlate with clinical resistance to specific antiretroviral drugs. Results are generally interpreted using rules-based algorithms. The phenotype test measures the inhibitory concentration (50% or 90%) of drug needed to suppress the patient's virus and compares them to values seen with a pansensitive ("wild type") strain. Changes of greater than 2.5- to 4-fold are reliably detected. Results are generally categorized as being sensitive, resistant, or intermediate (with significant fold-change "cutoffs" varying by drug). Genotype testing is more readily available, faster, and less costly than phenotype testing; however, it provides only an indirect measure of susceptibility and cannot evaluate the impact of interactions between mutations. Both tests examine only the predominant viral strain and may miss resistant "quasi-species" that constitute less than 25% of the total viral population. Because of these limitations, HIV resistance tests are useful in identifying drugs to which the virus is resistant but may be of limited help in predicting which ones will be effective. For both types of resistance testing, expert consultation is recommended for clinicians with limited experience.

What Are Long-Term Treatment Complications?

Long-term treatment complications associated with combination antiretroviral therapy include lipodystrophy syndrome, hepatotoxicity, peripheral neuropathy, lactic acidosis, premature bone loss, and avascular necrosis of the hips (see Chapter 6). Lipodystrophy syndrome consists of body morphology changes (deposition of fat in abdomen, breasts, and neck; loss of fat in face and extremities), metabolic complications (hyperlipidemia, glucose intolerance/diabetes mellitus), or both. Its epidemiology and pathogenesis are not fully understood, and its optimal management is unknown. An evolving literature suggests that patients on antiretroviral therapy may be at increased risk for coronary artery disease. Hepatotoxicity may occur with any antiretroviral drug but most often has been described with NNRTIs—especially nevirapine. Peripheral neuropathy has been reported in association with certain drugs (ddI, d4T, ddC) and HIV infection itself. Asymptomatic mild-to-moderate lactic acidemia is common in patients on NRTI-based regimens. Symptomatic lactic acidosis with a variety of manifestations (peripheral neuropathy, pancreatitis, myopathy, steatosis with liver failure) has less commonly been described. The mechanism of action is NRTI interference with DNA polymerase in mitochondria. A venous lactate level is recommended in patients on NRTI-based regimens who have unexplained constitutional or gastrointestinal symptoms. Premature bone loss (osteopenia/osteoporosis) and avascular necrosis of the hips also have been reported in HIV-infected patients on antiretroviral therapy. The etiology of these bone abnormalities is uncertain.

Prophylaxis of Opportunistic Infections

Pneumocystis jiroveci (carinii) Pneumonia (PCP)

Despite advances in the management of HIV disease, PCP remains a serious complication. PCP prophylaxis has been shown to decrease morbidity and mortality (see Chapter 7). The risk of developing PCP becomes significant when the patient's CD4 count falls to 200 cells/mm^3 and increases progressively as it gets lower.

An algorithmic approach to PCP prophylaxis is presented in Figure 3-1. Effective drugs for PCP prevention include trimethoprim-sulfamethoxazole (TMP-SMX), dapsone, aerosol pentamidine (AP), and atovaquone. All HIV-infected patients whose CD4 count is less than 200 cells/mm^3 or who have a prior history of PCP should receive prophylaxis. Consideration should be given to starting prophylaxis in patients with higher CD4 counts who have a history of thrush or persistent unexplained fever.

The drug of choice for PCP prophylaxis is TMP-SMX. The recommended dosage is one double-strength tablet per day, although there is evidence supporting the use of reduced-dose regimens (single strength per day or double strength three times per week) in patients unable to tolerate the standard dose.

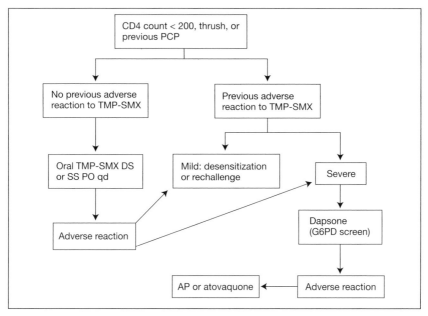

Figure 3-1. Approach to prophylaxis of *Pneumocystis jiroveci (carinii)* pneumonia (PCP). AP = aerosol pentamidine; DS = double-strength; G6PD = glucose-6-phosphate dehydrogenase; SS = single-strength; TMP-SMX = trimethoprim-sulfamethoxazole.

Table 3-1.   Comparison of PCP Prophylaxis Regimens

Issue	TMP-SMX	Dapsone	AP	Atovaquone
Efficacy	High	Moderate	Moderate	Moderate
Toxicity	Moderate	Low-Moderate	Low	Low
Cost	Low	Low	High	Very high
Toxoplasmosis protection	Yes	Yes*	No	?
Bacterial infection protection	Yes	?	No	No
Risk of extrapulmonary pneumocystosis	No	No	Yes	No

AP = aerosol pentamidine; TMF-SMX = trimethoprim-sulfamethoxazole.
* In conjunction with weekly pyrimethamine.

TMP-SMX is preferred to dapsone because of increased efficacy and protection against conventional bacterial infections (Table 3-1). It is preferred to AP because of increased efficacy, lower cost, protection against toxoplasmosis and conventional bacterial infections, and lower risk of extrapulmonary pneumocystosis. It is preferred to atovaquone because of increased efficacy and lower cost. Twenty-five percent to 50% of patients with HIV infection will develop toxicity to TMP-SMX. The most common side effects include fever, rash, liver function test abnormalities, and leukopenia. Strategies for managing mild reactions include discontinuation of the drug, resuming it at the same or lower dose at a later date, or using a desensitization protocol by gradually increasing doses over several days (see Table 7-2 in Chapter 7). For symptom management of mild drug reactions, acetaminophen and an antihistamine are often effective.

Dapsone, 100 mg/d taken orally, is recommended as the alternative agent in patients who cannot tolerate TMP-SMX. A G6PD qualitative assay should be performed before starting dapsone. Side effects may include fever, rash, liver function test abnormalities, leukopenia, and hemolytic anemia, especially in G6PD-deficient patients. For patients who cannot tolerate dapsone, AP is recommended (300 mg/month by Respirgard II jet nebulizer using 6 mL of sterile water delivered at 6 L/min from a 50-psi compressed-air source until the reservoir is dry, usually over 45 minutes). Active TB should be ruled out with a PPD, chest x-ray, and other studies as warranted before initiating AP. Measures should be in place to prevent TB transmission in the context of AP administration. These include use of individual rooms or booths with negative-pressure ventilation, air exhaust to the outside, scheduling to permit air exchange before use by another patient, use of particulate respirators by workers administering the drug, and forbidding patients to return to waiting areas until their coughing subsides.

Primary prophylaxis for PCP can be safely discontinued in patients whose CD4 cell count rises above 200/mm^3 for 3 months on combination antiretroviral therapy. Secondary prophylaxis (maintenance therapy) in patients with a history of PCP can also be stopped in this context.

Mycobacterium avium Complex (MAC) Infection

Mycobacterium avium complex is a slow-growing bacterium that is an important cause of disseminated infection in patients with advanced HIV disease. The risk of developing MAC infection becomes significant when the patient's CD4 count falls to 50 cells/mm^3 and increases progressively as it gets lower. Prophylactic therapy has been shown to be effective in preventing MAC infection, with the risk reduced by one-half in most studies (see Chapter 7).

Prophylaxis is recommended in all patients with a CD4 count of less than 50 cells/mm^3. Effective drugs for MAC prevention include azithromycin and clarithromycin; their usual oral dosages are 1200 mg/wk and 500 mg twice daily, respectively. Rifabutin, which had been used in the past, is less effective and has many drug interactions.

Primary MAC prophylaxis can be safely discontinued in patients whose CD4 cell count rises above 100/mm^3 for 3 months on combination antiretroviral therapy. Secondary prophylaxis (maintenance therapy) in patients with established MAC infection can be discontinued if patients who have completed 12 months of antimicrobial therapy are asymptomatic and their CD4 count has risen above 100/mm^3 for 6 months.

Tuberculosis

Tuberculosis is a significant cause of morbidity and mortality in HIV-infected patients (see Chapter 9). The risk of developing active TB in patients with HIV disease who are infected with *Mycobacterium tuberculosis* is approximately 10% each year compared with a 10% lifetime risk in immunocompetent hosts. TB may present with extrapulmonary manifestations in advanced HIV disease, and lack of reactivity to skin tests is more common in this context. Diagnosis and treatment may be delayed because of these characteristics.

Screening for TB should be part of the initial assessment of HIV-infected patients and repeated annually in high-risk patients if the previous test result is negative (see Chapter 7). Testing is performed with a PPD (intermediate strength, 5TU) administered intracutaneously and read at 48 to 72 hours. The routine use of control agents (e.g., *Candida*, tetanus toxoid, mumps) is not recommended because of their lack of standardization. A positive PPD in an HIV-infected patient is defined as 5 mm or more of induration.

Prophylactic antimicrobial therapy is recommended for HIV-infected patients regardless of age with any of the following: 1) positive PPD, 2) history of a positive PPD and no documentation of a standard course of prophylaxis, or 3) recent exposure to active pulmonary TB. Prophylaxis is not recommended in HIV-infected patients with a negative PPD who have historical risk factors for TB exposure. These include injection-drug use, alcoholism, homelessness, incarceration, having lived in a shelter or institution, and having originated from, or lived in, a country endemic for TB. A chest x-ray should be obtained for all patients with a positive PPD to rule out active pulmonary TB before initiating antimicrobial prophylaxis. If extrapulmonary disease is clinically suspected, appropriate studies to establish the diagnosis also should be performed.

The standard prophylactic regimen consists of isoniazid (INH; 300 mg/d) given with pyridoxine (50 mg/d) or directly observed therapy of INH 900 mg plus pyridoxine 100 mg, both taken twice weekly. Treatment is continued for 9 months. Hepatotoxicity to INH is uncommon in patients younger than 35 years but increases with advancing age. Other common side effects include fever and rash. The drug should be discontinued if clinical stigmata of hepatitis develop or if liver transaminases increase to greater than five times baseline. Rifampin (RIF; 600 mg/d) for 4 to 12 months is an alternative prophylactic regimen. RIF plus pyrazinamide for 2 months is no longer recommended because of significant hepatotoxicity. Expert consultation is recommended in the prophylaxis of multidrug-resistant (MDR) TB strains.

Other Pathogens

Primary prophylaxis is recommended for toxoplasmosis in patients with a positive IgG serology and CD4 count of less than 100 cells/mm³ (see Chapter 7). Either TMP-SMX or dapsone in conjunction with weekly pyrimethamine is useful for toxoplasmosis prevention. Oral ganciclovir has

Table 3-2.   Opportunistic Infection Prophylaxis Stratified by CD4 Cell Count

| Infection | CD4 Cell Count | | |
	> 200/mm³	200-50/mm³	< 50/mm³
Tuberculosis*	Isoniazid	Isoniazid	Isoniazid
PCP	None	TMP-SMX	TMP-SMX
Toxoplasmosis†	None	TMP-SMX	TMP-SMX
Fungal‡	None	Fluconazole	Fluconazole
HSV‡	None	Acyclovir	Acyclovir
MAC	None	None	Azithromycin
CMV	None	None	(Oral ganciclovir)

CMV = cytomegalovirus; GCV = ganciclovir; HSV = herpes simplex virus; MAC = *Mycobacterium avium* complex; PPD = purified protein derivative of tuberculin; TMP-SMX = trimethoprim-sulfamethoxazole.
* In patients with positive PPD.
† Prophylaxis indicated in patients with CD4 count < 100/mm³ and positive serology; alternative therapy is dapsone and pyrimethamine.
‡ Secondary prophylaxis only.

been demonstrated to be effective for primary prophylaxis of CMV infection but is not often prescribed because of concerns about toxicity and cost (see Chapter 7). Secondary prophylaxis with appropriate drugs is often necessary for candidiasis and HSV infection in advanced HIV disease.

Opportunistic infection prophylaxis recommendations stratified by CD4 cell count are summarized in Table 3-2.

Health Care Maintenance Issues

Immunizations

Patients with HIV disease are at increased risk for a variety of infections that can potentially be prevented by using available vaccine preparations. Immunizations should be given as early in the course of HIV disease as possible for optimal effect. Patients with relatively preserved immune function are more likely to respond to vaccine challenge than those who are significantly immunocompromised. Initiation of combination antiretroviral therapy in patients with advanced HIV disease prior to administering vaccines may be beneficial.

In general, live pathogen vaccines (e.g., varicella, MMR, oral polio, Flumist) should be avoided in HIV-infected patients unless the benefits clearly outweigh the risks. However, killed or inactivated vaccines are considered safe in this population. Although influenza and other vaccine preparations have been shown to stimulate HIV replication and to increase viral load transiently, this phenomenon does not seem to have an impact on disease progression.

Specific immunization recommendations are presented in Table 3-3. Pneumococcal vaccine should be administered to all HIV-infected patients

Table 3-3. Immunization Recommendations for HIV-Infected Adults

Vaccine	Status	Dose/Regimen	Comments
Pneumococcal vaccine	Recommended	0.5 mL IM	Administer to patients with CD4 cell count ≥ 200/mm³. Consider booster dose 5 years after initial immunization if given in context of low CD4 count.
Hepatitis B vaccine	Recommended in selected settings; see comments	Engerix B 20 µg or Recombivax HB 10 µg IM given at 0, 1, and 6 months; also available in combination with hepatitis A vaccine as Twinrix	Administer to patients without serologic evidence of past or present hepatitis B infection. Vaccinated patients should be tested for HBsAb response after the third dose; nonresponders should receive booster injection.
Hepatitis A vaccine	Recommended in selected settings; see comments	1 mL IM with revaccination in 6-12 months; also available in combination with hepatitis B vaccine as Twinrix	Administer to men who have sex with men and to patients with chronic hepatitis C infection. Serologic testing before vaccination is not necessary.
Haemophilus influenzae, type B, vaccine	Consider in selected settings; see comments	0.5 mL IM	Administer to asplenic patients and those with history of recurrent Haemophilus infection.
Influenza vaccine	Recommended; see comments	0.5 mL IM annually	Especially important in patients at high risk for exposure to or morbidity from influenza. There is evidence that the vaccine may transiently promote HIV replication.
Tetanus toxoid	Same as for patient without HIV infection	Td 0.5 mL IM	Td booster is recommended every 10 years.
Polio vaccine	OPV contraindicated; eIPV should be given if indicated	0.5 mL SC; three doses over 6-12 months for primary immunization	OPV has not proven harmful when given to asymptomatic HIV-infected patients, but eIPV is preferred.

with a CD4 cell count of 200/mm^3 or greater. Some experts recommend a booster dose 5 years after immunization. Hepatitis B immunization series should be administered to patients who have a negative screening serologic test for this infection. Hepatitis A vaccine should be given to MSM and to patients with chronic hepatitis B or C infection. It should also be considered in injection-drug users, in whom outbreaks have been described. Influenza vaccine is recommended for all HIV-infected patients by the CDC and is especially important in people with historical risk factors for exposure to the virus or who have conditions associated with increased morbidity from influenza infection. Routine use of *Haemophilus* B vaccine is not recommended, but asplenic patients and those with history of recurrent *Haemophilus* infection should receive it.

Cervical Cancer Screening

HIV disease is associated with an increased risk of cervical dysplasia and cancer in women (see Chapters 10 and 11). Most patients who develop these conditions have a previous history of HPV infection, which also causes genital warts. The risk of developing cervical dysplasia is greatest in women with advanced HIV disease. Pap smear has been demonstrated to be a useful screening test in this context.

A pelvic examination and Pap smear should be performed as part of the initial evaluation of all HIV-infected women. It should be repeated 6 months later and, if normal, repeated at 12-month intervals thereafter. Colposcopy is not recommended as a screening test in this population. More frequent Pap smears (every 4 to 6 months) are recommended in the following settings: 1) if endocervical component is absent, 2) if there is a history of HPV infection, or 3) after treatment for any cervical lesion. Women with abnormal Pap smear results showing cellular atypia or any degree of cervical dysplasia should be referred to a gynecologist for further diagnostic evaluation. In general, colposcopy and biopsy are performed.

Anal Cancer Screening

In addition to causing cervical dysplasia and cancer, several serotypes of HPV have been associated with anal squamous cell dysplasia and cancer in HIV-infected men and women. Some clinicians recommend baseline and 6-month anal Pap smears in patients with evidence of anogenital HPV infection, as well as subsequent annual screening in those with a CD4 cell count of less than 500/mm^3, although there are no published consensus guidelines at this time. Standard protocols for managing anal dysplasia are being developed. In general, anoscopy with biopsy is performed, followed by surgical or liquid nitrogen ablation where indicated.

Sexually Transmitted Diseases

Patients with HIV infection should be screened for other STDs at intake and periodically thereafter if they remain at risk. Emphasis should be placed on prevention. Genital ulcer diseases, such as syphilis and HSV, predispose to the transmission and acquisition of HIV infection.

Other Conditions

Age-appropriate screening for other conditions (e.g., breast, colon, and prostate cancers) should be performed in patients with HIV disease. Baseline mammography usually is advised in women at 40 years of age and repeated annually thereafter. In general, colonoscopy every 10 years is recommended in patients over 50 years of age, with hemoccult testing of stool in interval years. Digital prostate examination is generally performed annually in men over 50 years of age. The use of prostate-specific antigen (PSA) testing to screen for prostate cancer remains controversial.

Psychiatric Disorders

The most common psychiatric diagnoses in patients with HIV disease are adjustment disorder, major depression, anxiety disorder, and substance abuse. Psychological symptoms may be part of an organic syndrome warranting medical intervention. Sometimes, a clinical distinction can be made between early HIV-related neurocognitive disorder (manifested by withdrawal, apathy, avoidance of complex tasks, and mental slowing) (see Chapter 8) and depression (manifested by low self-esteem, irrational guilt, and vegetative symptoms). Neuropsychological testing or an empiric trial of antidepressant therapy may be indicated in more subtle instances.

Adjustment disorder with a depressed or anxious mood can occur frequently, and may be severe enough to warrant psychotherapy or pharmacologic treatment. Stressors may include: 1) any of the psychological issues associated with a potentially life-threatening illness; 2) stigmatization that threatens the patient's status in society; 3) uncertainty about the course of the disease; and 4) difficulty in obtaining adequate health care or financial resources.

Informing patients about support groups and AIDS service organizations within the community is an important aspect of primary care. "Buddies" through AIDS service organizations can provide long-term emotional support that may otherwise be unavailable to patients who are estranged from family or friends.

Other Issues

Complementary Medical Therapies

Complementary or alternative medical therapies are commonly used by HIV-infected patients in conjunction with conventional treatments. Patients may not volunteer such information unless it is requested specifically. The safety and efficacy of alternative medical therapies for HIV disease are not well established. In addition, drug interactions may be a concern with PIs and other medications.

Clinical Trials

Participation in clinical trials should be encouraged for HIV-infected patients in therapeutic areas in which the optimal management is unknown. Good communication between research staff and the primary care clinician is important to ensure coordination of care.

Substance Abuse

Some HIV-infected patients have a history of recurrent substance abuse involving alcohol, cocaine, crystal methamphetamine, or opiates (see Chapter 11). Clinicians should recognize that the stress of being HIV-seropositive or of developing symptomatic HIV disease may lead to substance abuse relapse. Fostering sobriety is an important component of care. In the active drug user, substance abuse treatment may take priority over the management of HIV disease.

Personal Finances

Assessment of the patient's financial situation and insurance status also should be part of the intake process, with attention given to ascertaining eligibility for health care, general relief, disability, and housing programs.

Legal Issues

A variety of legal issues can take on dramatic significance for persons with HIV disease, especially in the context of a long-term homosexual relationship. Ill patients may need to anticipate transfer in custody of their children. They should also be encouraged to arrange for others to make medical judgments on their behalf in case of severe illness by executing an advance directive for health care, a durable power of attorney, or both. Many AIDS service organizations assist patients in executing legal instruments and resolving custody issues.

Food, Animal, and Travel Safety

Caution in food preparation and handling is important given the vulnerability to infections that accompanies immunodeficiency. Using plastic or glass rather than wooden cutting boards may decrease the chance of bacterial contamination. Microwaved foods should be allowed to stand for a few minutes after cooking to ensure that heat is evenly distributed. Because of the risk of salmonellosis, raw egg products should not be consumed (including homemade Caesar salad dressing). Raw seafood (e.g., sashimi, sushi, oysters), poultry, and meat (e.g., steak tartare) should be avoided because of the potential for transmission of bacteria and protozoa. All produce should be cleaned before eating.

Patients should be reminded to wash their hands after bathroom use or after contact with animals or soil. They should not drink water from an untested source. Care should be exercised in the selection and handling of domestic animals. Foreign travel plans should be discussed in advance with a knowledgeable health care provider, and immunizations and prophylactic antimicrobial therapies should be administered as appropriate.

KEY POINTS

- In addition to history and physical examination, the initial evaluation of HIV-infected patients should include assessment of their knowledge of the disease and their emotional state.
- Baseline laboratory studies are performed to screen for occult disease and to guide drug usage, to determine HIV disease status, and to look for evidence of concurrent infections. The CD4 cell count and viral load are essential for staging and guiding therapeutic decisions.
- Antiretroviral therapy is generally indicated if: 1) the patient is symptomatic; 2) CD4 cell count is < 350 to 200/mm^3; or 3) the patient is pregnant. Antiretroviral therapy should be considered in the asymptomatic patient with CD4 count > 350/mm^3 and a viral load greater than 100,000 copies/mL. The most common regimens used are 2 NRTIs plus NNRTI and 2 NRTIs plus PI (often boosted). Factors that may have a negative impact on adherence should be reviewed and addressed before initiation of therapy.
- All HIV-infected patients, regardless of whether they are receiving antiretroviral therapy, should be monitored with laboratory tests at least every 3 to 4 months. HIV resistance testing, which may include genotypic and/or phenotypic profiling, is indicated when the viral load is not maximally suppressed in patients on antiretroviral therapy.
- Significant complications have been associated with long-term combination antiretroviral therapy. These include: 1) lipodystrophy

syndrome (body fat redistribution, hyperlipidemia, glucose intolerance); 2) lactic acidosis (peripheral neuropathy, pancreatitis, myopathy, steatosis); 3) premature bone loss (osteopenia and osteoporosis); 4) avascular necrosis of hips; and 5) possibly an increased risk of atherosclerotic disease.

- Opportunistic infection (OI) prophylaxis for PCP is indicated if CD4 count is less than 200/mm^3; TMP-SMX is the drug of choice. Prophylaxis for toxoplasmosis is indicated in patients with positive toxoplasmosis serology if CD4 count is less than 100/mm^3; TMP-SMX is the drug of choice. Prophylaxis for MAC infection is indicated if CD4 count is less than 50/mm^3; azithromycin is the drug of choice. OI prophylaxis can often be safely discontinued for many infections following immune reconstitution with antiretroviral therapy.
- Routine health care maintenance issues in HIV-infected patients include immunizations (pneumococcal, hepatitis B, hepatitis A, and influenza), periodic screening for concurrent infections (syphilis, other STDs, and TB), regular Pap smears in women, and other age- and sex-appropriate screening studies.

SUGGESTED WEB SITES

Aegis (www.aegis.com).

AIDS Education and Training Centers National Resource Center (www.aids-ed.org).

AIDSinfo: Department of Health and Human Services (www.aidsinfo.nih.gov).

The Body (www.thebody.com).

Centers for Disease Control and Prevention (www.cdc.gov/hiv/pubs/facts.htm).

HIV InSite (hivinsite.ucsf.edu).

Johns Hopkins AIDS Service (www.hopkins-aids.edu).

National HIV/AIDS Clinicians' Consultation Center (www.ucsf.edu/hivcntr).

SUGGESTED READINGS

Aberg JA, Gallant JE, Anderson J, et al. Primary care guidelines for the management of persons infected with human immunodeficiency virus: recommendations of the HIV Medicine Association of the Infectious Diseases Society of America. Clin Infect Dis. 2004;39:609-29.

Barrios A, Rendón A, Negredo E, Barreiro P, Garcia-Benayas T, Labarga P, et al. Paradoxical CD4+ T-cell decline in HIV-infected patients with complete virus suppression taking tenofovir and didanosine. AIDS. 2005;19:569-75.

Bartlett JG, ed. Hopkins HIV Report. Bimonthly publication of Johns Hopkins University AIDS Service, Baltimore, MD.

Centers for Disease Control and Prevention. Guidelines for the use of antiretroviral agents in HIV-infected adults and adolescents. Ann Intern Med. 2002;137:381-433. (Available as a living document on AIDSinfo: Department of Health and Human Services Web site at www.aidsinfo.nih.gov.)

Centers for Disease Control and Prevention. Public Health Service Task Force recommendations for the use of antiretroviral drugs in pregnant women infected with HIV-1 for maternal health and for reducing perinatal HIV-1 transmission in the United States. (Available as a living document on AIDSinfo: Department of Health and Human Services Web site at www.aidsinfo.nih.gov.)

Centers for Disease Control and Prevention. Revised recommendations for HIV testing of adults, adolescents, and pregnant women in health-care settings. MMWR. 2006;55 (RR-14):1-17.

Hammer SM. Clinical practice. Management of newly diagnosed HIV infection. N Engl J Med. 2005;353:1702-10.

Hecht FM, Grant RM. Resistance testing in drug-naive HIV-infected patients: is it time? [Editorial]. Clin Infect Dis. 2005;41:1324-5.

Hirsch MS, Brun-Vézinet F, D'Aquila RT, Hammer SM, Johnson VA, Kuritzkes DR, et al. Antiretroviral drug resistance testing in adult HIV-1 infection: recommendations of an International AIDS Society-USA Panel. JAMA. 2000;283:2417-26.

Mellors JW, Muñoz A, Giorgi JV, Margolick JB, Tassoni CJ, Gupta P, et al. Plasma viral load and CD4+ lymphocytes as prognostic markers of HIV-1 infection. Ann Intern Med. 1997;126:946-54.

Ryan DP, Compton CC, Mayer RJ. Carcinoma of the anal canal. N Eng J Med. 2000;342: 792-800.

Sax PE, ed. AIDS Clinical Care. Monthly publication of the Massachusetts Medical Society; Waltham.

Sax PE, Islam R, Walensky RP, et al. Should resistance testing be performed for treatment-naive HIV-infected patients? A cost-effectiveness analysis. Clin Inf Dis. 2005;41:1316-23.

Schambelan M, Benson CA, Carr A, et al. Management of metabolic complications associated with antiretroviral therapy for HIV-1 infection: recommendations of an International AIDS Society-USA panel. J Acquir Immune Defic Syndr. 2002;31:257-75.

Smith DM. Incidence of HIV superinfection following primary infection. JAMA. 2004; 292:1177-8.

U.S. Public Health Service/Infectious Disease Society of America. Guidelines for the prevention of opportunistic infections in persons infected with human immunodeficiency virus. Ann Intern Med. 2002;137:435-77. (Available as a living document on AIDSinfo: Department of Health and Human Services Web site at www.aidsinfo.nih.gov.)

Yeni PG, Hammer SM, Carpenter CC, et al. Antiretroviral treatment for adult HIV infection in 2002: updated recommendations of the International AIDS Society–USA Panel. JAMA. 2002;288:222-35.

Chapter 4

Antiretroviral Therapy

MARISSA B. WILCK, MBChB
PAUL E. SAX, MD

The widespread adoption of combination antiretroviral therapy (ART) in 1996 changed the course of HIV disease. Triple-drug therapy has led to a marked reduction in AIDS-related opportunistic infections (OIs) and deaths. For many patients who are able to access ART, HIV disease has become a chronic medical condition, with the focus of management shifted toward simplifying drug regimens, fostering adherence, and reducing long-term toxicity. With the expansion of existing drug classes and the development of new ones, the complexity of treatment has significantly increased.

This chapter addresses the goals of antiretroviral therapy, indications for therapy and timing of its initiation, determinants of virologic success, selection of an initial antiretroviral regimen, treatment interruption, when and how to modify therapy, antiretroviral therapy in pregnancy, and investigational drugs. Because of the rapidly changing nature of practice in this area, clinicians with limited experience should seek consultation.

Goals of Therapy

The goals of ART are to prevent and, when possible, reverse HIV disease progression, which results in significantly decreased morbidity and mortality. Maximal viral suppression and an increased CD4 cell count are the surrogate laboratory markers of success.

Indications for, and Timing of, Therapy

Despite advances in ART and a number of longitudinal studies addressing the issue of optimal timing of treatment, controversy exists regarding the "golden moment" to initiate therapy. As with all chronic diseases, the benefits of therapy must be carefully weighed against its toxicity. This is especially true for HIV infection, which has an asymptomatic phase that may last for many years. Furthermore, consideration of the patient's readiness and ability to take medications is paramount, because viral resistance may rapidly develop if they are taken inconsistently.

Guidelines from the Department of Health and Human Services (DHHS) and the International AIDS Society (IAS)-USA Panel for when to start treatment are summarized in Table 4-1. Advantages and disadvantages of early versus delayed treatment are shown in Table 4-2. These issues are reviewed in detail below.

Table 4-1.   Initiation of Antiretroviral Therapy in Patients with Chronic HIV Infection

Clinical Category	CD4 Cell Count	HIV Viral Load	IAS-USA Guidelines	DHHS Guidelines
AIDS-defining illness or severe symptoms	Any value	Any value	Treat	Treat
Asymptomatic	<200/mm^3	Any value	Treat	Treat
Asymptomatic	200-350/mm^3	Any value	Consider treatment	Offer treatment
Asymptomatic	350-500/mm^3	>100,000 copies/mL	Consider treatment*	Consider treatment
Asymptomatic	<350/mm^3	<100,000 copies/mL	Counseling	Defer treatment

* IAS-USA guidelines also recommend considering treatment if CD4 cell count is declining rapidly (>100/mm^3 per year).

Table 4-2.   Benefits and Risks of Early versus Delayed Initiation of Antiretroviral Therapy in Asymptomatic HIV-Infected Patients

Therapy	Benefits	Risks
Early	• Control of viral replication easier to achieve and maintain • Delay or prevention of immune system decline • Lower risk of resistance with complete viral suppression • Possible decreased risk of HIV transmission	• Drug-related reduction in quality of life • Greater cumulative drug-related adverse effects • Earlier development of drug resistance if there is suboptimal viral suppression • Limitation of future antiretroviral options
Delayed	• Avoidance of negative effects on quality of life • Avoidance of drug-related toxicities • Delayed development of drug resistance • Preservation of future drug options	• Possible risk of irreversible immune system depletion • Possible greater difficulty in suppression of viral replication • Possible increased risk of HIV transmission

Symptomatic Disease

The presence of symptomatic HIV disease is a clear indication to start therapy. Included in this category are all patients with a diagnosis of AIDS based on a history of an opportunistic disease and those without AIDS who have a significant complication, such as recurrent oral or vaginal candidiasis, cervical or anal dysplasia, or profound thrombocytopenia, which is attributable to HIV disease. Treatment is indicated in this group regardless of CD4 cell count and viral load.

Controversy exists over the optimal time to start therapy in the context of an active OI. The benefits of starting ART are more apparent when there is limited or no effective treatment for the OI. Examples of such infections include cryptosporidiosis, microsporidiosis, progressive multifocal leukoencephalopathy, and drug-resistant candidiasis, as well as HIV-related neurologic complications. With OIs for which there is effective therapy, such as *Pneumocystis jiroveci* pneumonia (formerly *Pneumocystis carinii* pneumonia [PCP]), toxoplasmosis, and cryptococcosis, many clinicians defer starting ART until that condition has stabilized. The reasons behind this decision are to avoid overlapping drug toxicities and concern for precipitation of the immune reconstitution syndrome. A clinical trial comparing early versus delayed therapy in this setting is in progress.

CD4 Cell Count

A key step in determining when to start treatment is the assessment of the patient's risk of progression to AIDS. The absolute CD4 count is the most reliable predictor of it in conjunction with the plasma HIV RNA level (see Figure 1-5 in Chapter 1).

Treatment should optimally be started before the CD4 count falls below 200 cells/mm^3. Multiple cohort studies have demonstrated that survival in patients who start with this degree of immune dysfunction is worse than in those who start earlier, even with optimal adherence and achievement of viral suppression.

For patients with asymptomatic infection and a CD4 count above 200 cells/mm^3, the decision of when to start treatment is less clear. Some cohort studies have suggested improved immunologic recovery and a survival benefit in persons initiating therapy when the CD4 count is as high as 350 cells/mm^3. Based on these data, strong consideration for treatment should be given to patients with a CD4 cell count between 200/mm^3 and 350/mm^3, with additional factors such as HIV viral load and patient willingness to start therapy also taken into account.

The CD4 percentage (CD4/total lymphocyte count) is generally not used in determining when to start ART. One study found the CD4 percentage is no better a predictor of HIV disease progression than the absolute count alone. In another study, a CD4 percentage less than 17 was a strong predictor of progression to AIDS among patients with an absolute count of greater than 350 cells/mm³.

Viral Load

Although not a primary indicator for treatment initiation, the viral load may provide supplemental information to aid in this decision. High viral loads, especially over 100,000 copies/mL, are associated with a more rapid decrease in CD4 count and clinical disease progression. It may thus be reasonable to initiate therapy in patients with CD4 counts in the 200 to 500 cells/mm³ range when the viral load is greater than 100,000 copies/mL.

Pregnancy

There is a strong correlation between maternal viral load at time of delivery and perinatal transmission of HIV. However, HIV transmission may occur even when the maternal viral load is undetectable. As a result, all HIV-infected pregnant women should receive ART even if they otherwise do not meet clinical or laboratory criteria. Further discussion of this issue is found below and in Chapter 11.

Acute HIV Infection

At least half of patients with acute HIV infection are symptomatic (see Chapter 1). Diagnosis is confirmed when the HIV antibody test is negative (or the ELISA is positive with an indeterminate Western blot) in the presence of a high-titer (>1,000,000 copies/mL) viral load. Because symptoms of acute HIV infection are nonspecific, it often goes unrecognized. However, when diagnosed, the question of whether to initiate ART should be raised.

The rationale for treatment of acute HIV infection is as follows:

- Alteration of viral set point, which can affect the rate of disease progression
- Reduction in rate of viral mutation and evolution with suppression of viral replication
- Preservation of immune function
- Reduction in the risk of viral transmission

On the other hand, treatment of acute HIV infection also has potential risks:

- Adverse effects on quality of life from drug toxicity
- Development of drug resistance if ART fails to suppress viral replication, thereby limiting future treatment options
- Possible need to continue therapy indefinitely

A small case series of patients given ART during acute infection suggested that it preserved HIV-specific CD4 responses, thereby leading to immunologic control of HIV after treatment was interrupted. Follow-up of these patients, however, has shown that this effect is not durable. While the benefits of ART for acute HIV infection are unproven, many clinicians offer treatment in this setting, especially if the patient is very symptomatic, or they refer patients for participation in a clinical trial. The optimal duration of therapy is uncertain.

Determinants of Virologic Success

As noted above, ART that leads to an undetectable viral load is most likely to result in immunologic recovery and the prevention of HIV disease progression. Several factors affect the likelihood of durable viral suppression. These include the patient's immunologic status, viral load, drug resistance, medication adherence, potency of ART, and pharmacokinetic issues.

Immunologic Status

A baseline CD4 count of greater than 200 cells/mm^3 has been associated in several studies with a higher likelihood of virologic suppression and immune reconstitution; by contrast, a count of less than 50/mm^3 has been shown to correlate with a lower probability. In the 2NN study, which compared efavirenz (EFV)- and nevirapine (NVP)-based regimens, all patients with lower baseline CD4 counts had a reduced virologic response.

Viral Load

In general, a higher baseline viral load (>100,000 copies/mL) has been associated with a reduced virologic response and a longer time required to achieve viral suppression. However, studies using the nonnucleoside reverse-transcriptase inhibitor (NNRTI) EFV or the boosted protease inhibitor (PI) lopinavir/ritonavir (LPV/RTV) have shown equal activity at all viral load strata, perhaps relating to their favorable pharmacokinetic properties. A response of 0.72 log decrease as early as 1 week into ART has also been shown to correlate with long-term viral suppression. The week 8 viral load level is another predictor.

Drug Resistance

The highest likelihood of achieving and maintaining viral suppression is seen in ART-naïve patients, with studies showing on-treatment success rates of 80% to 90% compared with 35% to 75% in treatment-experienced patients. Hence, the initial regimen carries the highest probability of prolonged viral suppression. Drug resistance most commonly arises after prior nonsuppressive regimens; it may also be seen as a result of transmission of resistant virus from one patient to another. In the United States, the estimated prevalence of drug resistance in treatment-naïve patients is approximately 14%. Therefore, obtaining a resistance test in newly diagnosed patients is recommended.

Medication Adherence

The importance of ART adherence to virologic response is critical. A striking example of this principle is illustrated by a study that showed a viral suppression rate of 80% in patients taking more than 95% of prescribed doses compared with less than 50% in those taking fewer doses. More recent studies of drugs with longer half-lives show that somewhat lower rates of adherence may be associated with treatment success but that it is still an important factor.

The frequency of poor adherence and treatment discontinuation is significantly higher in observational settings than in clinical trials. The Multicenter AIDS Cohort Study found that being African-American, no recent outpatient visit, lower income, use of more than three antiretroviral drugs, and being depressed predicted worse adherence. Critical components of care of patients starting ART include understanding the barriers to adherence, choosing drugs that will be least "disruptive," education about drug side effects and long-term toxicities, and implementation of strategies to improve adherence.

Once a decision is made to initiate ART, an obvious, but often overlooked, consideration is the patient's readiness to begin it. Starting therapy is never an emergency, and time spent preparing a patient generally results in a better outcome. In many practices, patients who are newly diagnosed undergo a formal evaluation by an HIV case manager to gather information on health insurance, family and work situation, history of substance abuse and/or domestic violence, and other factors that may make treatment more problematic.

Potency of Antiretroviral Therapy

All the DHHS preferred regimens are considered to be comparably potent. Older treatment strategies, such as triple nucleoside reverse-transcriptase inhibitor (NRTI) therapy and the use of early generation PIs, are less likely to achieve viral suppression even with optimal adherence.

Pharmacokinetic Issues

The optimal antiretroviral drug will maintain tissue and/or plasma levels above the concentration required for inhibition of the virus for a prolonged period of time. This characteristic can diminish the risk of resistance and allow more "forgiveness" when adherence is imperfect. Examples of such medications are EFV and LPV/RTV. Further discussion of this topic can be found in Chapter 5.

Selection of Initial Antiretroviral Regimen

There are currently 4 classes and 22 approved drugs for the treatment of HIV infection. All recommended regimens consist of at least three active drugs. The two main components of this regimen are:

1. An NRTI "backbone" consisting of lamivudine (3TC) or emtric-itabine (FTC) and one additional agent
   plus
2. A PI (often with RTV) or an NNRTI

The preferred antiretroviral regimens for initiation of therapy are shown in Table 4-3. It is common for the PI component to be given with low-dose RTV. Ritonavir is a potent inhibitor of cyp3A4 metabolism and, when given in a low dose, increases plasma levels of the other PIs but does not exert antiviral activity. Use of RTV in this manner is sometimes referred to as RTV "boosting." Of the PIs currently in widespread use, only nelfinavir (NFV) lacks an RTV-boosting option. Antiretroviral regimens and components that are not recommended are presented in Table 4-4.

Selection of the optimal regimen is individualized based on an understanding of patient preferences related to dosing frequency, pill burden, and potential drug toxicities. The four main decisions about selection of therapy can be summarized as follows:

1. Which NRTI should be paired with 3TC or FTC?
2. Should a PI-based or NNRTI-based regimen be used?
3. If a PI-based regimen, which one? Should it be RTV-boosted?
4. If an NNRTI-based regimen, should it be EFV or NVP?

Characteristics of NRTIs, NNRTIs, and PIs are shown in Tables 4-5, 4-6, and 4-7, respectively. NNRTIs and PIs have many potential drug interactions with each other and with other medications. Some drugs may require dosage adjustment or be contraindicated for coadministration (Table 4-8).

Treatment Options

The Nucleoside "Backbone"
DHHS-preferred combinations include: 1) zidovudine (ZDV) with 3TC; and 2) tenofovir (TDF) with FTC; alternatives include: 1) abacavir (ABC) with 3TC; and 2) didanosine (ddI) with FTC or 3TC. The choice of which combination to use is made according to the potency, side effect profile, and dosing schedule of the drugs.

Text continues on page 84.

Table 4-3.   Antiretroviral Components Recommended for HIV Infection in Treatment-Naïve Patients

A combination antiretroviral regimen in treatment-naïve patients generally contains
1 NNRTI + 2 NRTIs or a single or ritonavir-boosted PI + 2 NRTIs.

Selection of a regimen for an antiretroviral-naïve patient should be individualized based on virologic efficacy, toxicities, pill burden, dosing frequency, drug interaction potential, and co-morbid conditions. Components listed below are designated as preferred when clinical trial data suggest optimal and durable efficacy with acceptable tolerability and ease of use. Alternative components are those that show efficacy but have disadvantages compared with the preferred agents. In some cases, for an individual patient, a component listed as alternative may actually be preferred. Clinicians initiating antiretroviral therapy in an HIV-infected pregnant woman should refer to the specific DHHS guidelines.

To Construct an Antiretroviral Regimen, Select 1 Component from Column A + 1 from Column B

	Column A		Column B	
	(NNRTI or PI Options in alphabetical order)		*(Dual-NRTI Options in alphabetical order)*	
Preferred Components	NNRTI- efavirenz[1]	or PI Atazanavir + ritonavir Fosamprenavir + ritonavir (2×/day) Lopinavir/ritonavir[2] (2×/day) (co-formulated)	Preferred Components	Tenofovir/emtricitabine[3] (co-formulated) Zidovudine/lamivudine[3] (co-formulated)
Alternative to Preferred Components	NNRTI - nevirapine[4]	or PI Atazanavir[5] Fosamprenavir Fosamprenavir + ritonavir (1×/day) Lopinavir/ritonavir (1×/day) (co-formulated)	Alternative to Preferred Components	Abacavir/lamivudine[3] (co-formulated) Didanosine + (emtricitabine or lamivudine)

[1] Efavirenz is not recommended for use in first trimester of pregnancy or in sexually active women with child-bearing potential who are not using effective contraception.
[2] The pivotal study that led to the recommendation of lopinavir/ritonavir as a preferred PI component was based on twice-daily dosing. A smaller study has shown similar efficacy with once-daily dosing but also showed a higher incidence of moderate-to-severe diarrhea (16% vs. 5%).
[3] Emtricitabine may be used in place of lamivudine and vice versa.
[4] Nevirapine should not be initiated in women with CD4 count >250 cells/mm^3 or in men with CD4 count >400 cells/mm^3 because of increased risk of symptomatic hepatic events in these patients.
[5] Atazanavir must be boosted with ritonavir if used in combination with tenofovir.
Source: Department of Health and Human Services. Guidelines for the Use of Antiretroviral Agents in HIV-1 Infected Adults and Adolescents. Available as a "living document" at http://www.aidsinfo.nih.gov.

Table 4-4.   Antiretroviral Regimens and Components Not Recommended

	Rationale	Exception
Antiretroviral Regimens Not Recommended		
Monotherapy with NRTI or NNRTI	• Rapid development of resistance • Inferior antiretroviral activity when compared with combination of three or more antiretrovirals	• Pregnant women with pretreatment HIV RNA <1000 copies/mL using ZDV monotherapy for prevention of perinatal HIV transmission, not for HIV treatment for the mother*; however, combination therapy is generally preferred
Dual-NRTI regimens	• Rapid development of resistance • Inferior antiretroviral activity when compared with combination of three or more antiretrovirals	
Triple-NRTI regimens except for abacavir/zidovudine/lamivudine or possibly tenofovir + zidovudine/lamivudine	• High rate of early virologic non-response seen when triple NRTI combinations, including ABC/TDF/3TC or TDF/ddI/3TC, were used as initial regimen in treatment-naïve patients • Other 3-NRTI regimens have not been evaluated	• Abacavir/zidovudine/ lamivudine and possibly tenofovir + zidovudine/ lamivudine
Antiretroviral Components Not Recommended		
Amprenavir oral solution in pregnant women, children <4 yrs old, patients with renal or hepatic failure, and patients on metronidazole or disulfiram	• Oral liquid contains large amount of the excipient propylene glycol, which may be toxic in patients at risk	• No exception
Amprenavir + fosamprenavir	• Amprenavir is the active antiviral for both drugs; combined use has no benefit and may increase toxicities	• No exception
Amprenavir oral solution + ritonavir oral solution	• The large amount of propylene glycol used as a vehicle in amprenavir oral solution may compete with ethanol (the vehicle in oral ritonavir solution) for the same metabolic pathway for elimination; this may lead to accumulation of either one of the vehicles	• No exception
Atazanavir + indinavir	• Potential additive hyperbilirubinemia	• No exception

(cont'd)

Table 4-4.   Antiretroviral Regimens and Components Not Recommended (*cont'd*)

	Rationale	Exception
Antiretroviral Components Not Recommended (*cont'd*)		
Didanosine + stavudine	• High incidence of toxicities, including peripheral neuropathy, pancreatitis, and hyperlactatemia • Reports of serious, even fatal, cases of lactic acidosis with hepatic steatosis with or without pancreatitis in pregnant women*	• When no other antiretroviral options are available and potential benefits outweigh risks*
Didanosine + zalcitabine	• Additive peripheral neuropathy	• No exception
Efavirenz in first trimester of pregnancy or in women with significant child-bearing potential*	• Teratogenic in nonhuman primates	• When no other antiretroviral options are available and potential benefits outweigh risks*
Emtricitabine + lamivudine	• Similar resistance profile • No potential benefit	• No exception
Lamivudine + zalcitabine	• In vitro antagonism	• No exception
Nevirapine initiation in treatment-naïve women with CD4 >250 cells/mm³ or in treatment-naïve men with CD4 >400 cells/mm³	• Higher incidence of symptomatic (including serious and even fatal) hepatic events in these patient groups	• Only if benefits clearly outweigh risks
Saquinavir as single protease inhibitor	• Poor oral bioavailability • Inferior antiretroviral activity when compared with other protease inhibitors	• No exception
Stavudine + zalcitabine	• Additive peripheral neuropathy	• No exception
Stavudine + zidovudine	• Antagonistic effect on HIV	• No exception

*When constructing an antiretroviral regimen for an HIV-infected pregnant woman, consult the specific DHHS guidelines.
Source: Department of Health and Human Services. Guidelines for the Use of Antiretroviral Agents in HIV-1 Infected Adults and Adolescents. Available as a "living document" at http://www.aidsinfo.nih.gov.

Certain NRTIs should not be used together. Examples include: 1) NRTIs with very similar mechanisms of action, metabolism, or resistance patterns (e.g., ZDV and stavudine [d4T]), which are both thymidine analogues; FTC and 3TC, the former being a fluorinated analogue of the latter); 2) NRTIs with similar toxicity profiles (e.g., ddI and d4T, both of which cause peripheral neuropathy, lactic acidosis, and pancreatitis); and 3) combinations with inferior efficacy demonstrated in clinical trials (e.g., TDF and ddI, which may be related to TDF's inhibition of purine nucleoside phosphorylase, an enzyme involved in the breakdown of ddI).

Text continues on page 100.

Table 4-5. Characteristics of Nucleoside Reverse-Transcriptase Inhibitors (NRTIs)

Generic Name (abbreviation)/ Trade Name	Formulation	Dosing Recommendations	Food Effect	Oral Bioavailability	Serum Half-Life	Intracellular Half-Life	Elimination	Adverse Events
Abacavir (ABC)								
Ziagen	300 mg tablets or 20 mg/mL oral solution	300 mg two times/day or 600 mg once daily	Take without regard to meals; alcohol increases abacavir levels 41%; abacavir has no effect on alcohol	83%	1.5 hours	12-26 hours	• Metabolized by alcohol dehydrogenase and glucuronyl transferase • Renal excretion of metabolites 82% • Trizivir and Epzicom not for patients with CrCl < 50 mL/min	• Hypersensitivity reaction, which can be fatal • Symptoms may include fever, rash, nausea, vomiting, malaise or fatigue, loss of appetite, and respiratory symptoms such as sore throat, cough, shortness of breath
Trizivir	ABC 300 mg + ZDV 300 mg + 3TC 150 mg	1 tablet two times/day						
Epzicom	ABC 600 mg + 3TC 300 mg	1 tablet once daily						
Didanosine (ddI) Videx EC	125, 200, 250, 400 mg; buffered tablets (non-EC) are no longer available	• Body weight ≥ 60 kg: 400 mg once daily EC capsule; with TDF: 250 mg/day • Body weight < 60 kg: 250 mg daily EC capsule; with TDF: 200 mg/day	Levels decrease 55%; take ½ hour before or 2 hours after meal	30-40%	1.5 hours	>20 hours	• Renal excretion 50% • Dosage adjustment in renal insufficiency	• Pancreatitis, peripheral neuropathy, nausea • Lactic acidosis with hepatic steatosis (rare but potentially life-threatening toxicity associated with use of NRTIs)

(cont'd)

Table 4-5.   Characteristics of Nucleoside Reverse-Transcriptase Inhibitors (NRTIs) (cont'd)

Generic Name (abbreviation)/ Trade Name	Formulation	Dosing Recommendations	Food Effect	Oral Bioavailability	Serum Half-life	Intracellular Half-life	Elimination	Adverse Events
Emtricitabine (FTC)				93%	10 hours	>20 hours	• Renal excretion • Dosage adjustment in renal insufficiency • Atripla not for patients with CrCl < 50 mL/min • Truvada not for patients with CrCl < 30 mL/min	• Minimal toxicity; lactic acidosis with hepatic steatosis (rare but potentially life-threatening toxicity with use of NRTIs) • Hyperpigmentation/skin discoloration
Emtriva	200 mg hard gelatin capsule or 10 mg/mL oral solution	200 mg capsule once daily or 240 mg (24 mL) oral solution once daily	Take without regard to meals					
Atripla	FTC 200 mg + EFV 600 mg + TDF 300 mg	One tablet once daily						
Truvada	FTC 200 mg + TDF 300 mg	One tablet once daily						
Lamivudine (3TC)				86%	5-7 hours	18-22 hours	• Renal excretion • Dosage adjustment in renal insufficiency • Combivir, Trizivir, and Epzicom not for patients with CrCl < 50 mL/min	• Minimal toxicity; lactic acidosis with hepatic steatosis (rare but potentially life-threatening toxicity with use of NRTIs)
Epivir	150 and 300 mg tablets or 10 mg/mL oral solution	150 mg two times/day or 300 mg daily	Take without regard to meals					
Combivir	3TC 150 mg + ZDV 300 mg	1 tablet two times/day						
Epzicom	3TC 300 mg + ABC 600 mg	1 tablet once daily						
Trizivir	3TC 150 mg + ABC 300 mg + ZDV 300 mg	1 tablet two times/day						

Drug	Formulation	Dosage	Food	Bioavailability		Half-life	Comments	Adverse Effects
Stavudine (d4T) Zerit	15, 20, 30, 40 mg capsules or 1 mg/mL oral solution	• Body weight >60 kg: 40 mg two times/day; • Body weight <60 kg: 30 mg two times/day	Take without regard to meals	86%	1.0 hour	7.5 hours	• Renal excretion 50% • Dosage adjustment in renal insufficiency	• Peripheral neuropathy • Lipodystrophy • Pancreatitis • Lactic acidosis with hepatic steatosis: higher incidence than with other NRTIs • Hyperlipidemia • Rapidly progressive ascending neuromuscular weakness (rare)
Tenofovir Disoproxil Fumarate (TDF) Viread	300 mg tablet	1 tablet once daily	Take without regard to meals	25% in fasting state; 39% with high-fat meal	17 hours	>60 hours	• Renal excretion • Dosage adjustment in renal insufficiency • Atripla not for patients with CrCl < 50 mL/min • Truvada not for patients with CrCl < 30 mL/min	• Asthenia, headache, diarrhea, nausea, vomiting, and flatulence; renal insufficiency; lactic acidosis with hepatic steatosis (rare but potentially life-threatening toxicity with use of NRTIs)
Atripla	TDF 300 mg + EFV 600 mg + FTC 200 mg	1 tablet once daily						
Truvada	TDF 300 mg + FTC 200 mg							

(cont'd)

Table 4-5.   Characteristics of Nucleoside Reverse-Transcriptase Inhibitors (NRTIs) (cont'd)

Generic Name (abbreviation)/ Trade Name	Formulation	Dosing Recommendations	Food Effect	Oral Bioavailability	Serum Half-life	Intracellular Half-life	Elimination	Adverse Events
Zalcitabine (ddC) HIVID	0.375, 0.75 mg tablets	0.75 mg three times/day	Take without regard to meals	85%	1.2 hours	N/A	• Renal excretion 70% • Dosage adjustment in renal insufficiency	• Peripheral neuropathy • Stomatitis • Lactic acidosis with hepatic steatosis (rare but potentially life-threatening toxicity with use of NRTIs) • Pancreatitis
Zidovudine (AZT, ZDV) Retrovir	100 mg capsules, 300 mg tablets, 10 mg/mL IV solution, 10 mg/mL oral solution	300 mg two times/day or 200 mg three times/day	Take without regard to meals	60%	1.1 hours	7 hours	• Metabolized to AZT glucuronide (GAZT) • Renal excretion of GAZT • Dosage adjustment in renal insufficiency • Combivir and Trizivir not for patients with CrCl < 50 mL/min	• Bone marrow suppression: macrocytic anemia or neutropenia • Gastrointestinal intolerance, headache, insomnia, asthenia • Lactic acidosis with hepatic steatosis (rare but potentially life-threatening toxicity associated with use of NRTIs)
Combivir	ZDV 300 mg + 3TC 150 mg	1 tablet two times/day						
Trizivir	ZDV 300 mg + ABC 300 mg + 3TC 150 mg	1 tablet two times/day						

Source: Department of Health and Human Services. Guidelines for the Use of Antiretroviral Agents in HIV-1 Infected Adults and Adolescents. Available as a "living document" at http://www.aidsinfo.nih.gov.

Table 4-6.   Characteristics of Non-Nucleoside Reverse-Transcriptase Inhibitors (NNRTIs)

Generic Name (abbreviation)/ Trade Name	Formulation	Dosing Recommendations	Food Effect	Oral Bioavailability	Serum Half-life	Elimination	Adverse Events
Delavirdine (DLV) Rescriptor	100 or 200 mg tablets	400 mg 3 times/day; 4 100 mg tablets can be dispersed in ≥3 oz of water to produce slurry; 200 mg tablets should be taken as intact tablets; separate dose from antacids by 1 hour	Take without regard to meals	85%	5.8 hours	• Metabolized by cytochrome P450 (3A inhibitor); 51% excreted in urine (<5% unchanged), 44% in feces	• Rash* • Increased serum transaminases • Headache
Efavirenz (EFV) Sustiva	50, 100, 200 mg capsules or 600 mg tablets	600 mg daily on an empty stomach, at or before bedtime	High-fat/ high-caloric meals increase peak plasma concentrations of capsules by 39% and tablets by 79%; take on an empty stomach	Data not available	40-55 hours	• Metabolized by cytochrome P450 (3A mixed inducer/ inhibitor) • No dosage adjustment in renal insufficiency if EFV is used alone • Atripla not for patients with CrCl < 50 mL/min	• Rash* • Central nervous system symptoms† • Increased serum transaminases • False-positive cannabinoid test • Teratogenic in monkeys
Atripla	EFV 600 mg + FTC 200 mg + TDF 300 mg	1 tablet once daily					

(cont'd)

Table 4-6.   Characteristics of Non-Nucleoside Reverse-Transcriptase Inhibitors (NNRTIs) (cont'd)

Generic Name (abbreviation)/ Trade Name	Formulation	Dosing Recommendations	Food Effect	Oral Bioavailability	Serum Half-life	Elimination	Adverse Events
Nevirapine (NVP) Viramune	200 mg tablets or 50 mg/5 mL oral suspension	200 mg daily for 14 days, then 200 mg PO two times/day	Take without regard to meals	>90%	25-30 hours	• Metabolized by cytochrome P450 (3A inducer); 80% excreted in urine (glucuronidated metabolites; <5% unchanged); 10% in feces	• Rash including Stevens-Johnson syndrome* • Symptomatic hepatitis, including fatal hepatic necrosis[‡]

* During clinical trials, NNRTI was discontinued because of rash among 7% of patients taking nevirapine, 4.3% of patients taking delavirdine, and 1.7% of patients taking efavirenz. Rare cases of Stevens-Johnson syndrome have been reported with the use of all three NNRTIs, the highest incidence with nevirapine.

[†] Adverse events can include dizziness, somnolence, insomnia, abnormal dreams, confusion, abnormal thinking, impaired concentration, amnesia, agitation, depersonalization, hallucinations, and euphoria. Overall frequency of any of these symptoms associated with use of efavirenz was 52%, as compared with 26% among control subjects; 2.6% of those persons on efavirenz discontinued the drug because of these symptoms; symptoms usually subside spontaneously after 2–4 weeks.

[‡] Symptomatic, sometimes serious, and even fatal hepatic events (accompanied by rash in approximately 50% of cases) occur with significantly higher frequency in treatment-naïve female patients with pre-nevirapine CD4 count >250 cells/mm³ or in treatment-naïve male patients with pre-nevirapine CD4 count >400 cells/mm³. Nevirapine should not be initiated in these patients unless the benefit clearly outweighs the risk. This toxicity has not been observed when nevirapine is given as single doses to mothers or infants for prevention of mother-to-child HIV transmission.

Source: Department of Health and Human Services. Guidelines for the Use of Antiretroviral Agents in HIV-1 Infected Adults and Adolescents. Available as a "living document" at http://www.aidsinfo.nih.gov.

Table 4-7. Characteristics of Protease Inhibitors (PIs)

Generic Name/ Trade Name	Formulation	Dosing Recommendations	Food Effect	Oral Bioavailability	Serum Half-life	Route of Metabolism	Storage	Adverse Events
Amprenavir (APV) Agenerase	50 mg capsules or 15 mg/mL oral solution (capsules and solution *not* interchangeable on mg per mg basis) Note: APV 150 mg capsule is no longer available; consider using fosamprenavir in these patients.	1400 mg two times/day (oral solution) Note: APV and RTV oral solution should not be co-administered because of competition of the metabolic pathway of the two vehicles.	• High-fat meal decreases blood concentration 21% • Can be taken with or without food, but high fat meal should be avoided	Not determined in humans	7.1–10.6 hours	• Cytochrome P450 3A4 inhibitor, inducer, and substrate • Dosage adjustment in hepatic insufficiency recommended	Room temperature (up to 25°C or 77°F)	• GI intolerance, nausea, vomiting, diarrhea • Rash • Oral paresthesias • Hyperlipidemia • Increased serum transaminases • Fat maldistribution • Hyperglycemia • Possible increased bleeding episodes in pts with hemophilia Note: Oral solution contains propylene glycol; contraindicated in pregnant women, children <4 years old, patients with hepatic or renal failure, & patients treated with disulfiram or metronidazole
Atazanavir (ATV) Reyataz	100, 150, 200 mg capsules	• 400 mg once daily • If taken with efavirenz or tenofovir: RTV 100 mg + ATV 300 mg once daily	• Administration with food increases bioavailability • Take with food; avoid taking with antacids	Not determined	7 hours	• Cytochrome P450 3A4 inhibitor and substrate • Dosage adjustment in hepatic insufficiency recommended	Room temperature (up to 25°C or 77°F)	• Indirect hyperbilirubinemia • Prolonged PR interval; 1st degree symptomatic AV block in some pts • Use with caution in pts with underlying conduction defects or on concomitant medications that can cause PR prolongation

(cont'd)

Table 4-7.   Characteristics of Protease Inhibitors (PIs) (cont'd)

Generic Name/ Trade Name	Formulation	Dosing Recommendations	Food Effect	Oral Bioavailability	Serum Half-life	Route of Metabolism	Storage	Adverse Events
Atazanavir (ATV) Reyataz (cont'd)								• Hyperglycemia • Fat maldistribution • Possible increased bleeding episodes in pts with hemophilia
Darunavir (DRV) Prezista	300 mg tablet	DRV 600 mg + RTV 100 mg twice daily	Food ↑ C_{max} & AUC by 30%, administer with food	Absolute bioavailability: DRV alone - 37%; w/ RTV - 82%	15 hours (when combined with RTV)	Cytochrome P450 3A4 inhibitor and substrate	Room temperature (up to 25°C or 77°F)	• Skin rash (7%) - DRV has a sulfonamide moiety; Stevens-Johnson syndrome and erythema multiforme have been reported. • Diarrhea, nausea • Headache • Hyperlipidemia • Increased serum transaminases • Hyperglycemia • Fat maldistribution • Possible increased bleeding episodes in pts with hemophilia
Fosamprenavir (fAPV) Lexiva	700 mg tablet	ARV-naïve patients: • fAPV 1400 mg bid or • (fAPV 1400 + RTV 200 mg) qd or • (fAPV 700 mg + RTV 100 mg) bid PI-experienced pts (qd not recommended): • (fAPV 700 mg + RTV 100 mg) bid	No significant change in amprenavir pharmacokinetics in fed or	Not established	7.7 hours (amprenavir)	• Amprenavir is a cytochrome P450 3A4 inhibitor, inducer, and substrate • Dosage adjustment in hepatic insufficiency recommended	Room temperature (up to 25°C or 77°F)	• Skin rash (19%) • Diarrhea, nausea, vomiting • Headache • Hyperlipidemia • Increased serum transaminases • Hyperglycemia • Fat maldistribution • Possible increased bleeding episodes in pts with hemophilia

Drug	Formulation	Dosing	Bioavailability	Food	Half-life	Metabolism	Storage	Adverse effects
Fosamprenavir (fAPV) Lexiva (cont'd)		Coadministration w/ EFV (fAPV boosted only): • (fAPV 700 mg + RTV 100 mg) bid or • (fAPV 1400 mg + RTV 300 mg) qd						
Indinavir Crixivan	200, 333, 400 mg capsules	• 800 mg q8h • With RTV: IDV 800 mg + RTV 100 or 200 mg| q12h	65%	• Unboosted IDV levels decrease by 77% • Take 1 hour before or 2 hours after meals; may take with skim milk or low-fat meal • RTV-boosted IDV: take with or without food	1.5-2 hours	• Cytochrome P450 3A4 inhibitor (less than ritonavir) • Dosage adjustment in hepatic insufficiency recommended	Room temperature 15-30°C (59-86°F); protect from moisture	• Nephrolithiasis • GI intolerance, nausea • Indirect hyperbilirubinemia • Hyperlipidemia • Headache, asthenia, blurred vision, dizziness, rash, metallic taste, thrombocytopenia, alopecia, hemolytic anemia • Hyperglycemia • Fat maldistribution • Possible increased bleeding episodes in pts with hemophilia
Lopinavir + Ritonavir (LPV/RTV) Kaletra	• Each tablet contains LPV 200 mg + RTV 50 mg • Oral solution: Each 5 mL contains LPV 400 mg + RTV 100 mg Note: Oral solution contains 42% alcohol	• LPV 400 mg + RTV 100 mg (2 tablets or 5 mL) twice daily or LPV 800 mg + RTV 200 mg (4 tablets or 10 mL) once daily Note: Once-daily dosing recommended only for treatment-naïve pts; not for patients receiving EFV, NVP, fAPV, or NFV	Not determined in humans	• Tablet: No food effect; take with or without food • Oral solution: Moderately fatty meal ↑ LPV AUC & Cmin by 80% & 54%, respectively; take with food	5-6 hours	Cytochrome P450 3A4 inhibitor and substrate	• Tablet is stable at room temperature • Oral solution is stable at 2-8°C until date on label; stable when stored at room temperature (up to 25°C or 77°F) for 2 months	• GI intolerance, nausea, vomiting, diarrhea (higher incidence with once-daily than twice-daily dosing) • Asthenia • Hyperlipidemia (esp. hypertriglyceridemia) • Increased serum transaminases • Hyperglycemia • Fat maldistribution

(cont'd)

Table 4-7. Characteristics of Protease Inhibitors (PIs) (cont'd)

Generic Name/ Trade Name	Formulation	Dosing Recommendations	Food Effect	Oral Bioavailability	Serum Half-life	Route of Metabolism	Storage	Adverse Events
Lopinavir + Ritonavir (LPV/RTV) Kaletra (*cont'd*)		With EFV or NVP: For treatment-experienced pts: • LPV 600 mg + RTV 150 mg (3 oral tablets twice daily *or* • LPV 533 mg + RTV 133 mg (6.7 mL oral solution) twice daily with food						• Possible increased bleeding episodes in patients with hemophilia
Nelfinavir (NFV) Viracept	250 or 625 mg tablets or 50 mg/g oral powder	1250 mg two times/day or 750 mg three times/day	• Levels increase 2-3 fold • Take with meal or snack	20-80%	3.5-5 hours	Cytochrome P450 3A4 inhibitor and substrate	Room temperature 15-30°C (59-86°F)	• Diarrhea • Hyperlipidemia • Hyperglycemia • Fat maldistribution • Possible increased bleeding episodes in patients with hemophilia • Increased serum transaminases

Ritonavir (RTV) Norvir	100 mg capsules or 600 mg/7.5 mL solution	• 600 mg q 12 h* (when ritonavir is used as sole PI) • As pharmacokinetic booster for other PIs - 100 mg—400 mg per day—in 1-2 divided doses	• Levels increase 15% • Take with food if possible; this may improve tolerability	Not determined	3-5 hours	Cytochrome P450 (3A4 > 2D6; potent 3A4 inhibitor)	• Refrigerate capsules • Capsules can be left at room temperature (up to 25°C or 77°F) for ≤30 days; • Oral solution should *not* be refrigerated	• GI intolerance, nausea, vomiting, diarrhea • Paresthesias: circumoral and extremities • Hyperlipidemia, esp. hypertriglyceridemia • Hepatitis • Asthenia • Taste perversion • Hyperglycemia • Fat maldistribution • Possible increased bleeding episodes in patients with hemophilia
Saquinavir (SQV) Invirase	200 mg hard gel capsules or 500 mg tablets	Unboosted SQV not recommended With RTV: • (RTV 100 mg + SQV 1000 mg) two times/day	Take within 2 hours of a meal when taken with RTV	4% erratic (when taken as sole PI)	1-2 hours	Cytochrome P450 3A4 inhibitor and substrate	Room temperature 15-30°C (59-86°F)	• GI intolerance, nausea and diarrhea • Headache • Increased serum transaminases • Hyperlipidemia • Hyperglycemia • Fat maldistribution • Possible increased bleeding episodes in patients with hemophilia
Tipranavir (TPV) Aptivus	250 mg capsules	• 500 mg twice daily with ritonavir 200 mg twice daily • Unboosted tipranavir is *not* recommended	• Take both TPV & RTV with food • Bioavailability increased with high-fat meal	Not determined	6 hours after single dose of TPV/RTV	• TPV: Cytochrome P450 3A4 inducer and substrate	• Refrigerated capsules are stable until date on label • If stored at room temperature (up to 25°C or 77°F), must be used within 60 days	• Hepatotoxicity: clinical hepatitis including hepatic decompensation has been reported, monitor closely, esp. in patients with underlying liver disease

(cont'd)

Table 4-7. Characteristics of Protease Inhibitors (PIs) (cont'd)

Generic Name/ Trade Name	Formulation	Dosing Recommendations	Food Effect	Oral Bioavailability	Serum Half-life	Route of Metabolism	Storage	Adverse Events
Tipranavir (TPV) Aptivus (cont'd)						• Net effect when combined with RTV: CYP 3A4 inhibitor and CYP 2D6 inhibitor		• Skin rash: TPV has a sulfonamide moiety, use with caution in patients with known sulfonamide allergy • Rare cases of fatal and non-fatal intracranial hemorrhage have been reported; most patients had underlying co-morbidity such as brain lesion, head trauma, recent neurosurgery, coagulopathy, hypertension, alcoholism, or were on medication with increase risk for bleeding • Hyperlipidemia (esp. hypertriglyceridemia) • Hyperglycemia • Fat maldistribution • Possible increased bleeding episodes in patients with hemophilia

* Dose escalation for ritonavir when used as sole PI: Days 1 and 2: 300 mg two times; days 3-5: 400 mg two times; days 6-13: 500 mg two times; day 14: 600 mg two times.
Source: Department of Health and Human Services. Guidelines for the Use of Antiretroviral Agents in HIV-1 Infected Adults and Adolescents. Available as a "living document" at http://www.aidsinfo.nih.gov.

Table 4-8.   Drugs That Should Not Be Used with PIs or NNRTIs

Drug Category[a]	Calcium Channel Blocker	Cardiac	Lipid-Lowering	Anti-mycobacterial[‡]	Anti-histamine[‡]	Gastroin-testinal[ʃ]	Neuro-leptic	Psychotropic	Ergot Alkaloids	Herbs	Other
						Protease Inhibitors					
Amprenavir[*] and Fosamprenavir	Bepridil	—	Simvastatin, lovastatin	Rifampin, rifapentine	Astemizole, terfenadine	Cisapride	Pimozide	Midazolam,[Σ] triazolam	Dihydroergotamine, ergotamine[‡] (various forms), ergonovine, methylergonovine	St. John's wort	Delavirdine,[***] fluticasone,[***] oral contraceptives
Atazanavir	Bepridil	—	Simvastatin, lovastatin	Rifampin, rifapentine	Astemizole, terfenadine	Cisapride, proton pump inhibitors	Pimozide	Midazolam,[Σ] triazolam	Dihydroergotamine, ergotamine[‡] (various forms), ergonovine, methylergonovine	St. John's wort	Fluticasone,[***] indinavir, irinotecan
Darunavir	—	—	Simvastatin, lovastatin	Rifampin, rifapentine	Astemizole, terfenadine	Cisapride	Pimozide	Midazolam,[Σ] triazolam	Dihydroergotamine, ergotamine[‡] (various forms), ergonovine, methylergonovine	St. John's wort	Carbamazepine, phenobarbital, phenytoin, fluticasone[***]
Indinavir	—	Amiodarone	Simvastatin, lovastatin	Rifampin, rifapentine	Astemizole, terfenadine	Cisapride	Pimozide	Midazolam,[Σ] triazolam	Dihydroergotamine, ergotamine[‡] (various forms), ergonovine, methylergonovine	St. John's wort	Atazanavir
Lopinavir/ ritonavir[**]	—	Flecainide, propafenone	Simvastatin, lovastatin	Rifampin, rifapentine	Astemizole, terfenadine	Cisapride	Pimozide	Midazolam,[Σ] triazolam	Dihydroergotamine, ergotamine[‡] (various forms), ergonovine, methylergonovine	St. John's wort	Fluticasone[***]
Nelfinavir	—	—	Simvastatin, lovastatin	Rifampin, rifapentine	Astemizole, terfenadine	Cisapride	Pimozide	Midazolam,[Σ] triazolam	Dihydroergotamine, ergotamine[‡] (various forms), ergonovine, methylergonovine	St. John's wort	

(cont'd)

Table 4-8.   Drugs That Should Not Be Used with PIs or NNRTIs (cont'd)

Drug Category[a]	Calcium Channel Blocker	Cardiac	Lipid-Lowering	Anti-mycobacterial[‡]	Anti-histamine[b]	Gastrointestinal[b]	Neuro-leptic	Psychotropic	Ergot Alkaloids	Herbs	Other
Ritonavir	Bepridil	Amiodarone, flecainide, propafenone, quinidine	Simvastatin, lovastatin	Rifapentine	Astemizole, terfenadine	Cisapride	Pimozide	Midazolam,[Σ] triazolam	Dihydroergotamine, ergotamine[‡] (various forms), ergonovine, methylergonovine	St. John's wort	Voriconazole (with RTV ≥ 400 mg bid), fluticasone,[***] alfuzosin
Saquinavir	—	—	Simvastatin, lovastatin	Rifampin, rifabutin,[Δ] rifapentine	Astemizole, terfenadine	Cisapride	Pimozide	Midazolam,[Σ] triazolam	Dihydroergotamine, ergotamine[‡] (various forms), ergonovine, methylergonovine	St. John's wort, garlic supplements	Fluticasone[***]
Tipranavir	Bepridil	Amiodarone, flecainide, propafenone, quinidine	Simvastatin, lovastatin	Rifampin, rifapentine	Astemizole, terfenadine	Cisapride	Pimozide	Midazolam,[Σ] triazolam	Dihydroergotamine, ergotamine[‡] (various forms), ergonovine, methylergonovine	St. John's wort	Fluticasone[***]
Non-Nucleoside Reverse-Transcriptase Inhibitors											
Delavirdine	—	—	Simvastatin, lovastatin	Rifampin, rifapentine,[‡] rifabutin	Astemizole, terfenadine	Cisapride H2-blockers, proton pump inhibitors	—	Alprazolam, midazolam,[Σ] triazolam	Dihydroergotamine, ergotamine[‡] (various forms), ergonovine, methylergonovine	St. John's wort	Amprenavir, fosamprenavir, carbamazepine, phenobarbital, phenytoin

(cont'd)

Non-Nucleoside Reverse-Transcriptase Inhibitors (cont'd)

Efavirenz	—	—	—	Rifapentine‡	Astemizole, terfenadine	Cisapride	—	Midazolam,Σ triazolam	Dihydroergotamine, Ergotamine‡ (various forms), ergonovine, methylergonovine	St. John's wort
Nevirapine	—	—	—	Rifampin, rifapentine‡	—	—	—	—	St. John's wort	Voriconazole

* Certain listed drugs are contraindicated based on theoretical considerations. Thus, drugs with narrow therapeutic indices and suspected metabolic involvement with P450-3A, 2D6, or unknown pathways are included in this table. Actual interactions may or may not occur among patients.

‡ HIV-infected patients treated with rifapentine have a higher rate of TB relapse than those treated with other rifamycin-based regimens; an alternative agent is recommended.

Δ Rifabutin may be used with saquinavir only if it is combined with ritonavir.

Σ Midazolam can be used with caution as a single dose and given in a monitored situation for procedural sedation.

† This likely is a class effect.

∂ Astemizole and terfenadine are not marketed in the U.S. The manufacturer of cisapride has a limited-access protocol for patients meeting specific clinical eligibility criteria.

* Each mL of amprenavir oral solution has 46 IU vitamin E. Patients should be cautioned to avoid supplemental doses of vitamin E. Multivitamin products containing minimal amounts of vitamin E are acceptable.

** In one small study, higher doses of RTV (additional 300 mg bid) or a double dose of LPV/RTV offset rifampin-inducing activity of LPV. Of note, 28% of subjects discontinued because of increases in LFTs. The safety of this combination is still under evaluation. Further studies are needed.

*** Concomitant use of fluticasone and ritonavir results in significantly reduced serum cortisol concentrations. Coadministration of fluticasone and ritonavir or any ritonavir-boosted PI regimen is not recommended unless potential benefit outweighs risk of systemic corticosteroid side effects. Fluticasone should be used with caution and alternatives considered if given with an unboosted PI regimen.

Suggested Alternatives:

Cerivastatin (no longer marketed in the United States), simvastatin, lovastatin: Pravastatin and fluvastatin have the least potential for drug interactions (except for pravastatin with darunavir/ritonavir); atorvastatin should be used with caution, using the lowest possible starting dose and monitoring closely; no pharmacokinetic data or safety data are available for coadministration of rosuvastatin with antiretroviral drugs.

Rifabutin: clarithromycin, azithromycin (MAC prophylaxis); clarithromycin, azithromycin, ethambutol (MAC treatment)

Astemizole, terfenadine (no longer marketed in the United States): desloratadine, loratadine, fexofenadine, cetirizine

Midazolam, triazolam: temazepam, lorazepam

Source: Department of Health and Human Services. Guidelines for the Use of Antiretroviral Agents in HIV-1 Infected Adults and Adolescents. Available as a "living document" at http://www.aidsinfo.nih.gov.

Two NRTIs Plus a PI

DHHS-preferred combinations include: 1) atazanavir (ATV) with RTV boosting; 2) fosamprenavir (FPV) with RTV boosting; and 3) LPV with RTV boosting; alternatives include ATV and FPV.

PI-based regimens have the greatest amount of clinical data supporting their efficacy in reducing HIV-related complications and prolonging survival. Virologic suppression rates of 75% to 90% at 48 weeks are noted in studies using a viral load cutoff of less than 500 copies/mL, and 50% to 70% in those using a cutoff of less than 20 to 50 copies/mL. Disadvantages of the older PIs (e.g., saquinavir [SQV], RTV, indinavir [IDV]) include frequent dosing, high pill burden, food restrictions, and gastrointestinal and metabolic side effects. Some of the more recently approved PIs (e.g., LPV/RTV, ATV, FPV) are easier to dose and have improved toxicity profiles.

The main advantages of PI-based regimens are their virologic, immunologic, and clinical efficacy, durability, and higher genetic barrier to resistance compared with NNRTIs. The main disadvantages are their higher pill burdens, more frequent gastrointestinal side effects, and long term drug toxicities, particularly insulin resistance and hyperlipidemia.

Ritonavir-boosting of PI-based regimens leads to significantly higher plasma levels of the boosted PI, in some cases reducing pill burden and allowing for once-daily administration. A potential disadvantage of this approach is an increase in the toxicity of the boosted compound. For example, RTV-boosted IDV leads to higher trough concentrations and allows for twice-daily dosing; however, studies consistently show a higher rate of IDV-related toxicity (e.g., nephrolithiasis, hyperlipidemia) compared with unboosted IDV.

Several options for initial PI-based therapy are recommended by both the DHHS and IAS treatment guidelines. In the DHHS guidelines, LPV/RTV is the preferred PI for treatment-naïve patients given its virologic potency and high barrier to resistance. In 2005, it was reformulated from a capsule to a tablet that has no food restrictions, improved pharmacokinetic predictability, decreased gastrointestinal side effects, and a lower pill burden. The primary metabolic side effect of LPV/RTV is hyperlipidemia.

Atazanavir requires only once-daily dosing and may be given boosted or unboosted. A consistent finding in clinical studies has been a relatively neutral effect on lipid parameters; metabolic studies also show no evidence of glucose intolerance, which distinguishes it from other PIs. Prospective clinical trials demonstrate equal efficacy of unboosted ATV and EFV or NFV. In a trial of 358 treatment experienced patients, boosted ATV appeared virologically and immunologically non-inferior to LPV/RTV. A head-to-head trial of boosted ATV vs. LPV/RTV in treatment-naïve patients has not been performed. Atazanavir requires acidic environment for complete absorption, and administration to persons on proton pump inhibitors is contraindicated. H2 receptor blockers can be used if ATV is taken at least two hours before. A predictable side effect of ATV is an increased unconjugated bilirubin level, the degree of which varies from patient to patient. However, in clinical trials of ATV, jaundice was rarely of sufficient concern to cause discontinuation of the drug.

Fosamprenavir is the prodrug of amprenavir, with improved tolerability and lower pill burden. In a 48-week trial of 249 patients, 66% of the FPV group and 51% of the NFV group achieved a viral load of < 400 copies/mL. The improved virologic suppression in the FPV group was especially apparent at high baseline viral loads. Fosamprenavir can also be given boosted with RTV in a once-daily regimen in treatment-naïve patients; however, in a clinical trial of PI-experienced patients who were randomized to receive twice-daily LPV/RTV, once-daily boosted FPV, or twice-daily boosted FPV, the once-daily FPV group had a lower rate of viral suppression. As a result, once-daily administration should be avoided in PI-experienced patients.

Tipranavir (TPV) has in vitro activity against many PI-resistant strains. Compared with currently available PIs, it showed enhanced activity in prospective clinical trials of patients with extensive baseline PI resistance. Tipranavir has a more complex drug interaction profile than other PIs, requires a higher dose of RTV boosting (200 mg twice-daily), and has been associated with hyperlipidemia, hepatotoxicity (especially in patients with chronic viral hepatitis), and intracranial hemorrhage. As such, its use should be restricted to highly treatment-experienced patients.

Darunavir (DRV) also has in vitro activity against many PI-resistant viruses. In a prospective trial in patients with three-class resistance, an optimized background regimen selected on the basis of HIV-resistance testing was compared with regimens with various doses of RTV-boosted DRV. All the treatment arms receiving DRV had better responses, as measured by viral load reduction, the proportion of patients achieving an undetectable viral load, and CD4 count responses. DRV has been associated with rash, gastrointestinal side effects, and hyperlipidemia.

Nelfinavir is no longer considered a first-line medication as it is inferior to LPV/RTV- and EFV-containing regimens. A potential benefit is that treatment failure on NFV-containing regimens often selects for the D30N mutation, which confers little cross-resistance with other PIs, allowing for the subsequent use of boosted PIs. Unboosted IDV or SQV, and RTV alone, are not recommended as initial therapy because of dosing inconvenience, gastrointestinal intolerance, and/or poor bioavailability.

Two NRTIs Plus an NNRTI

The DHHS-preferred drug is EFV, and NVP is the alternative choice. The use of 2 NRTIs plus a NNRTI has gained increased popularity as an alternative to a PI-based regimen, with randomized trials showing equivalent or better efficacy. The lower pill burden, decreased gastrointestinal toxicity, and reduced metabolic complications all contribute to improved adherence. Although a prospective randomized controlled clinical trial comparing EFV and a boosted PI has not been performed, two such studies are in progress.

There are three available NNRTIs, with EFV and NVP most often prescribed. Delavirdine (DLV) is infrequently used because of its toxicity profile, drug interactions, and thrice-daily dosing. Some cohort studies have suggested that EFV is more potent than NVP. These drugs were compared in an industry-sponsored prospective randomized trial in treatment-naïve patients. The four study arms consisted of once-daily EFV, once- and twice-daily NVP, and the combination of EFV and NVP. All study subjects also received d4T and 3TC. The EFV arm subjects had a lower overall rate of treatment failure, but the difference between the EFV and NVP arms was not statistically significant. Notably, the combination EFV and NVP arm had greater toxicity and conferred no additional antiviral benefit.

Based on these data, in general, EFV is preferred over NVP for initial therapy because of its efficacy, low pill burden, and favorable toxicity profile. Its long half-life allows for once-daily administration and perhaps a higher degree of "forgiveness" with variable dosing schedules or missed doses. The main side effects of EFV are neuropsychiatric symptoms (sleep disturbance, dizziness, and mood alteration) and rash. These side effects peak with initial therapy and usually, but not invariably, resolve over a few weeks. Rash occurs in approximately 20% of patients and is often mild enough to allow continued dosing. However, severe rash, including Stevens-Johnson syndrome, can occur, and therapy should be stopped in this setting. In animal studies of EFV, central nervous system abnormalities have been demonstrated in monkey fetuses. Since licensure of the EFV, four cases of central nervous system defects have been retrospectively identified in children born to mothers receiving it during the first trimester. As such, the drug is considered pregnancy category D, which denotes evidence of risk to human fetuses. EFV should therefore be avoided in women of childbearing potential who are interested in becoming pregnant or who are not consistently using birth control.

Nevirapine is preferred in pregnant women and in those likely to become pregnant. Its side effects include rash and hepatic dysfunction, both of which can sometimes be severe. Liver function tests should be monitored closely during the initial phases of treatment. Patients who experience a significant rash and/or increased liver function tests shortly after beginning NVP should have the drug promptly discontinued. In general, NVP should be avoided in women with a CD4 count of greater than 250 cells/mm^3 and in men with a CD4 count of greater than 400 cells/mm^3 because of an increased risk of severe toxicity reported in these groups.

Triple Nucleoside Therapy

The main advantages of triple nucleoside therapy are sparing of the PI and NNRTI drug classes, fewer drug interactions, and availability of the coformulated tablet containing ZDV, 3TC, and ABC. A comparative trial of ZDV, 3TC, and ABC with an IDV-containing regimen showed similar viral suppression overall. However, lower rates of suppression were seen in the triple nucleoside arm when the baseline viral load was greater than 100,000 copies/mL. This combination was further evaluated in a randomized trial comparing it with EFV-containing regimens. The study was stopped after an analysis at 32 weeks showed higher virologic failure for the triple nucleoside arm compared with the EFV-containing regimens (21% vs. 11% respectively), as well as a shorter time to virologic failure. This difference was observed regardless of initial viral load or CD4 count. Based on these studies, triple nucleoside regimens should not be prescribed as first-line therapy unless exceptional circumstances prevent the use of all other drug classes.

Enfuvirtide

Enfuvirtide acts by binding to the HIV envelope glycoprotein 41 and interfering with viral entry. This mechanism of action is distinct from the other three drug classes, and, as such, there is no cross-resistance. A large, nonabsorbable peptide, enfuvirtide must be given by subcutaneous injection twice daily. Almost all users experience injection site reactions, which is the most common side effect, and these have necessitated discontinuation of the drug in 4.4% of patients in trial settings. The Biojector, a needleless injection system that reduces the discomfort of injection, is currently being tested in clinical studies. Two trials comprising 995 treatment-experienced patients compared the addition of enfuvirtide to an optimized regimen of 3 to 5 drugs guided by HIV resistance testing to an optimized regimen alone. At 24 weeks in the TORO 1 study, the mean viral load decrease from baseline was 1.696 log10 copies/mL in the enfuvirtide group vs. 0.764 log10 copies/mL in the control group. The CD4 count increased by 76 cells/mm^3 and 32 cells/mm^3, respectively. Similar findings were evident in TORO 2, and these effects were sustained at 48 weeks. Enfuvirtide has been reserved for use in highly treatment-experienced patients because of its expense and need for subcutaneous administration. Characteristics of enfuvirtide are presented in Table 4-9.

Treatment Interruption

Several different rationales for treatment interruption of ART have been proposed:

- As a means of "auto-vaccination," with the theory that exposure to rebounding virus induces a more robust immune response
- As a way of reducing drug toxicity and cost
- As "pulse therapy," with treatment continued only until the CD4 count reaches a safe level and then discontinued until it declines to a threshold where therapy is again warranted
- As a way of increasing the success of salvage therapy by allowing the regrowth of wild-type virus

Table 4-9. Characteristics of Enfuvirtide

Generic Name/ Trade Name	Formulation	Dosing Recommendations	Bioavailability	Serum Half-life	Route of Metabolism	Storage	Adverse Events
Enfuvirtide Fuzeon	• Injectable, in lyophilized powder • Each single-use vial contains 108 mg of enfuvirtide to be reconstituted with 1.1 mL of sterile water for injection delivery of approximately 90 mg/1 mL	90 mg/1 mL SC two times/day	84.3% (SC compared with IV)	3.8 hours	Expected to undergo catabolism to its constituent amino acids, with subsequent recycling of the amino acids in the body pool	• Store at room temperature (up to 25°C or 77°F) • Reconstituted solution should be stored under refrigeration at 2°C to 8°C (36°F to 46°F) and used within 24 hours	• Local injection site reactions in almost 100% of patients: pain, erythema, induration, nodules and cysts, pruritus, ecchymosis • Increased rate of bacterial pneumonia • Hypersensitivity reaction (<1%); symptoms may include rash, fever, nausea, vomiting, chills, rigors, hypotension, or increased serum transaminases; rechallenge is not recommended

Source: Department of Health and Human Services. Guidelines for the Use of Antiretroviral Agents in HIV-1 Infected Adults and Adolescents. Available as a "living document" at http://www.aidsinfo.nih.gov.

While all of these approaches can be theoretically justified, clinical trials have found no benefit to treatment interruption strategies, and, in some cases, they have been harmful. For example, in the CPCRA study, patients with drug-resistant virus were randomized to start a new regimen immediately or to do so after a 16-week treatment interruption to allow regrowth of wild-type virus. Before the study was completed, the data safety and monitoring board terminated it because of more rapid HIV disease progression in the interruption group. Studies with long-cycle scheduled interruptions have been associated with increased antiretroviral drug resistance, and a large trial of CD4 count-driven intermittent therapy was recently discontinued because of a higher rate of disease progression in the interruption group. Given these concerns, except in the setting of drug toxicity, treatment interruption cannot be advocated at this time in clinical practice.

Monitoring of CD4 Cell Count and Viral Load

Upon establishing a diagnosis of HIV infection, two measurements of the CD4 count and viral load on separate occasions should be obtained to ensure an accurate baseline. Measurements should not be done within 4 weeks of intercurrent infections or immunizations. CD4 counts decreased by more than 30% from baseline or a decline of more than 3% in baseline CD4 percentage is considered a significant change. There is a variability of 0.3 log (three- to five-fold) in the viral load assay, meaning that differences between sequential values must meet this threshold to be considered significant. It has been noted that viral loads may be higher when plasma preparation tubes rather than EDTA tubes are used to collect specimens, and only the latter are recommended. Because of the increasing prevalence of resistant viral strains in the community, an HIV genotype test is also now recommended prior to initiation of ART.

In the untreated patient, CD4 counts and HIV viral loads should be measured every 3 to 6 months. In patients beginning ART, these measurements should be done at baseline before initiation of therapy and repeated in 2 to 4 weeks. In ART–naïve patients, viral loads should decrease approximately 1.5 to 2 log by week 8, and viral suppression should be achieved in most patients by 24 weeks. Patients with a baseline viral load greater than 100,000 copies/mL may take as long as 48 weeks to achieve suppression. Once a patient is on a stable regimen, these laboratory tests should be monitored every 3 to 4 months.

When to Modify Therapy

Changing therapy during the course of HIV treatment is common and may be necessary because of treatment failure or drug toxicity. Subcategories of treatment failure include virologic failure, immunologic failure, and clinical disease progression. These conditions are not mutually exclusive.

Virologic Failure

Virologic failure refers to a failure to reach an undetectable HIV viral load or the occurrence of virologic rebound. Specific criteria include the following:

- Less than 1 log reduction by 8 weeks or 0.5 to 0.75 log reduction in viral load by 4 weeks after initiating therapy.
- Failure to suppress viral load to undetectable levels within 4 to 6 months of starting therapy. The degree of initial decrease in viral load and overall trend in decreasing viremia should be considered before changing therapy. In patients with very high baseline viral loads (>100,000 copies/mL) that stabilize after 6 months of therapy at a level of less than 10,000 copies/mL, an immediate change in therapy may not be warranted as long as the trajectory is downward.
- Repeated detection of virus in plasma after initial suppression to an undetectable level suggesting the development of resistance. The degree of viremia must be considered. It may be reasonable to consider close, short-term observation in a patient whose viral load increases from undetectable to a low level (50 to 5000 copies/mL). Some patients in this category will show progressively increased viral loads and eventually require a change in therapy; others will achieve resuppression of the viral load on the same regimen. The occurrence of transient low-level viremia, sometimes termed a *blip,* has not been correlated with subsequent risk of virologic failure.
- Any reproducibly significant increase (>3-fold) from the nadir viral load not caused by intercurrent infection, vaccination, or change in test methodology.

Immunologic Failure

Immunologic failure refers to declining CD4 counts as measured on at least two separate occasions. Criteria for significant declines in the CD4 count and CD4 percentage are described above. The optimal management of patients who achieve virologic suppression but whose CD4 count either plateaus or declines is not known. Factors associated with this paradoxical response in studies have included older age, hepatitis C coinfection, treatment with an NNRTI-based regimen, and the use of TDF and ddI in combination.

Clinical Disease Progression

Clinical disease progression refers to the development of HIV-related opportunistic diseases or death. In the current era, HIV-related OIs occur most often in patients not taking ART either because of poor medication adherence or their late presentation for care. It is important to recognize that not all HIV-related OIs that occur after starting ART are related to treatment failure. In particular, some patients with advanced HIV disease (CD4 count $< 100/mm^3$) with a subclinical OI develop symptoms in this setting because of an enhanced immunologic response to the pathogen. Immune reconstitution syndrome has been described with *Mycobacterium avium* complex infection, tuberculosis, cytomegalovirus infection, hepatitis B and C infections, cryptococcosis, and histoplasmosis. Its time of onset is typically within weeks to a few months of starting or resuming ART.

How to Modify Therapy

Virologic Failure

It is important to recognize that patients with virologic failure often continue to have substantial immunologic and clinical benefits from ART. The most likely explanations for this apparent paradox are a continued antiviral effect of some drugs despite the presence of resistance and a reduction in the virulence of some resistant HIV isolates compared with wild-type strains. When changes in ART are made for virologic failure, HIV resistance testing can help guide the selection of new drugs (see Chapter 5). In general, introduction of at least two new active agents is recommended.

This "disconnect" between a detectable HIV viral load on the one hand and a stable or even rising CD4 count on the other makes selecting the optimal time to switch therapy difficult. An aggressive approach of switching therapy promptly at the first sign of virologic failure has the advantage of reducing the risk of accumulating additional resistance mutations; however, it also could lead to the earlier exhaustion of treatment options. A more cautious approach of deferring a switch until the CD4 count begins to fall takes advantage of the continued antiviral activity of a failing regimen but may lead to more resistance mutations developing over time, possibly reducing the success of subsequent regimens.

In the absence of a clinical trial comparing early versus delayed switching of ART, we advocate the more aggressive approach in patients who are on their first regimen and in those with limited evidence of drug resistance. Once adherence is adequately addressed, such individuals will have a high likelihood of subsequent treatment success. The opposite approach should be taken for patients who are clinically stable but have a history of multiple prior drug regimen failures and evidence of drug resistance to multiple classes. In such individuals, clinicians should continue the "failing" regimen until at least two fully active new drugs are available. For example, the release of TPV, which has activity against many PI-resistant viruses, permitted some patients with multidrug resistant HIV to achieve virologic suppression when it was combined with enfuvirtide.

When a patient has evidence of drug resistance to all classes such that there are fewer than two active agents available for a new regimen, ART should be continued because it continues to exert antiviral and immuno-logic benefits in some instances. Based on studies of selective drug dis-continuation, there are certain principles behind selecting an appropriate "holding" regimen: 1) it should always include 3TC or FTC; 2) it should never contain an NNRTI, as this class of drugs does not continue to exert an antiviral effect once resistance is established; and 3) selection of specific drugs from the PI and NRTI classes should be based on tolerability. The goal of ART in this setting is to maintain the patient in a state of good health pending the development of effective new drugs.

Drug Toxicity

When a patient has an undetectable viral load but needs to make a change in the antiretroviral regimen because of drug toxicity, a single substitution within the same class is generally acceptable as long as there is no prior history of resistance to the new drug. As examples, a patient receiving d4T who experiences lipoatrophy can have an alternative NNRTI such as TDF or ABC substituted without risking virologic failure, and a patient with marked hyperlipidemia on LPV/RTV may show improvement by substitut-ing ATV. A switch outside of the same class because of drug toxicity may be riskier but also effective in some instances.

Inconvenience of Regimen

As noted above, an adherence assessment is essential prior to commencing ART. Currently, several effective combinations offer convenient once- or twice-daily dosing without food restrictions. Patients on older, more cum-bersome regimens can often be switched to easier options with little risk of drug toxicity. Ideally, these switches should be made within a drug class. For example, a patient receiving IDV at the original dose of 800 mg every 8 hours on an empty stomach may benefit from switching to one of the newer PIs that can be given once daily.

Antiretroviral Therapy in Pregnancy

There are two main treatment goals in the HIV-infected woman who is pregnant or planning to become pregnant: 1) maximizing maternal health by reducing the risk of HIV disease progression; and 2) preventing trans-mission of HIV to the fetus while minimizing exposure to potentially toxic medications. Therefore, an experienced HIV clinician should be involved in the care of such patients. See Chapter 11 for further discussion of this subject.

Although the landmark study that used ZDV monotherapy demon-strated a reduction in perinatal transmission in both the mother and newborn, the current standard of care is to use combination therapy during pregnancy with the goal of achieving an undetectable viral load. Rates of perinatal transmission are less then 2% for HIV-infected women with an undetectable viral load on ART.

In general, antiretroviral regimens chosen for pregnant women should contain 2 NRTIs plus either a PI or NVP, with pretreatment HIV genotype testing guiding the choice of drugs. Based on extensive clinical experience and the absence of maternal or fetal toxicity, the preferred NRTI combination is ZDV plus 3TC; ddI and d4T should be avoided because of an increased risk of maternal lactic acidosis and hepatic steatosis, as well as their potential deleterious effect on the developing nervous system of the newborn. For the PI, NFV or LPV/RTV is preferred; both drugs may have reduced plasma levels during pregnancy, but this observation has not been shown to influence treatment outcome. As noted above, EFV is contraindicated in pregnancy because of its potential for teratogenicity, and NVP should be avoided in women with a CD4 count of greater than 250 cells/mm^3 because of toxicity concerns.

In asymptomatic women with a CD4 count greater than 350 cells/mm^3, ART can be safely deferred until the second trimester. Treatment can then be discontinued after delivery if it was indicated only for prevention of perinatal transmission. Women already receiving ART when they become pregnant should continue on it, with modification of the regimen to avoid potentially teratogenic drugs (e.g. EFV) and dangerous combinations (e.g. ddI and d4T).

Elective caesarian delivery resulted in a five-fold decrease in transmission over perinatal ZDV monotherapy. However, in the era of effective combination ART, the additional benefit of caesarian section must be weighed against its risks. An elective caesarian section, prior to labor or rupture of membranes, is recommended only in women with a viral load above 1000 copies/mL.

HIV is found in breast milk, and breast feeding is estimated to confer an additional 16% increased risk of transmission when the mother is untreated. Some antiretroviral drugs also get into breast milk and may help decrease its viral load. However, if there is a safe, alternative form of nutrition for the newborn, HIV-infected women should be advised against breast feeding.

Investigational Antiretroviral Drugs

TMC-125 (etravirine), an experimental NNRTI, and MK-0518, (raltegravir) an integrase inhibitor, are currently available through expanded-access programs (Table 4-10). Both drugs may be approved for use in 2007. Promising other drugs in existing classes include D-d4FC (NRTI), TMC-278 (NNRTI), and brecanavir (PI). Antiretroviral drugs with novel mechanisms of action would presumably have limited or no cross-resistance with older

Table 4-10.   Investigational Antiretroviral Drugs Available Through Expanded Access Program

Drug	TMC-125 (Etravirine)	MK-0518 (Raltegravir)
Source	• 1-866-889-2074 • TMC125EAP@i3research.com • http://www.tibotec.com	http://www.earmrk.com
Class	Non-nucleoside reverse-transcriptase inhibitor (NNRTI)	Integrase inhibitor
Dose	TMC-125 200 mg twice daily + optimized background therapy (based on prior history and resistance testing)	MK-0518 400 mg twice daily + optimized background therapy (based on prior history and resistance testing)
Enrollment criteria	• >18 years old • Limited or no treatment options because of virologic failure or intolerance to multiple ART regimens • Unable to use currently approved NNRTIs because of resistance and/or intolerance • Have received therapy with each of the 3 major ART classes • Have received 2 different PI-based regimens • Primary NNRTI resistance can be included if experienced with at least 2 classes of ART (PI, NRTI) • Have not participated in TMC-125 studies • *Consult expanded access protocol for exclusion criteria*	• ≥16 years old • Limited or no treatment options available because of resistance (documented resistance to ≥ 1 drug in each of the 3 major ART classes or intolerance to multiple antiretroviral regimens • Not achieving adequate virologic suppression on current regimen • At risk for immunologic progression • Clinically stable • Have not received MK-0518 in a clinical trial • Have CrCl >30 mL/min • *Consult expanded access protocol for exclusion criteria*

Source: Department of Health and Human Services. Guidelines for the Use of Antiretroviral Agents in HIV-1 Infected Adults and Adolescents. Available as a "living document" at http://www.aidsinfo.nih.gov.

classes and be especially useful in treatment-experienced patients. CCR5 antagonists act by binding reversibly to this chemokine receptor (see Chapter 1), preventing entry of R5 tropic viruses into the cell. Several studies demonstrate that drugs with this mechanism of action induce a significant reduction in the viral load. Maraviroc, the CCR5 antagonist that is furthest in development, may be approved for use in 2007. However, obstacles to the development of CCR5 antagonists include the presence of dual-tropic viruses in patients with advanced HIV disease, as well as the theoretical concern of acting on a cellular rather than viral target. Drug development has also been slowed by hepatotoxicity in one candidate (aplaviroc) and limited potency when compared with EFV in another (vicriviroc). Other drugs that interfere with viral integrase (GS-9137) and maturation (PA-457) are also in development.

KEY POINTS

- Since the advent of effective combination ART in 1996, there has been a marked reduction in deaths from AIDS-related OIs.
- Disease-free survival is prolonged when patients receive ART that results in viral suppression.
- Antiretroviral therapy is generally indicated if: 1) the patient is symptomatic; 2) CD4 cell count is < 350 to $200/mm^3$; or 3) the patient is pregnant. Antiretroviral therapy should be considered in: 1) the asymptomatic patient with CD4 count $> 350/mm^3$ with a viral load greater than 100,000 copies/mL; and 2) the patient who has seroconverted within the past six months. Recommended ART regimens consist of at least three active drugs, including: 1) a dual NRTI "backbone" consisting of 3TC or FTC and one additional agent; and 2) a PI (often "boosted" with RTV) or an NNRTI.
- ART should be modified in the event of treatment failure: 1) when the viral load does not reach an undetectable level or becomes detectable on therapy; 2) when a significant decline in the CD4 count ($>30\%$ from baseline or $>3\%$ percentage) is noted; or 3) when clinical disease progression occurs. If ART is changed because of virologic failure, HIV resistance testing can help guide the selection of new drugs. In general, introduction of at least two new active agents is recommended.
- ART may also need to be modified sometimes because of drug toxicity. In this instance, a single substitution from the same class as the offending drug is recommended.
- ART is recommended in all pregnant HIV-infected women starting in the second trimester. While most drugs appear safe during pregnancy, EFV, ddI, and d4T should be avoided.

SUGGESTED READINGS

AIDS Clinical Trials Group 384 Team. Comparison of sequential three-drug regimens as initial therapy for HIV-1 infection. N Engl J Med. 2003;349:2293-303.

Campbell TB, Shulman NS, Johnson SC, Zolopa AR, Young RK, Bushman L, et al. Antiviral activity of lamivudine in salvage therapy for multidrug-resistant HIV-1 infection. Clin Infect Dis. 2005;41:236-42.

Clifford DB, Evans S, Yang Y, Acosta EP, Goodkin K, Tashima K, et al. Impact of efavirenz on neuropsychological performance and symptoms in HIV-infected individuals. Ann Intern Med. 2005;143:714-21.

Connor EM, Sperling RS, Gelber R, Kiselev P, Scott G, O'Sullivan MJ, et al. Reduction of maternal-infant transmission of human immunodeficiency virus type 1 with zidovudine treatment. Pediatric AIDS Clinical Trials Group Protocol 076 Study Group. N Engl J Med. 1994;331:1173-80.

Department of Health and Human Services. Guidelines for the Use of Antiretroviral Agents in HIV-1-Infected Adults and Adolescents. Available as a living document as www.aidsinfo.nih.gov.

El-Sadr W, Neaton J, for the SMART Study Investigators. Episodic CD4-guided use of antiretroviral therapy is inferior to continuous therapy: results of the SMART study. Thirteenth Conference on Retroviruses and Opportunistic Infections, Denver, abstract 106LB, 2006.

European Collaborative Study. Mother-to-child transmission of HIV infection in the era of highly active antiretroviral therapy. Clin Infect Dis. 2005;40:458-65.

Losina E, Islam R, Pollock AC, Sax PE, Freedberg KA, Walensky RP. Effectiveness of antiretroviral therapy after protease inhibitor failure: an analytic overview. Clin Infect Dis. 2004;38:1613-22.

Lyles RH, Muñoz A, Yamashita TE, Bazmi H, Detels R, Rinaldo CR, et al. Natural history of human immunodeficiency virus type 1 viremia after seroconversion and proximal to AIDS in a large cohort of homosexual men. Multicenter AIDS Cohort Study. J Infect Dis. 2000;181:872-80.

Matthews GV, Sabin CA, Mandalia S, Lampe F, Phillips AN, Nelson MR, et al. Virological suppression at 6 months is related to choice of initial regimen in antiretroviral-naive patients: a cohort study. AIDS. 2002;16:53-61.

Mofenson LM, Lambert JS, Stiehm ER, Bethel J, Meyer WA 3rd, Whitehouse J, et al. Risk factors for perinatal transmission of human immunodeficiency virus type 1 in women treated with zidovudine. Pediatric AIDS Clinical Trials Group Study 185 Team. N Engl J Med. 1999;341:385-93.

Moore RD, Keruly JC, Gebo KA, Lucas GM. An improvement in virologic response to highly active antiretroviral therapy in clinical practice from 1996 through 2002. J Acquir Immune Defic Syndr. 2005;39:195-8.

Nettles RE, Kieffer TL, Kwon P, Monie D, Han Y, Parsons T, et al. Intermittent HIV-1 viremia (Blips) and drug resistance in patients receiving HAART. JAMA. 2005;293:817-29.

O'Brien ME, Clark RA, Besch CL, Myers L, Kissinger P. Patterns and correlates of discontinuation of the initial HAART regimen in an urban outpatient cohort. J Acquir Immune Defic Syndr. 2003;34:407-14.

Palella FJ Jr., Cole SR, Chmiel JS, Riddler SA, Visscher B, Dobs A, et al. Anthropometrics and examiner-reported body habitus abnormalities in the multicenter AIDS cohort study. Clin Infect Dis. 2004;38:903-7.

Paredes R, Mocroft A, Kirk O, Lazzarin A, Barton SE, van Lunzen J, et al. Predictors of virological success and ensuing failure in HIV-positive patients starting highly active antiretroviral therapy in Europe: results from the EuroSIDA study. Arch Intern Med. 2000;160:1123-32.

Ratnam I, Chiu C, Kandala NB, Easterbrook PJ. Incidence and risk factors for immune reconstitution inflammatory syndrome in an ethnically diverse, HIV type 1-infected cohort. Clin Infect Dis. 2006;42:418-27.

Sax PE, Islam R, Walensky RP, Losina E, Weinstein MC, Goldie SJ, et al. Should resistance testing be performed for treatment-naive HIV-infected patients? A cost-effectiveness analysis. Clin Infect Dis. 2005;41:1316-23.

Sterling TR, Chaisson RE, Keruly J, Moore RD. Improved outcomes with earlier initiation of highly active antiretroviral therapy among human immunodeficiency virus-infected patients who achieve durable virologic suppression: longer follow-up of an observational cohort study. J Infect Dis. 2003;188:1659-65.

Study 934 Group. Tenofovir DF, emtricitabine, and efavirenz vs. zidovudine, lamivudine, and efavirenz for HIV. N Engl J Med. 2006;354:251-60.

Study Team of the Terry Beirn Community Programs for Clinical Research on AIDS. Structured treatment interruption in patients with multidrug-resistant human immunodeficiency virus. N Engl J Med. 2003;349:837-46.

Swiss Cohort Study. Response to first protease inhibitor- and efavirenz-containing antiretroviral combination therapy. The Swiss HIV Cohort Study. AIDS. 2001;15:1793-800.

TORO 1 Study Group. Enfuvirtide, an HIV-1 fusion inhibitor, for drug-resistant HIV infection in North and South America. N Engl J Med. 2003;348:2175-85.

2NN Study Group. The effect of baseline CD4 cell count and HIV-1 viral load on the efficacy and safety of nevirapine or efavirenz-based first-line HAART. AIDS. 2005;19:463-71.

2NN Study Group. Comparison of first-line antiretroviral therapy with regimens including nevirapine, efavirenz, or both drugs, plus stavudine and lamivudine: a randomised open-label trial. Lancet. 2004;363:1253-63.

van Leeuwen R, Katlama C, Murphy RL, Squires K, Gatell J, Horban A, et al. A randomized trial to study first-line combination therapy with or without a protease inhibitor in HIV-1-infected patients. AIDS. 2003;17:987-99.

Wang C, Vlahov D, Galai N, Bareta J, Strathdee SA, Nelson KE, et al. Mortality in HIV-seropositive versus HIV-seronegative persons in the era of highly active antiretroviral therapy: implications for when to initiate therapy. J Infect Dis. 2004;190:1046-54.

Chapter 5

Antiretroviral Pharmacokinetics, Resistance Testing, and Therapeutic Drug Monitoring

EDWARD P. ACOSTA, PharmD
JOHN G. GERBER, MD
DANIEL R. KURITZKES, MD

Combination antiretroviral therapy has reduced the morbidity and mortality of HIV infection. However, disease progression may still occur over time as the effectiveness of the drug regimen diminishes. Treatment failure, which manifests as an increasing viral load, is attributable to a variety of factors, including inadequate medication adherence, insufficient drug potency, pharmacokinetic attributes, and the emergence of drug-resistant virus.

Heterogeneity in the response to antiretroviral drugs has been attributed to pharmacologic, virologic, immunologic, and behavioral differences among patients. Advances in molecular diagnostic techniques have led to the development of assays for HIV resistance testing that are available to most clinicians. Quantifying the pharmacologic contribution to differences in response by therapeutic drug monitoring (TDM) remains an important objective. Data on antiretroviral drug dose- and concentration-effect relationships continue to accumulate.

This chapter reviews the pharmacokinetics and pharmacodynamics of antiretroviral drugs, addresses the current status of genotypic and phenotypic resistance testing in the management of HIV infection, and explores the potential role of TDM. The clinical use of antiretroviral drugs is discussed in Chapter 4.

Clinical Pharmacology of Antiretroviral Drugs

Nucleoside and Nucleotide Reverse-Transcriptase Inhibitors

Nucleoside reverse-transcriptase inhibitors (NRTIs) are the cornerstones of most antiretroviral regimens. The NRTIs are 3'-modified deoxynucleosides that require intracellular phosphorylation to become activated. Specific cellular host enzymes are responsible for this process. Once activated, the phosphorylated moiety is incorporated into the growing DNA strand by HIV reverse transcriptase (RT), thereby preventing further reverse transcription. Thymidine analogs (zidovudine [ZDV] and stavudine [d4T]) are preferentially phosphorylated in activated cells, whereas lamivudine (3TC) and didanosine (ddI) are preferentially phosphorylated in resting cells. As ZDV and d4T compete for the same activating enzymes, their coadministration results in clinically significant antagonism. Abacavir (ABC) is a guanosine-derived NRTI. It has a slightly different activation pathway from the other NRTIs in that it requires an additional step to form carbovir monophosphate, which is then converted to the active compound, carbovir triphosphate. Although the plasma half-life ($T_{1/2}$) of most NRTIs is relatively short (1 to 2 hours), the long intracellular half-lives of the active triphosphate forms of these drugs allows them to be dosed once or twice a day (Table 5-1). With the exception of ZDV and ABC, the NRTIs are primarily excreted unchanged by the kidneys. As a result, drug interactions are uncommon with this class.

Nonnucleoside Reverse-Transcriptase Inhibitors

Nonnucleoside reverse-transcriptase inhibitors (NNRTIs) have contributed significantly to the development of simplified antiretroviral regimens because their pharmacokinetic profiles allow once- or twice-daily administration (Table 5-2). Unlike the nucleoside analogs, NNRTIs do not require intracellular activation. The three currently available NNRTIs are metabolized by the liver via the cytochrome P450 (CYP 450) enzyme system; CYP 3A4 is the isozyme primarily responsible. Because this inducible isozyme is also involved in the metabolism of many other agents, significant drug interactions are common. Both efavirenz (EFV) and nevirapine (NVP) induce CYP 3A4, whereas delavirdine (DLV) inhibits it.

Protease Inhibitors

The advent of protease inhibitors (PIs) represented a major advance in the treatment of HIV infection. HIV protease is an enzyme responsible for posttranslational cleavage of viral polyprotein precursors into smaller, mature proteins. PIs block this action, leading to the production of immature noninfectious virions. PIs are large, lipophilic, organic bases that are moderately to highly bound to plasma proteins. Most are also metabolized by CYP 450 enzymes and have the potential for significant drug interactions.

Protein binding, particularly to alpha-1 acid glycoprotein (AAG), is an important characteristic of the PIs because only the free fraction of a drug is able to elicit its pharmacologic action. Moreover, the greater the free fraction of a drug, the better it is able to distribute into other tissues such as the central nervous system. In general, for drugs that are more than 90% protein-bound, the free fraction is susceptible to fluctuations in plasma

Table 5-1. Pharmacokinetic Characteristics of Nucleoside/Nucleotide Reverse-Transcriptase Inhibitors

Drug	Adult Dose	T_{max} (h)	C_{max} (µg/mL)	AUC_τ (µg·h/mL)	$T_{1/2}$ (h)	Intracellular Triphosphate $T_{1/2}$ (h)
Zidovudine	300 mg bid	0.75	1.19	1.38	0.71	7-10
Didanosine	200 mg bid	0.89	1.05	1.92	1.42	12-24
	400 mg qd	0.67	1.475	2.516	1.64	—
Didanosine EC	400 mg qd	2.0	9.3	2.432	1.6	—
Stavudine	40 mg bid	1.0	0.52	1.26	1.51	3-4
Lamivudine	150 mg bid	1.6 ± 0.7	2.1 ± 0.82	17.1 ± 6.5	6.1 ± 1.9	8-12
	300 mg qd	2.2 ± 1.3	3.5 ± 0.85	16.6 ± 4.2	7.9 ± 3.4	—
Abacavir	300 mg bid	0.89 ± 0.31	2.17 ± 0.47	5.47 ± 1.38	0.85 ± 0.22	3.3
Emtricitabine	200 mg qd	1-2	1.8 ± 0.7	10 ± 3.1	10	39
Tenofovir	300 mg qd	2.3	3.26	3.02	14.4	>60

See *Physicians' Desk Reference* for drug dosing guidelines and pharmacokinetic data references. AUC = area-under-the curve for the dosing interval specified under adult dose; EC = enteric-coated capsule formulation.

Table 5-2.   Pharmacokinetic Characteristics of Non-Nucleoside Reverse-Transcriptase Inhibitors[*]

Drug	IC_x (µg/mL)	Adult Dose	T_{max} (h)	C_{max} (µg/mL)	C_{min} (µg/mL)	AUC_τ (µg•h/mL)	$T_{1/2}$ (h)	% PB
Delavirdine	IC_{50} = 0.017	60 mg bid	1.2 ± 0.3	15 (7.8-30)	5.9 (0.7-11.9)	115 (40-222)	5.8 (2-11)	~98
Nevirapine[†]	IC_{50} = 0.003-0.03	400 mg qd	1.5 (1.0-2.4)	6.7 (6.0-8.6)	2.9 (2.3-4.1)	101.8 (92.6-145.3)	21.5 (15-32.8)	~60
Efavirenz[†]	IC_{90-95} = 0.0005-0.008	600 mg qd	2.0 (1.5-3.0)	3.6 (2.6-5.4)	1.8 ± 1.0	54.8 (33-67)	35.8 (18.1-50.6)	>99

See *Physicians' Desk Reference* for drug dosing guidelines and pharmacokinetic data references. IC_x = Concentration of drug needed to inhibit x% of viral replication in vitro; AUC_τ = area-under-the curve for the dosing interval; % PB = percent of drug protein-bound.

[*] Values are mean ± standard deviation or median (range) where available.

[†] Reported as median (interquartile range).

protein concentrations; a small increase in plasma protein levels may cause a decrease in the free drug concentration. This principle is important for drugs bound primarily to AAG because there is a large degree of intrapatient variability in AAG concentrations. Moreover, because AAG is an acute phase reactant, chronic diseases (inflammatory or infectious) can alter AAG concentrations.

For most PIs, antiviral activity is correlated with the plasma minimum concentration (C_{min}). Ideally, the drug concentration should be maintained several-fold above the 50% inhibitory concentration (IC_{50}) for HIV throughout the dosing interval (Figure 5-1). However, there is considerable inter- and intrapatient variability in PI absorption and clearance (Table 5-3). Deviations from the prescribed dosing schedule, including recommendations regarding administration with or without food, can result in a C_{min} that falls below the IC_{50} of the viral strain. Such "gaps" in drug exposure may permit resumption of HIV replication, leading ultimately to the emergence of resistant virus and treatment failure.

Standard PI therapy for HIV infection typically requires administration of multiple oral doses at frequent intervals. Because most PIs are CYP 3A4 substrates, their pharmacokinetics can be altered by coadministration of a CYP 3A4 inhibitor. The PI ritonavir (RTV) is a potent CYP 3A4 inhibitor that slows the metabolism of most PIs. Coadministration of low doses of RTV with therapeutic doses of one or more PIs can be used to enhance their pharmacologic effects (Table 5-4). These regimens generally involve less frequent dosing schedules with lower pill burdens, both of which may improve adherence to antiretroviral therapy. Pharmacologic enhancement

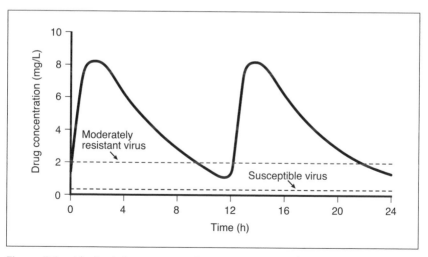

Figure 5-1. Idealized drug concentration over time curve for an antiretroviral agent dosed twice daily. C_{min} at 12 h is adequate to inhibit a susceptible virus with an IC_{50} of 0.2 μM, but inadequate to inhibit a moderately resistant virus with an IC_{50} of 2.0 μM.

Table 5-3. Pharmacokinetic Characteristics of Protease Inhibitors

Drug	IC_x (µg/mL)	Adult Dose	T_{max} (h)	C_{max} (µg/mL)	C_{min} (µg/mL)	AUC_t (µg•h/mL)	$T_{1/2}$ (h)	% PB
Amprenavir	IC_{50} = 0.006-0.040	1200 mg bid	1.9 ± 1.0	5.36 ± 3.32	0.28 ± 0.15	18.5 ± 11.7	8.9 ± 1.8	90%
Fosamprenavir	IC_{50} = 0.006-0.040	1400 mg bid	1.3	4.82	0.35	16.5	7.7	90%
Atazanavir	IC_{50} = 0.0014-0.004	400 mg qd	2.0	2.3 ± 1.6	0.12 ± 0.13	14.9 ± 13.5	6.5 ± 2.6	86%
Indinavir	IC_{95} = 0.015-0.061	800 mg q8h	0.8 ± 0.3	7.75 ± 2.48	0.15 ± 0.11	18.8 ± 7.0	1.8 ± 0.4	60%
Nelfinavir	IC_{95} = 0.004-0.111 IC_{95} = 1.0*	750 mg tid	2.8 ± 1.0	2.9 ± 1.3	1.3 ± 0.7	16.3 ± 7.7	4.0 ± 0.6	>98%
Ritonavir	IC_{50} = 0.003-0.110 IC_{90} = 2.1*	600 mg bid	3.3 ± 2.2	11.2 ± 3.6	3.03 ± 2.13	60.8 ± 23.4	4.0 ± 1.0	>99%
Saquinavir	IC_{90} = 0.003-0.054	1200 mg tid	2.5 ± 0.5	2.05	0.18	18.11	ND	~97%

Based on data from Acosta EP, Kakuda TN, Brundage RC, Anderson PL, Fletcher CV. Pharmacodynamics of HIV-1 protease inhibitors. Clin Infect Dis. 2000;30(S2): S151-S159. See *Physicians' Desk Reference* for drug dosing guidelines and pharmacokinetic data references. IC_x = concentration of drug needed to inhibit x% of viral replication *in vitro*; AUC = area-under-the curve for the dosing interval; % PB = percent of drug bound to plasma protein; ND = no data available.

* Adjusted for plasma protein binding in vitro

Table 5-4.   Pharmacokinetic Characteristics of Ritonavir-Boosted Protease Inhibitors

Drug	Dose Regimen	T_{max} (h)	C_{max} (µg/mL)	C_{min} (µg/mL)	AUC_τ (µg•h/mL)	$T_{1/2}$ (h)
fAPV/RTV	1400/200 mg qd	2.1	7.24	1.45	69.4	—
	700/100 mg bid	1.5	6.1	2.12	79.2	—
ATV/RTV	300/100 mg qd	3.0	4.4 ± 2.6	0.64 ± 0.62	46.1 ± 30.4	8.6 ± 2.3
TPV/RTV**	500/200 mg bid	3.0	129 ± 27	21.5 ± 10.1	428 ± 124	6.0
IDV/RTV	800/100 mg bid	1.4	8.9	1.3	46.6	3.5
	800/200 mg bid	2.9 ± 1.1	7.7 ± 3.4	1.2 ± 1.2	47.8 ± 21.8	2.5 ± 1.0
SQV/RTV	1000/100 mg bid	3 (2.5-4)	5.3 (3.9-6.6)	0.07 (0.04-0.15)	35.5 (28.9-50.2)	3.6 (3.0-5.3)
	1600/100 mg qd	6	8.9 ± 4.7	0.6 ± 0.4	87.4 ± 42.7	4.3
LPV/RTV*	400/100 mg bid	4.2	9.8 ± 3.7	5.5 ± 2.7	92.6 ± 36.8	9.9
APV/RTV	600/100 mg bid	1 (0.5-2.0)	7.1 (5.1-9.9)	1.9 (1.3-2.8)	32.1 (24.0-42.8)	6.9
	1200/200 mg qd†	—	8.2	0.9	49.8	—

See *Physicians' Desk Reference* for drug dosing guidelines and pharmacokinetic data references. Values are mean ± SD or median (range) where available. AUC = area-under-the curve for the dosing interval specified under adult dose.

* Increasing the dose of LPV/RTV to 533 mg/133 mg bid in HIV-infected patients receiving EFV produced similar concentrations to those achieved with LPV/RTV 400 mg/100 mg bid in the absence of EFV.

† Geometric mean

** Data are for males; females have increased TPV exposure.

with RTV can also partially compensate for CYP 3A4 induction by other antiretroviral drugs, such as EFV or NVP, which tend to lower PI concentrations. Furthermore, the higher C_{min} achieved with RTV-enhanced regimens may produce better antiretroviral responses, even in patients whose viral strains exhibit reduced PI susceptibility.

Antiretroviral Drug Resistance

Pathogenesis

The high error rate of HIV RT and the rapid replication of the virus result in genetic diversity over time. Because of an error frequency of approximately 10^{-5} per replication cycle, a genome size of nearly 10,000 nucleotides, and a minimum of 10^7 to 10^8 rounds of replication per day, each individual mutation could, in theory, be represented many times in the quasispecies. Specific double mutations are less common, however, and specific triple mutations are relatively rare.

When drugs that inhibit HIV replication are subtherapeutically administered, the resulting evolutionary pressure selects for resistant strains. Drug-resistant variants develop at a rate proportionate to the frequency of preexisting variants and their relative growth advantage in the presence of a drug. For some drugs, including 3TC, NVP, and EFV, drug-resistant viruses may emerge in a matter of weeks because of the selection of point mutations that confer up to 1,000-fold resistance. For other drugs, such as ZDV and most PIs, high-level resistance requires the step-wise acquisition of multiple mutations. Consequently, resistance to these drugs tends to develop over months instead of weeks.

Mechanisms of Resistance

Because new data continuously add to the list of mutations known to influence HIV drug susceptibility and treatment response, the reader is urged to consult the excellent Web sites devoted to drug resistance for up-to-date information (e.g., www.hiv.lanl.gov, www.iasusa.org, and hivdb.stanford.edu). Appendix II summarizes our current understanding of the clinical significance of these mutations.

Although a detailed discussion of specific drug-resistance mutations is beyond the scope of this chapter, several basic principles are worth noting. Mutations that confer antiretroviral drug resistance do so by a variety of mechanisms. These include altered drug binding, improved enzyme efficiency, alterations in the enzyme substrate, and nucleoside excision. Most drug-resistance mutations result in the production of a viral protein with reduced affinity for one or more drugs. This mechanism is the basis for resistance to 3TC, ddI, the NNRTIs, and the PIs. In many cases these mutations also impair enzyme function, resulting in a virus that is less fit than wild-type. Additional mutations, sometimes referred to as "secondary" or "compensatory," may emerge that improve the catalytic efficiency of the enzyme and restore viral fitness. Other mutations may alter the enzyme target (e.g., mutations in the cleavage sites of the gag-pol polyprotein precursor) to compensate for reduced substrate affinity of drug-resistant protease.

A unique mechanism implicated in resistance to ZDV and other NRTIs involves nucleoside excision, also known as primer unblocking. The nucleoside analog inhibitors of RT are all dideoxynucleosides. Once incorporated into a growing DNA chain, they act as chain terminators, thereby halting reverse transcription. Removal of this terminal dideoxynucleoside monophosphate relieves the blockade and allows reverse transcription to proceed. Mutations selected by ZDV or d4T confer resistance by increasing the rate of nucleoside excision. Although these mutations accelerate excision of ZDV and d4T to the greatest extent, they affect all nucleoside and nucleotide RT inhibitors somewhat. Therefore, these mutations (previously referred to as *thymidine analog mutations* [TAMs]) are referred to as *nucleoside excision mutations.*

NRTI Resistance

Because individual NRTIs select for distinct mutations in RT, patterns of resistance were previously thought to be drug-specific. It is now clear, however, that mutations to ZDV confer broad cross-resistance within this class. Studies show a strong correlation between ZDV susceptibility and susceptibility to every other NRTI. The extent of nucleoside resistance correlates significantly with the number of accumulated TAMs.

Two additional sets of mutations can confer multinucleoside resistance: the Q151M complex and the insertion mutations at codon 69. These mutations, which are found in 2% to 6% of resistant isolates, are less common than TAMs. The Q151M complex most often emerges in patients treated with a thymidine analog plus ddI, but can be selected by ZDV or d4T plus zalcitabine (ddC). The Q151M mutation, in concert with mutations at codons 62, 75, 77, and 116, confers resistance to all of the currently available NRTIs, with the exception of tenofovir (TDF). Similarly, insertion mutations at codon 69, when associated with TAMs at codons 210 and 215, confer broad resistance to nucleoside and nucleotide reverse-transcriptase inhibitors.

The nonthymidine NRTIs select for mutations that confer more limited cross-resistance. For example, ABC, TDF, and ddC each select for the K65R mutation; this mutation also confers resistance to ddI, but not to ZDV or d4T. Similarly, ddI and ABC select for the L74V mutation, which confers resistance to ddC, but not to TDF or the thymidine analogs. The 184V mutation, which confers high-level resistance to 3TC, is also selected by ABC. However, clinical studies show that the response to ABC is not significantly diminished by the presence of the 184V mutation alone. Mutations at codons 65, 74, and 184 share the property of enhancing viral susceptibility to the thymidine analogs. These mutations also reduce viral fitness to varying degrees.

NNRTI Resistance

Mutations that confer resistance to NNRTIs are present in two clusters in the RT gene at codons 100 to 108 and 179 to 236. The most common changes involve a K103N mutation (selected by NVP, DLV, and EFV), and a Y181C mutation (selected by NVP and DLV). Additional mutations accumulate after initial emergence of K103N or Y181C, suggesting continued remodeling and adaptation of RT under the selective pressure of NNRTI therapy. As a rule, resistance to one NNRTI generally results in resistance to the entire class, particularly when the K103N mutation has been selected. However, there are exceptions. For example, HIV isolates that carry the Y181C mutation remain susceptible to EFV in vitro, but the use of EFV after NVP failure generally leads to prompt emergence of EFV resistance. Likewise, the G109A mutation is associated with resistance to EFV and NVP. The major NNRTI resistance mutations have little effect on viral fitness and, as a consequence, persist in the population for many months after interruption of antiretroviral therapy.

PI Resistance

Despite the small size of the protease gene (99 amino acids), multiple mutations at numerous codons have been associated with resistance. Many of these mutations map to the substrate-binding site and directly interfere with binding of PIs. Additional (secondary) mutations map to other regions of the protease and improve the activity of mutant proteases without directly affecting inhibitor binding. Resistance to PIs emerges rapidly when these drugs are administered at inadequate doses or as part of suboptimal regimens. For some PIs (e.g., saquinavir, nelfinavir), the level of resistance conferred by single mutations is sufficient to compromise activity; for others (e.g., indinavir, lopinavir/ritonavir), step-wise accumulation of multiple mutations is required to generate high-level resistance. Although primary mutations are usually drug-specific, a similar set of secondary mutations is selected by most PIs, leading ultimately to broad cross-resistance within the class.

A unique class of PI resistance mutations has been identified at cleavage sites in the gag-pol polyprotein precursor, which is the substrate of HIV protease. Cleavage site mutations do not, themselves, produce drug resistance but compensate for alterations in protease activity that result from primary and secondary resistance mutations in the enzyme.

Interpreting the significance of protease mutants is made difficult by the polymorphisms found in genes from HIV isolates of PI-naïve patients. In one study, variation was noted in nearly 48% of protease codons compared with the wild-type sequence, including substitutions usually associated with PI resistance. The significance of these polymorphisms in determining treatment outcome remains uncertain. Another difficulty in the interpretation of PI resistance is the relationship between drug susceptibility and achievable plasma concentrations. In the case of PIs that can be administered with or without RTV boosting (e.g., atazanavir), two different cut-offs are needed.

Entry Inhibitor Resistance

Resistance to enfuvirtide, an entry inhibitor, is mediated by substitutions at amino acids 36 to 45 of gp4 within the first heptad repeat to which the drug binds. The substitutions most frequently associated with resistance include G36D, S, V, or E; V38A, E, or M; Q40H; N42T; and N43D. Although genotypic and phenotypic testing for enfuvirtide resistance is available, its clinical utility may be limited.

Viral Fitness and Replication Capacity

Viral fitness and replication capacity are closely related, yet distinct, properties. As applied to HIV, viral fitness refers to the relative ability of two or more different isolates to replicate under particular conditions (e.g., in the presence of 3TC). Although drug-resistant variants are more fit than wild-type viruses in the presence of a drug, they are often significantly less fit than wild-type virus in the absence of a drug and replaced by wild-type if antiretroviral therapy is interrupted. By contrast, replication capacity refers to the amount of virus produced in a given period (e.g., per round of replication or per day). As drug resistance mutations alter the function of the viral enzyme or protein in which they occur, most reduce viral replication capacity to some extent. Thus, a drug-resistant virus might be substantially more fit than wild-type in the presence of drug but have markedly reduced replication capacity. For this reason, a "failing" antiretroviral drug regimen may nevertheless maintain plasma viremia at levels below the pretreatment baseline. Viral fitness can be assessed by growth competition assays, in which the relative replication of two or more viral species is tested in the same culture. Viral replication capacity can be measured by a modification of the phenotypic resistance assay. At present, the clinical utility of these assays remains undefined.

Resistance Testing

Genotypic and Phenotypic Assays

Advances in technology have made drug-resistance testing a practical tool in the management of HIV-infected patients. The viral genotype or phenotype can be determined from plasma samples using commercially available automated assays. A growing body of data from retrospective and prospective studies provides evidence to support the clinical utility of these tests in guiding antiretroviral management decisions in patients with treatment failure.

Genotypic assays for drug resistance determine the nucleotide sequence and, by inference, the predicted amino acid sequence of the protease and RT genes. Phenotypic assays, on the other hand, measure the susceptibility of HIV to inhibition by a particular drug by determining the amount required to suppress virus production in vitro by 50%, 90%, or 95% (IC_{50}, IC_{90}, or IC_{95}, respectively). Both types of such assays depend upon amplification of HIV protease and RT genes from viral RNA in plasma by means of RT-coupled polymerase chain reaction (RT-PCR). In the case of genotypic assays, the protease-RT amplicons can then be subjected to automated DNA sequencing by a variety of techniques, probed by hybridization-based assays (e.g., line probe assay), or tested by further PCR using selective priming or selective nucleotide addition (e.g., point mutation assay). The TruGene HIV-1 Genotyping Kit and OpenGene DNA Sequencing System and the ViroSeq HIV-1 Genotyping System have been approved for clinical use by the Food and Drug Administration.

In the case of phenotypic assays, the amplified protease and RT sequences are cloned into a plasmid from which these genes have been deleted. The resulting plasmids carry patient protease and RT sequences in a uniform HIV backbone. Transfection of these plasmids into permissive cells results in production of recombinant virus, which can be assayed for drug susceptibility. Modification of this assay to introduce envelope sequences in place of protease and RT allows measurement of susceptibility to enfuvirtide and other entry inhibitors. Three phenotypic tests are available for clinical use: Antivirogram from Virco, PhenoSense from Monogram Biosciences, and Phenoscript from VIRalliance. In addition, a database-driven interpretation of genotypic data that derives a predicted phenotype ("virtual phenotype") is also available from Virco (VircoType).

Genotypic and phenotypic resistance assays provide complementary information. Both have unique advantages and disadvantages, but also share certain limitations. For example, currently available assays are relatively insensitive to the presence of minority species in the virus population. In addition, technical limitations in the RT-PCR step required to amplify protease and RT genes make it difficult to obtain reliable results when the plasma HIV RNA level is less than 1,000 copies/mL.

Genotypic assays have the relative advantage of being faster and easier to perform, resulting in quicker turn-around times and lower cost than phenotypic assays. In addition, sentinel mutations may be detectable by genotypic assay before a shift in drug susceptibility becomes apparent. A major limitation of genotypic assays is the difficulty in predicting the consequences of mutational interactions on drug susceptibility. This situation is illustrated best by the variable effect of 3TC resistance on resistance to ZDV. Polymorphisms and mutations at numerous loci not directly involved in drug resistance appear to modulate the expression of dual resistance to ZDV and 3TC. Likewise, the extent of cross-resistance among drugs within a class can be difficult to predict on the basis of a genotype alone.

Phenotypic assays can provide susceptibility data even if the genetic basis of resistance to a particular drug has not yet been worked out. Another advantage of phenotypic assays is that clinicians are more familiar with interpreting data expressed as IC_{50} or IC_{90} compared with genotypic data. Phenotypic assays can determine the net effect of different mutations on drug susceptibility and cross-resistance. However, specific "break-points" for classifying isolates as sensitive or resistant have not been established for all antiretroviral drugs. A major disadvantage of phenotypic assays is their relatively limited availability and greater cost compared with genotypic assays. Another disadvantage of phenotypic assays is the time required to generate a result, which is still several weeks despite the advance of recombinant virus assays.

Effect of Protein Binding on Susceptibility

Protein binding must be taken into consideration when determining inhibitory concentrations. For example, if a drug is 98% protein-bound and has an IC_{95} of 0.10 µM with no AAG present, then the in vivo-adjusted IC_{95} must take into account physiologic concentrations of AAG. This effect on wild-type IC_{50} has been examined by adding 50% human serum to the culture system. As expected, the IC_{50} shifts only slightly for drugs with minimal protein binding (indinavir and NVP; 2- and 1.3-fold increases in susceptibility, respectively) compared with highly bound drugs (saquinavir and nelfinavir; 25- to 35-fold increases, respectively). The IC_{50} corrected for protein binding will more accurately reflect the plasma-trough concentration that should be maintained in a given patient.

Clinical Utility

Results from several randomized clinical trials support the use of resistance testing to help select antiretroviral therapy in patients on failing drug regimens (Table 5-5). The studies differ in several important design features, including the extent of previous treatment experience of the population, the particular resistance test employed, whether or not expert advice was provided in addition to test results, duration of follow-up, and the definition of virologic success or failure used as the primary endpoint. Therefore, it is not surprising that these studies have sometimes yielded contradictory results.

Three trials showed an advantage for genotypic testing compared with standard of care in selection of salvage regimens for patients on failing combination antiretroviral therapy. Patients in the genotypic arms of these studies had average declines in plasma HIV RNA levels that were significantly

Table 5-5.   Prospective Trials of Drug Resistance Testing

Study	Study Arm	HIV RNA (log₁₀ copies/mL)	% Below Detection
VIRADAPT	Genotype	−1.04	29%
	SOC	−0.46	14%
		($P = 0.01$)	($P = 0.017$)
GART	Genotype + EA	−1.19	55%
	SOC	−0.61	25%
		($P < 0.001$)	($P < 0.001$)
Havana	Genotype	−0.84	48.5%
	No genotype	−0.63	36.2%
		($P < 0.05$)	($P < 0.05$)
	Expert advice	−0.75	47.2%
	No expert advice	−0.73	37.4%
		($P = NS$)	($P = NS$)
ARGENTA	Genotype	−0.62	27%
	SOC	−0.38	12%
		($P = 0.12$)	($P = 0.01$)
VIRA 3001	Phenotype	−1.23	46%
	SOC	−0.87	34%
		($P = 0.005$)	($P = 0.079$)
NARVAL	Genotype	−0.95	44%
	Phenotype	−0.93	35%
	SOC	−0.76	36%
		($P = 0.215, 0.274$)	($P = 0.918, 0.120$)
CCTG 575	Phenotype	−0.71	48%
	SOC	−0.69	48%
		($P = NS$)	($P = NS$)
GenPheRex	Phenotype	−0.92	20%
	Virtual phenotype	−0.94	24%
		($P = NS$)	($P = NS$)
RealVirFen	Phenotype	−1.00	47%
	Virtual phenotype	−1.30	56%
		($P = 0.017$)	($P = 0.1$)
ERA	Genotype	−1.37	35%
	Genotype + Phenotype	−1.28	27%
		($P = 0.77$)	($P = 0.3$)

HIV RNA = change in plasma HIV RNA level from baseline; SOC = standard of care; EA = expert advice; NS = not significant.
Study publication abstracts can be accessed at www.pubmed.gov.

greater than patients in the standard-of-care arms over periods ranging from 8 to 24 weeks; they were also more likely to achieve plasma HIV RNA levels below the limits of detection. In a fourth trial, the advantages of genotypic testing proved to be short-lived. Further analysis demonstrated the importance of achieving adequate plasma drug levels for an optimal treatment response, even after taking into account the benefits of genotypic testing.

Expert advice also plays a significant role in the outcome of salvage therapy. In a study that compared the utility of genotypic resistance testing, expert advice, or both, genotyping and expert advice each resulted in significantly better virologic responses. However, the best response rates were observed in patients who received both genotyping and expert advice. These results suggest that, although expert advice is helpful, the availability of genotypic testing leads to further improvement in virologic outcome of salvage therapy.

Trials of phenotypic testing have produced mixed results. In a study of patients on their first failing PI-containing regimen, selection of salvage therapy guided by results of phenotypic testing resulted in significantly greater reduction in plasma HIV RNA level by week 16 compared with the standard of care. Other studies have failed to show a benefit of phenotypic testing. However, secondary analyses in some of these trials have shown an advantage of phenotyping in the subgroup of patients with a history of extensive prior antiretroviral therapy. Studies comparing phenotyping with the virtual phenotype have also yielded equivocal results, as did a study comparing genotyping alone with the combination of genotyping plus phenotyping.

The cost-effectiveness of resistance testing has been modeled using data from clinical trials together with data from the AIDS Cost and Services Utilization Survey and the 1998 Red Book to determine the cost of HIV-related care. The incremental increase in cost per quality-adjusted life-years compared favorably to the cost of prophylaxis against opportunistic infections such as disseminated *Mycobacterium avium* complex infection. Using the same model, the cost-effectiveness of resistance testing for patients with primary HIV infection was shown to increase in parallel with increasing rates of the transmission of drug-resistant strains.

In summary, prospective randomized trials provide evidence of at least short-term clinical benefit for both genotypic and phenotypic drug-resistance testing. Numerous factors contribute to determining the outcome of salvage therapy and complicate the design and interpretation of resistance testing studies. In the absence of data from comparative trials, there is insufficient evidence to support the use of one type of resistance testing over the other.

Recommendations

Drug-resistance testing is potentially useful in guiding antiretroviral therapy in several situations. These include choosing an initial treatment regimen, explaining and managing treatment failure, and tracking the prevalence of primary (transmitted) drug resistance. Expert consultation is recommended for clinicians with limited experience in this area.

Data suggest that HIV drug-resistance mutations are present in 10% to 15% of newly infected patients and can persist for a year or more in the absence of treatment. Transmission of multiple-resistant strains of HIV also has been documented. Screening for the presence of drug resistance before initiating antiretroviral therapy is sensible and cost-effective, particularly in areas of high HIV seroprevalence.

The strongest case for resistance testing can be made for patients in whom current therapy is failing. Retrospective and prospective studies have demonstrated the utility of resistance testing in choosing a salvage regimen. However, several important caveats should be kept in mind. First, treatment failure should be determined using standard criteria, such as a rising viral load and/or falling CD4 cell count. Second, because resistance testing is less reliable at lower viral loads, these assays generally should not be performed in patients with plasma HIV RNA levels of less than 1000 copies/mL. Third, resistance tests are no substitute for obtaining a thorough treatment history. Given the possibility of laboratory error, when a test result does not make sense in the context of a patient's treatment history, a repeat test or a test by an alternative technology may be warranted. Lastly, resistance testing is most reliable in detecting the presence or absence of resistance to drugs in the current failing regimen.

If resistance to a given drug is detected, it is reasonable to assume that further treatment with it is unlikely to be of significant benefit. In some cases, resistance testing may fail to detect resistance to drugs used in previous regimens. This is because, when treatment is interrupted, residual wild-type virus may overtake resistant virus and become the predominant species in the plasma within a matter of weeks. In this setting, resistant virus persists at a low but detectable level and may re-emerge if drugs to which the virus is resistant are used in a subsequent regimen. If resistance to a specific drug has ever been detected, it should not be reused in future regimens if possible. Thus, resistance testing is helpful in identifying drugs to be avoided, but the absence of apparent resistance to drugs used in the past does not guarantee their effectiveness.

Whether to use genotypic or phenotypic testing is a matter of convenience and cost. Genotypic testing is generally quicker and cheaper than phenotypic testing. It also may be more sensitive for detecting early evidence of drug resistance, particularly in the case of mixtures of wild-type and mutant virus. Although phenotypic testing is slower and more expensive, it is easier for most clinicians to interpret and may provide better data regarding cross-resistance within drug classes. Thus, genotypic testing may be sufficient in patients whose first or second regimen has failed, whereas phenotypic testing may be preferred in patients with numerous previous failed regimens.

Studies have shown that presence of ZDV resistance in maternal HIV-isolates reduces its efficacy in preventing perinatal transmission. Furthermore, because the risk of vertical transmission is related to maternal viral load, it is imperative that combination antiretroviral therapy be optimized in HIV-infected women who become pregnant. Resistance testing can play an important role in selecting an appropriate regimen in this setting.

The finding of drug resistance in the context of a rising plasma HIV RNA level is evidence that the regimen in question is no longer effective. Conversely, the complete absence of drug-resistance markers in a patient with a rising plasma HIV RNA level suggests poor adherence or inadequate potency of the regimen. In the case of poor adherence, factors such as toxicity or complexity of the regimen should be identified, and alternative agents should be considered.

Therapeutic Drug Monitoring

In general, a quantitative relationship exists between drug concentrations in blood or plasma and the therapeutic or toxic effect of the drug. This concentration-response relationship is used to define the range of concentrations at which the beneficial effect of a particular drug is maximized while its toxicities are minimized. Adjusting doses to maintain concentrations within a pre-established therapeutic range is commonly termed *therapeutic drug monitoring* (TDM) and should result in improved efficacy and less toxicity than simply prescribing a standard dose for all patients. This approach has been clearly useful for some drug classes, including antiarrhythmics, anticonvulsants, and aminoglycoside antibiotics.

Dose-response and concentration-response relationships exist for most antiretroviral drugs. What makes these relationships unique in the treatment of HIV infection is that combinations of drugs, all of which contribute to the response, are used therapeutically. Attention has focused on the role that inadequate plasma concentrations of PIs may play in treatment failure or resistance. Higher doses of PIs are associated with a more durable suppression of viral load, which would be expected to confer a lower probability of the emergence of drug-resistant virus. A considerable body of concentration-effect data is available for the NNRTIs and PIs. Some data are also available for the plasma concentrations of the nucleoside triphosphates. However, intracellular nucleoside triphosphate concentrations are much more difficult to measure, and concentration-response data have not been clearly established.

Application to Antiretroviral Drugs

Analytic, pharmacologic, and clinical criteria have been developed to help determine whether drugs in a particular therapeutic class are suitable for TDM. Analytic criteria include the availability of drug assays with high specificity and their ability to be performed on small sample volumes with reasonably rapid turnaround times. Pharmacologic criteria require that: 1) the drugs in question show significant interindividual pharmacokinetic variability; 2) adequate pharmacokinetic data are available; 3) a pharmacologic effect is proportional to the plasma drug concentration; 4) a narrow range exists between therapeutic and toxic drug concentrations; and 5) a constant pharmacologic effect exists over an extended period of time. The clinical criterion is whether studies have been performed defining therapeutic and toxic ranges of the drugs.

Analytic criteria have been met for most antiretroviral drugs. Sensitive and specific assays are available at reasonable cost for the PIs, NNRTIs, and NRTIs. Several of the pharmacologic criteria have been met as well. Substantial interpatient variability in achieved plasma concentrations is well documented for the PIs and NNRTIs. Defining the therapeutic range of these drugs has been difficult because of limitations in absorption and tolerability of some agents. It is likely that most drugs used in the treatment of HIV infection have a narrow range between the maximum tolerated dose and the systemic concentration required for durable viral suppression. Whether antiretroviral drugs exhibit a constant pharmacologic effect over an extended period of time depends on whether drug-resistant variants emerge.

Therapeutic ranges have not been established for all antiretroviral drugs, but concentration-response data are available for most of the PIs and NNRTIs. One issue is the uncertainty as to which pharmacokinetic parameter best defines the therapeutic and toxic exposures of the drugs. The lowest concentration of the drug (C_{min}) is monitored to determine efficacy primarily because it is the easiest to collect for both the patient and the investigator. Calculating an accurate area-under-the-curve (AUC) would require multiple phlebotomies over an extended period of time, which is unrealistic in a busy clinical setting. Both trough and peak (C_{max}) drug concentrations may provide useful information. However, correlation of the C_{min} with efficacy has not been prospectively validated for any of the antiretroviral drugs. The C_{max} of indinavir may approximate the risk of nephrotoxicity. Retrospective correlation of central nervous system toxicity with plasma concentrations of EFV has been attempted in a small group of subjects. Although this approach may be a suitable way to define a therapeutic drug range, prospective studies that validate these findings would strengthen the argument for TDM.

Because treatment of HIV infection requires the use of multiple drugs, monitoring only a single agent may not be appropriate under all circumstances. Both the efficacy and toxicity of PIs and NNRTIs may demonstrate synergy, antagonism, or additivity when combined with the various NRTIs. In addition, the presence of baseline minority drug-resistant mutations and the evolution of mutations over time can make establishing the concentration necessary for antiretroviral efficacy a moving target.

Clinical Utility

Prospective and retrospective studies have shown some clinical and virologic benefit of incorporating TDM into routine patient care. The first evidence that TDM could play a role in antiretroviral therapy management came from a randomized trial that compared concentration-controlled versus fixed-dose administration of ZDV monotherapy in treatment-naïve patients. Average ZDV intracellular triphosphate concentrations and CD4 cell count increases were significantly greater in patients assigned to the concentration-controlled dosing arm. Although ZDV is not currently used as monotherapy, data suggest that maintaining a targeted level of drug exposure and decreasing the variability of plasma concentrations may improve treatment response.

The importance of PI plasma concentrations was evaluated retrospectively in the Viradapt study, in which patients prospectively received genotypic-testing-guided therapy. Plasma concentrations of the PIs used in the study were measured serially over 12 months, and patients were categorized as those with "optimal" and "suboptimal" plasma PI concentrations. Patients with optimal PI concentrations had significantly greater reductions in plasma HIV-RNA levels. Multivariate analysis demonstrated that PI concentrations were an independent predictor. This study did not have medication adherence measures, and differences in adherence may have explained differences in plasma drug concentrations.

In a prospective TDM trial, patients were randomized to receive nelfinavir- or indinavir-based regimens, with or without TDM. Treatment failure was significantly more common in the non-TDM arms. Of note, control-arm patients who received nelfinavir were more likely to experience virologic failure, whereas those who received indinavir were more likely to show failure related to drug toxicity. These results suggest that TDM may be potentially helpful in the management of both efficacy and toxicity issues.

Another study evaluated concentration-controlled versus fixed-dose therapy with ZDV, 3TC, and indinavir in treatment-naïve patients. Dose changes in the concentration-controlled arm were implemented at week 4 based on intensive pharmacokinetic data collected at week 2. In the concentration-controlled dosing arm, dose adjustments were required in 44%, 31%, and 81% of patients receiving ZDV, 3TC, and indinavir, respectively. These patients were nearly twice as likely to have plasma HIV RNA levels of less than 50 copies/mL at 52 weeks compared with those in the fixed-dose arm. This study suggests that uniform dosing of antiretroviral drugs for HIV-infected patients may not be optimal.

One approach to integrating TDM and drug-resistance data involves calculating the C_{min}/IC_{50} ratio, also known as the inhibitory quotient (IQ). Intuitively, maintaining C_{min} above the IC_{50}, (e.g., an IQ significantly > 1) should increase the probability of producing a good virologic outcome. Retrospective analysis of treatment-experienced patients who received salvage therapy with indinavir/ritonavir showed that the IQ was a significant predictor of virologic response. Application of IQ to patient management is now being evaluated in randomized clinical trials.

Limitations

A number of factors may alter the concentration-response relationship of antiretroviral drugs, potentially confounding the interpretation of therapeutic levels. First, combinations of antiretroviral drugs can be synergistic, additive, or antagonistic. If synergy or additivity exists between classes of drugs, the concentration of each drug required to produce the half-maximum antiviral effect (EC_{50}) would decrease, and lower doses might produce the same effect when used in combination. Second, baseline plasma HIV RNA and CD4 count levels may affect concentration-response relationships. A third factor that alters these relationships is cross-resistance among drugs in the same class. As a result, higher plasma concentrations may be required to produce the desired antiviral effect. In many cases, concentrations higher than those safely achievable may be needed. A fourth factor is that variable adherence patterns may make establishing pharmacodynamic relationships difficult. Last, interlaboratory variability must be taken into account. A number of commercial diagnostic laboratories and academic institutions offer antiretroviral drug assays, but to date there are no cross-validation or quality-assurance/quality-control (QA/QC) programs to ensure their accuracy and reproducibility.

Recommendations

Until prospective randomized trials demonstrate the clinical utility of TDM, routine monitoring of antiretroviral drug levels cannot be recommended. Nevertheless, there are some situations in which clinicians may wish to consider TDM. For drugs with longer half-lives, such as EFV, NVP, and RTV-boosted PIs, TDM may be useful to assess adherence. A single sample drawn any time post-dose should be sufficient, and the result should be compared with known concentration-time data. However, plasma drug concentrations obtained during a clinic visit reflect only recent, not overall, adherence. In cases where malabsorption is suspected, obtaining a plasma level at the time of anticipated C_{max} can help establish this diagnosis.

TDM may also be useful in assessing drug interactions. For example, addition of a CYP 450 inducer, whether an antiretroviral agent or drug from another class, to a regimen can significantly alter plasma levels of the PIs. Measuring C_{min} at baseline and 7 to 14 days after addition of the new drug could help determine whether dosage adjustments are needed. Although pharmacologic enhancement of PIs by coadministration with RTV reduces interpatient variation in levels of the boosted PI, considerable variability remains. Determining the C_{min} of the boosted PI early in therapy might provide useful information regarding the adequacy of the regimen. Finally, certain drug-related toxicities, such as indinavir-induced nephrotoxicity, may be managed by cautious dose adjustment guided by TDM.

KEY POINTS

* Altered drug binding, improved enzyme efficiency, changes in the enzyme substrate, and nucleoside excision are some of the mechanisms by which mutations confer antiretroviral drug resistance. Most resistant mutations result in the production of a viral protein with reduced affinity for one or more drugs.
* Among NRTIs, mutations associated with thymidine analog resistance confer broad cross-resistance within the class; nonthymidine NRTIs select for mutations that lead to more limited cross-resistance.
* Viral fitness refers to the relative ability of two or more different isolates to replicate under particular conditions, while replication capacity refers to the amount of virus produced in a given period. The clinical utility of these tests is presently undefined.
* Drug-resistance testing can be used to determine the viral genotype or phenotype.
* Short-term clinical benefit for both genotypic and phenotypic drug-resistance testing has been demonstrated by prospective randomized trials, with stronger evidence for genotypic testing.
* Resistance testing is most useful for choosing an antiretroviral drug regimen for patients whose current therapy is failing. It is also recommended in pregnant women and in patients with newly diagnosed HIV infection.
* With therapeutic drug monitoring, doses are adjusted to maintain concentrations within a pre-established range. Monitoring antiretroviral therapy, however, is complicated by the fact that combinations of drugs, rather than a single agent, contribute to the observed treatment response.
* Although routine therapeutic drug monitoring is not recommended for patients receiving antiretroviral therapy because of the many factors that confound the interpretation of plasma levels, it may still be useful in certain clinical situations, such as assessing the significance of drug interactions.

SUGGESTED READINGS

Acosta EP, Kakuda TN, Brundage RC, Anderson PL, Fletcher CV. Pharmacodynamics of human immunodeficiency virus type 1 protease inhibitors. Clin Infect Dis. 2000;30(Suppl 2): S151-9.

Acosta EP, King JR. Methods for integration of pharmacokinetic and phenotypic information in the treatment of infection with human immunodeficiency virus. Clin Infect Dis. 2003;36:373-7.

Adult AIDS Clinical Trials Group 5055 Protocol Team. Comparison of two indinavir/ritonavir regimens in the treatment of HIV-infected individuals. J Acquir Immune Defic Syndr. 2004;37:1358-66.

Adult Pharmacology Committee of the AIDS Clinical Trials Group. Position paper on therapeutic drug monitoring of antiretroviral agents. AIDS Res Hum Retroviruses. 2002;18: 825-34.

Back D, Gatti G, Fletcher C, et al. Therapeutic drug monitoring in HIV infection: current status and future directions. AIDS. 2002;16(Suppl 1):S5–37.

Boffito M, Acosta E, Burger D, Fletcher CV, Flexner C, Garaffo R, et al. Current status and future prospects of therapeutic drug monitoring and applied clinical pharmacology in antiretroviral therapy. Antivir Ther. 2005;10:375-92.

Clavel F, Hance AJ. HIV drug resistance. N Engl J Med. 2004;350:1023-35.

Hirsch MS, Brun-Vézinet F, Clotet B, et al., and the International AIDS Society-USA Resistance Testing Guidelines Panel. Questions to and answers from the International AIDS Society-USA Resistance Testing Guidelines Panel. Top HIV Med. 2003;11:150-4.

Johnson VA, Brun-Vézinet F, Clotet B, et al. Update of the drug resistance mutations in HIV-1: Fall 2006. Top HIV Med. 2006;14:125-30.

Kappelhoff BS, Crommentuyn KM, de Maat MM, et al. Practical guidelines to interpret plasma concentrations of antiretroviral drugs. Clin Pharmacokinet. 2004;43:845–53.

King JR, Wynn H, Brundage R, Acosta EP. Pharmacokinetic enhancement of protease inhibitor therapy. Clin Pharmacokinet. 2004;43:291-310.

Morse GD, Catanzaro LM, Acosta EP. Clinical pharmacodynamics of HIV-1 protease inhibitors: use of inhibitory quotients to optimise pharmacotherapy. Lancet Infect Dis. 2006;6:215-25.

Plank R, Kuritzkes DR. An update on HIV-1 antiretroviral resistance. Curr Opinion HIV AIDS. 2006;1:417-23.

Chapter 6

Long-Term Treatment Complications

PATRICK W.G. MALLON, MBBCh, PhD
DAVID A. COOPER, MD, DSc
ANDREW CARR, MD

Although the introduction of combination antiretroviral therapy was a watershed event in the management of HIV disease, concern about long-term treatment complications has arisen over the past decade. These conditions include lipodystrophy, hepatic and renal toxicity, peripheral neuropathy, lactic acidemia and acidosis, and bone abnormalities. Although research has advanced our understanding of the pathogenetic mechanisms of these conditions, most appear to be multifactorial in origin. This chapter reviews the etiology, diagnosis, and management of long-term treatment complications associated with antiretroviral therapy.

Lipodystrophy

Description

Lipodystrophy describes a constellation of abnormalities of adipose tissue and lipid/glucose metabolism that develops in some HIV-infected patients on long-term antiretroviral therapy. Morphologic abnormalities include wasting of peripheral subcutaneous fat (face, limbs, and buttocks) and accumulation of central visceral fat (cervicodorsal region, breasts, and abdomen) (Box 6-1 and Figure 6-1). Discrete lipomata have also been described. Metabolic abnormalities include dyslipidemia, insulin resistance, diabetes mellitus, and lactic acidemia. The manifestations of lipodystrophy vary among patients and over time in individual patients.

The term "fat redistribution" has been used to describe the combined loss of peripheral fat and gain in central fat in patients with lipodystrophy. However, this term is inappropriate as it suggests that adipose tissue is "moved," when it is likely that these body fat changes reflect different pathological processes in two distinct tissue types.

Box 6-1. Features of Lipodystrophy

Lipoatrophy
- Loss of subcutaneous fat from face, arms, legs, buttocks

Central fat accumulation
- Visceral abdominal fat
- Breasts
- Neck
- Interscapular fat ("buffalo hump")

Dyslipidemia
- Increased total and LDL cholesterol
- Increased triglycerides (VLDL)
- Decreased HDL cholesterol

Insulin resistance
- Peripheral and hepatic insulin resistance
- Hyperinsulinemia
- Lipotoxicity (accumulation of lipids in nonadipose tissues)
- Type 2 diabetes mellitus

Lactic acidemia
- Anion gap metabolic acidosis
- May be symptomatic (fatigue, weight loss) or asymptomatic
- Associated with peripheral lipoatrophy
- Related to NRTI use

HDL = high density lipoprotein; LDL = low density lipoprotein; NRTI = nucleoside reverse-transcriptase inhibitor; VLDL = very low density lipoprotein.

Epidemiology and Natural History

The prevalence of lipodystrophy has ranged between 38% and 58% in study cohorts. This variability is likely the result of differences in the subjective criteria used to diagnose lipodystrophy, in treatment patterns and duration of exposure to antiretroviral therapy, and in the race, ethnicity, and gender of patients.

Prospective studies of patients initiating antiretroviral therapy have demonstrated that they gain lean mass (predominantly muscle) and fat (both centrally and peripherally) over the first 6 months, probably reflecting changing nutritional requirements and a reduction in the catabolic effects of HIV infection. Subsequently, patients experience a selective progressive loss of limb fat, which continues for at least 3 years (Figure 6-2). In a non-randomized prospective study, patients lost approximately 14% of their limb fat for every year of exposure to antiretroviral therapy after the first 6 months of treatment. In a randomized study, researchers reported the incidence of lipoatrophy to be 17% to 44% after 15 months. As with lipoatrophy, there is a wide variation in the severity of central fat-accumulation described in cohorts. There is also debate as to whether many

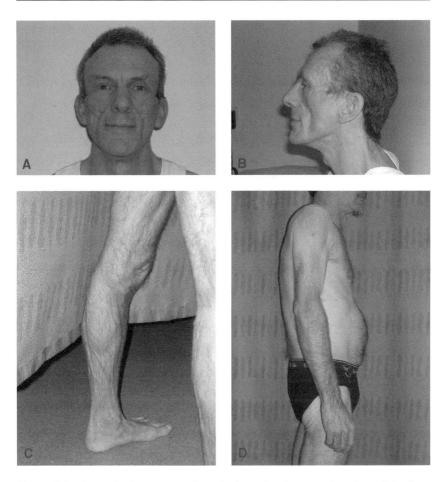

Figure 6-1.   Loss of adipose tissue from the buccal and temporal regions of the face. **A** and **B** are characteristics of lipodystrophy. Loss of fat from the limbs often leads to a striking muscular appearance, with protruding subcutaneous veins readily visible **(C).** Accumulation of adipose tissue in the abdominal region may also occur **(D)** with marked loss of adipose tissue over the gluteal region (note the skin folds).

cases of central fat accumulation are simply a result of the normal aging process made visibly worse by the loss of subcutaneous adipose tissue.

The prevalence and evolution of dyslipidemia, insulin resistance, and diabetes mellitus have been less well defined in this population, likely owing to the complexity of interactions between these metabolic derangements and specific drug exposures and changes in body composition. Studies in HIV-seronegative patients have demonstrated lipid abnormalities and altered insulin sensitivity to occur after only a few weeks of exposure to some antiretroviral drugs (Table 6-1).

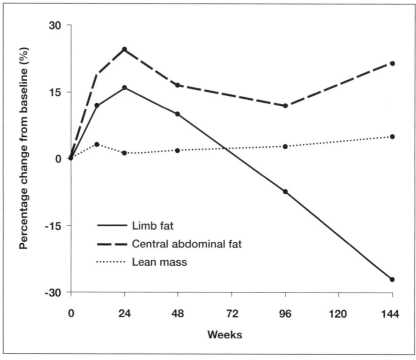

Figure 6-2. Changes in body composition observed in a cohort of patients initiating antiretroviral therapy for the first time (week 0). Body composition was measured by whole-body DEXA scanning. (Adapted with permission from Mallon P, et al. AIDS. 2003; 17:971-9.)

Risk Factors

Cross-sectional studies have identified several factors associated with development of lipodystrophy (Table 6-2). Prior or continuing protease inhibitor (PI) or nucleoside reverse-transcriptase inhibitor (NRTI) use and increased age are predictive. Less clear associations include male gender, pretreatment AIDS diagnosis, and greater CD4 cell count and viral load responses to antiretroviral therapy. Although lipodystrophy can develop in patients treated with PIs or NRTIs alone, the incidence is higher when these drug classes are used together. A prospective, randomized study identified a higher baseline CD4 cell count, higher baseline cholesterol and triglyceride concentrations, greater early changes in triglyceride concentrations, and NRTI used to be associated with subsequent development of lipoatrophy.

Cohort data show that factors such as gender, age, and baseline lipid values can alter the risk of developing lipodystrophy. The link between high baseline cholesterol and triglyceride values and lipoatrophy suggests a genetic component. Associations between morphologic and metabolic changes and certain genetic polymorphisms have been identified (Table 6-3). Studies

Table 6-1. Studies of Antiretroviral Toxicity in Healthy Volunteers

Drug (s)	Class	Duration of Exposure	N	Summary of Findings
Zidovudine/lamivudine Stavudine/lamivudine	NRTI	6 weeks	20	No change in cholesterol, triglycerides, insulin, glucose or body composition. Decreased mitochondrial RNA expression in subcutaneous adipose tissue at two weeks and peripheral blood monocytes at six weeks (Reference a).
Indinavir	PI	4 weeks	10	Increased fasting glucose, insulin and insulin resistance. No change in cholesterol, triglycerides or free fatty acids. No change in subcutaneous or visceral fat. Small decrease in total fat (Reference b).
Indinavir	PI	Single dose	6	Acute increase in insulin resistance (Reference c).
Ritonavir	PI	2 weeks	21	Increases in triglycerides, total and VLDL cholesterol and apolipoprotein B. Decreases in HDL cholesterol (Reference d).
Lopinavir/ritonavir	PI	4 weeks	10	Increased triglycerides, free fatty acids and VLDL cholesterol. No change in fasting glucose, insulin, total cholesterol or HDL cholesterol. Increased post-glucose tolerance test insulin and glucose (Reference e).
Atazanavir (ATV) Lopinavir/ritonavir (LPVr)	PI	5 days	30	LPVr induced more insulin resistance and higher triglycerides than ATV (Reference f).

HDL = high density lipoprotein; NRTI = nucleoside reverse-transcriptase inhibitor; PI = protease inhibitor; VLDL = very low density lipoprotein.
References: a. Mallon P, et al. J Infect Dis. 2005;191:1686-96. b. Noor M, et al. AIDS. 2001;15:11-18. c. Noor M, et al. AIDS. 2002;16:F1-F8. d. Purnell, et al. AIDS. 2000;14:51-7. e. Lee G, et al. AIDS. 2004;18:641-9. f. Noor M, et al. AIDS. 2004;18:2137-44.

Table 6-2. Factors Associated with Development of Lipodystrophy

Cohort	N	↑Age	Sex	PI Now	PI Duration	NRTI Now	NRTI Duration	NNRTI	CD4 Count	HIV RNA	AIDS Diagnosis	↑Lactate	↑Lipids	Insulin Resistance
Aquitaine	581	LA	LA	ns	+	ns	+	ns	−	−	+	ns	+	+
Australia	1348	+	LA	+	+	+	+	−	−	+	+	−	+	+
HOPS	1077	+	−	IDV	IDV	d4T	d4T	−	nadir	+	+	ns	+	ns
Italian	2250	−	−	+	+	+	+	−	−	+	−	+	ns	ns
Sydney	221	−	ns	+	+	+	+	−	−	−	−	+	+	+
Spanish	494	+	♀	−	−	−	−	−	+	+	−	ns	+	−
German	115	+	♂	LH	ns	+	ns	ns	−	+	ns	ns	LH	ns
French	685	+	−	+	+	d4T	ns	−	−	+	+	ns	+	ns
Swiss	1480	−	ns	+	+	+	+	−	ns	−	−	+	+	ns

'+' = associated with development of lipodystrophy; '−' = not associated with development of lipodystrophy; ns = not studied; d4T = stavudine; IDV = indinavir; LA = associated with development of predominant lipoatrophy; LH = associated with development of predominant lipohypertrophy; NNRTI = non-nucleoside reverse-transcriptase inhibitor; NRTI = nucleoside reverse-transcriptase inhibitor; PI = protease inhibitor; PI/NRTI "duration" = total length of exposure to stated class of drug; PI/NRTI "now" = subject on PI/NRTI-containing regimen at time of study.

Table 6-3. Pharmacogenomics and Lipodystrophy

Gene (s)	Polymorphism(s)/ Alleles	N	Percent Male	Region	Race/ Ethnicity	Summary of Findings
APOC3	455T/C 482C/T Intron 1 C/G SstI	626	89%	N. America	63% White 19% Black 18% Hispanic	Racial/ethnic differences in severity of dyslipidemia; Variant alleles protective against PI-induced dyslipidemia in Hispanic group
APOC3	455T/C 482C/T SstI	60	100%	Europe	—	All three polymorphisms positively associated with triglyceride concentrations
APOC3 APOE	455T/C 482C/T SstI ε2, ε4 alleles	329	79.3%	Europe	88% White 7% Black 3% Hispanic	High triglycerides with ritonavir treatment in individuals with APOC3 and APOE variants
SREBP1	322C/G	355	80%	International	57% White 25% Black 13% Hispanic	Presence of polymorphism not predictive of hyperlipidemia
SREBP1	322C/G	71	—	Europe	—	Less antiretroviral-associated increase in total cholesterol in patients with 322C/G
TNF-α	238G/A	191	100%	Australasia	100% White	Increased risk of progression to lipodystrophy in heterozygotes
TNF-α	238G/A	96	89%	Europe	100% White	Higher frequency of 238G/A polymorphism in patients with lipodystrophy
TNF-α	238G/A	329	79.3%	Europe	88% White 7% Black 3% Hispanic	No effect of TNFα polymorphism on development of lipoatrophy

show the prevalence and severity of dyslipidemia, particularly changes in the triglyceride level, to be affected by race, ethnicity, and the presence of polymorphisms or groups of polymorphisms in the gene for apolipoprotein C-III (apoC-III).

Pathogenesis

Lipodystrophy has a multifactorial etiology, with treatment variability, patient characteristics, and disease factors all contributing to its manifestations. However, current research points to antiretroviral therapy, specifically the use of certain PIs and NRTIs, as being the principal driving force behind the development of this syndrome. Although these drug classes, when used in combination, have a synergistic effect on the development of lipodystrophy, PIs have been most closely associated with dyslipidemia and insulin resistance, while NRTIs, particularly zidovudine (ZDV) and stavudine (d4T), have been implicated in the development of lipoatrophy and lactic acidemia.

The phenotype of lipodystrophy results from long-term disturbances in the metabolism of lipids and glucose. The handling of dietary fats and glucose by the body involves skeletal muscle, liver, and central and peripheral adipose tissue. Normal glucose and lipid metabolism relies on complex homeostatic relationships of dietary, hormonal, and organ/tissue factors. In patients with lipodystrophy, there is an overall disruption of these relationships, eventually giving rise to the spectrum of clinical abnormalities.

Lipoatrophy

Antiretroviral drug-induced insults to adipocyte function at the molecular level and the body's responses to them play important roles in the pathogenesis of lipoatrophy. Although PIs and NRTIs affect different metabolic pathways in adipocytes, they both decrease expression of the peroxisome proliferator-activated receptor gamma (PPAR-gamma), a nuclear receptor and transcription factor central to the transcription of lipid metabolism genes.

In vitro, PIs affect the expression of the transcription factor sterol regulatory element-binding protein-1 (SREBP-1). This sterol-responsive factor normally translocates to the nucleus, where it increases the expression of lipid metabolism genes. Localization of SREBP-1 to the nucleus is blocked by PIs, resulting in down-regulation of PPAR-gamma, decreased differentiation of adipocytes, and less accumulation of intracellular lipid.

NRTIs, particularly ZDV and d4T, cause depletion of mitochondria in adipocytes. Measurement of mitochondrial DNA (mtDNA) is commonly used as a surrogate marker of the number of mitochondria in a cell. In vitro, NRTIs inhibit the enzyme DNA polymerase-gamma (DNA pol-gamma) and also cause downregulation of mitochondrial RNA (mtRNA) expression. DNA pol-gamma and mtRNA are essential for the normal replication of mitochondria, and both are inhibited by NRTIs, leading to mtDNA depletion. Importantly, inhibition of mtRNA expression by NRTIs is accompanied by downregulation of PPAR-gamma, which helps explain not only how NRTI-induced mitochondrial dysfunction results in adipose tissue dysfunction but also the synergistic effects of NRTIs and PIs in the development of lipoatrophy.

Adipocyte toxicity induced by PIs and NRTIs results in cellular dysfunction and, in the case of mitochondrial toxicity, decreased oxidative capacity with the potential for increased free radical activity leading to cellular damage. Several studies of patients with lipodystrophy have shown infiltration of adipose tissue by macrophages, which is thought to be a response to this cellular damage. Subsequent release of powerful pro-inflammatory cytokines, such as tumor necrosis factor alpha (TNF-alpha), interferon gamma (IFN-gamma), and interleukin-6 (IL-6), by infiltrating macrophages may lead to additional loss of adipocytes and accelerate lipoatrophy. A similar cytokine-driven process is thought to underlie the loss of fat and lean mass observed in patients with advanced HIV disease suffering from "wasting syndrome."

Central Fat Accumulation
In contrast to subcutaneous fat, which is made up of predominantly "white fat," central fat is composed of "brown fat." White and brown fat are distinct tissues with very different functions, which may explain why antiretroviral therapy exposure leads to selective loss of white, but not brown, fat. White fat acts primarily as a storage tissue, whereas brown fat is involved in the generation of heat.

It is unlikely that age-related changes in body morphology are responsible for all cases of lipodystrophy-associated fat accumulation. An alternative explanation is that central adiposity occurs as part of a compensatory process for lipoatrophy, in which excess circulating lipids and glucose, which would normally be stored in peripheral adipose tissue, are taken up by other tissues. Development of a "buffalo hump," a manifestation of central fat accumulation associated with increased insulin resistance, is much more prevalent in HIV-infected patients with lipodystrophy than in the general adult population.

Dyslipidemia
The pathogenesis of dyslipidemia is complex, with HIV infection, antiretroviral drugs (particularly PIs), diet, and genetic factors all contributing to its development.

Studies in antiretroviral drug-naïve patients and recent seroconverters have shown that HIV infection itself can cause decreases in HDL cholesterol, total cholesterol, and triglyceride levels. The exact mechanism is unclear, although the decrease in HDL cholesterol may reflect disruption of reverse cholesterol transport in circulating monocytes and tissue macrophages. In vitro studies have shown that PIs affect expression of

molecules, such as CD36, which play an important role in reverse cholesterol transport and HDL cholesterol production.

Increased cholesterol and triglyceride levels are commonly seen in patients treated with ritonavir, which is used in small doses to pharmacologi-
cally "boost" the levels of other PIs. These changes can occur early in
therapy, predating any changes in body composition. Short-term treatment
of HIV-seronegative volunteers with ritonavir and lopinavir increased triglyceride levels after only a few weeks (see Table 6-1). This drug effect is
thought to involve disruption in hepatic lipoprotein production. In vitro,
hepatoma cells exposed to PIs produce excess apolipoprotein B (apoB)-
containing lipoproteins. This effect is possibly a consequence of reduced
metabolism of apoB particles resulting from PI-induced inhibition of the cellular proteasome, an intracellular complex of proteases that rapidly degrades
many proteins. Levels of apoC-III, which forms an important component of
triglyceride-rich lipoproteins, are also increased with exposure to PIs.

Once changes in body composition are established, increased cholesterol and triglyceride levels can be exacerbated by decreased clearance of
excess lipoproteins from the circulation. Subcutaneous adipose tissue normally acts as a buffer for dietary lipids. With the onset of lipoatrophy, there
is less available storage for circulating lipids.

Insulin Resistance

Insulin sensitivity is affected directly by some PIs (see Table 6-1) and indirectly
by disturbances in lipid metabolism and adipose tissue induced by PIs and
NRTIs. In HIV-seronegative volunteers, short-term exposure to indinavir and
lopinavir increases peripheral insulin resistance. This drug effect is thought to
be mediated through inhibition of the insulin-regulated glucose transporter,
GLUT-4, a molecule involved in insulin-mediated glucose uptake by cells.

As mentioned above, subcutaneous fat is a storage tissue for dietary
lipids and glucose. The onset of lipoatrophy removes this potential site,
leading to accumulation of excess lipids in other tissues and organs. Over
time, this accumulation of lipids results in insulin resistance. Studies in HIV-
infected patients have demonstrated close correlations between skeletal
muscle intracellular lipid content, lipoatrophy, and insulin resistance.

Subcutaneous adipose tissue secretes the hormones leptin and
adiponectin, both of which are involved in the regulation of insulin sensitivity. Lipoatrophic patients have low leptin levels. The importance of leptin and adiponectin levels in the development of insulin resistance in
patients with lipodystrophy has yet to be determined. However, in congenital lipodystrophies, leptin infusions improve insulin sensitivity.

Lactic Acidemia

Lipodystrophy has been reported in patients treated with NRTIs alone. In
such cases, lipoatrophy predominates in conjunction with lactic acidemia,
reflecting disruption of intracellular oxidative capacity from NRTI-induced
mitochondrial dysfunction.

Atherosclerotic Disease

With dyslipidemia, insulin resistance, and central fat accumulation being common manifestations of lipodystrophy, a principal concern is that patients on long-term antiretroviral therapy will experience increased morbidity from premature coronary artery and cerebrovascular disease. In addition, factors such as increased oxidative stress, cytokine production associated with HIV infection, increased blood pressure, and cigarette smoking among many cohorts of patients have the potential to contribute independently to accelerated atherosclerosis.

More light has been shed on this topic by the Data Collection of Adverse Events of Anti-HIV Drugs (DAD) study. This international multicenter cohort, which began in 1999, included approximately 23,500 HIV-infected patients. Its purpose was to monitor the number of cases and determine factors associated with acute myocardial infarction (AMI). More than 24% of those enrolled were female, and 56% were smokers. Initial results, published in 2003, showed an increased risk of AMI in HIV-infected patients who had traditional cardiovascular risk factors, such as older age, male gender, and a positive family history of coronary artery disease. Treatment with antiretroviral therapy was also associated with an increased risk of AMI, an effect which persisted when corrected for the above risk factors. Analysis suggested that some but not all of this risk was attributed to drug-induced dyslipidemia. While initial results could not determine the effect of individual drugs or drug classes on the risk of AMI, follow-up analysis has suggested that PIs are mainly responsible. Overall, the risk of AMI increased 17% per year during the first 4 to 6 years of antiretroviral therapy. While of concern, these data need to be considered in the context of the overall risks and benefits of treating HIV infection. The total mortality rate in the DAD study was 2%, with the death rate from AMI being only 0.13% compared with an annual mortality rate of 20% observed in HIV-infected populations prior to the advent of combination antiretroviral therapy.

In addition to atherosclerotic disease, other complications may arise as a result of the metabolic derangements of lipodystrophy. Severe hyperlipidemia is an independent risk factor for pancreatitis and central retinal vessel occlusion. Carpal tunnel syndrome is associated with diabetes mellitus and obesity and has been reported in patients treated with PIs.

Evaluation

Diagnosis and monitoring of lipodystrophy involves both subjective and objective measures. It is important to ask patients about changes in their physical appearance. However, subjective assessment by patients and physicians is sometimes discordant. Anthropometric measurements (e.g., waist-to-hip ratio) have been used clinically but provide low predictive value.

Several radiologic techniques have been used to assess body composition. Whole-body dual-energy x-ray absorptiometry (DEXA) scanning provides a weight-based assessment of total and regional body fat and lean mass. It can also be used to estimate bone mineral density. Although DEXA scanning accurately measures changes in limb, trunk, and abdominal fat, it has limited ability to differentiate subcutaneous from visceral fat, and it cannot measure fat deposition in the face (Figure 6-3, *A*).

Imaging technologies such as computed topography (CT) and magnetic resonance imaging (MRI) have also been used to measure specific body regions (Figure 6-3, *B*). Cross-sectional images of the central abdomen are performed using the lumbar vertebral bodies as anatomical landmarks.

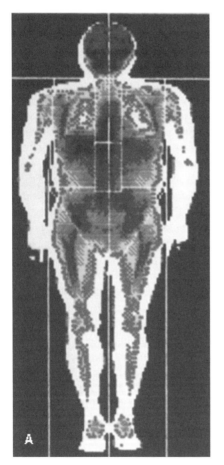
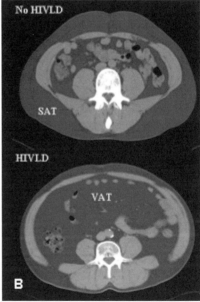

Figure 6-3. Techniques used to measure body composition include whole-body DEXA scanning **(A)** and cross-sectional computed tomography (CT) scanning of the abdomen **(B),** from which measurements of subcutaneous adipose tissue (SAT) and visceral adipose tissue (VAT) are made. **B** shows CT scans from two patients, one with and one without lipodystrophy. The patient with lipodystrophy has increased VAT and decreased SAT compared with the patient without lipodystrophy. (From Grinspoon S, Carr A. N Engl J Med. 2005;352:48-62; with permission. Copyright © 2005 Massachusetts Medical Society. All rights reserved.)

From these images, areas of subcutaneous and visceral adipose tissue can be measured, an average value can be calculated, and the ratio of visceral to subcutaneous fat (VAT:SAT) can be determined. Newer scanning technologies, including spiral CT and MRI, both of which can produce three-dimensional images of a body region, may be even more accurate and able to measure subtle changes in facial fat.

Assessment of metabolic abnormalities includes the measurement of fasting total cholesterol, HDL cholesterol, triglyceride, and glucose levels. If necessary for clinical purposes, insulin resistance can also be calculated from fasting glucose and insulin levels.

Using a combination of objective measures, a standardized case definition for lipodystrophy with a high degree of sensitivity and specificity has been developed (Table 6-4). This model has been adjusted for clinical settings in which imaging modalities are not available.

Management

Many therapeutic interventions have been used in the management of lipodystrophy with varying degrees of success. However, no single approach has been found to reverse the syndrome once it has become established. The major interventions and their outcomes are listed in Table 6-5. Nonpharmacologic interventions, including improved diet, increased exercise, and smoking cessation remain important components of care.

Therapeutic strategies to manage metabolic abnormalities in the general population appear to be less effective in the setting of lipodystrophy. Several factors may explain this finding. First, the presence of continued antiretroviral therapy may render conventional treatments less potent. An example is rosiglitazone of the thiazolidinedione class, which acts as a PPAR-gamma agonist. HIV-seronegative patients exposed to this drug respond with an increase in limb fat and improved insulin sensitivity. When

Table 6-4.   Lipodystrophy Case Definition

Body Composition	Metabolic Parameters	Patient Demographic Factors
• VAT:SAT ratio (CT)	• HDL cholesterol	• Gender
• Trunk fat: limb fat ratio (DEXA)	• Anion gap	• Age
• Leg fat percentage (DEXA)		• Duration of HIV infection
• Waist:hip ratio		• CDC category

Score attributed to each measurement; 79% sensitivity and 80% specificity for the presence of lipodystrophy. CDC = Centers for Disease Control and Prevention; CT = computed tomography; DEXA = dual-energy x-ray absorptiometry; HDL = high density lipoprotein; SAT = subcutaneous adipose tissue; VAT = visceral adipose tissue. (From Carr A, Emery S, Law M, et al. An objective case definition of lipodystrophy in HIV-infected adults: a case-control study. Lancet. 2003;361:726-35; with permission.)

Table 6-5.   Management Interventions for Lipodystrophy

Intervention	Peripheral Fat	Central Fat	Triglycerides	Cholesterol	Insulin Resistance	Lactate	Risk	Current Use	Q
Diet & exercise	→	→	No Δ	↓ LDL ↓ HDL	→	No Δ likely	↑ lipoatrophy	VAT accumulation	III
Switch PI to NNRTI/abacavir	No Δ or ↓	→	→	↓ LDL ↑ HDL	No Δ or ↓	No Δ likely	Virologic failure New toxicities	Hyperlipidemia	I
Switch PI to NNRTI	No Δ	No data	→	↓ LDL ↑ HDL	No Δ	No data	Virologic failure	Research	II
Switch tNRTI	↑	No Δ	No Δ / →	No Δ	Unclear	No Δ / →	Virologic failure New toxicities	Research	I/II
Metformin	→	→	No Δ	No Δ	→	No Δ	↑ lipoatrophy	Diabetes mellitus VAT accumulation	I
Glitazones	No Δ	No Δ	↑	↑	→	No Δ	Increased transasminases	Insulin resistance Hyperlipidemia	I
Fibrates	No Δ likely	No Δ likely	↓ ψ	No Δ	No Δ	No Δ likely	None	Hypertriglyceridemia	I
Statins	↑	No Δ	No Δ / →	↓ ψ	No Δ	No Δ likely	P450 interaction	Hypercholesterolemia	I/II
Growth hormone	No Δ	→	No Δ	→	↑	No data	Lipoatrophy	Research Hyperglycemia	I
GHRH	No Δ	→	No Δ	No Δ	No Δ	No data	New toxicities	Research	I
Localized injection*/ plastic surgery	Improved facial appearance	Transient ↓ buffalo hump	No Δ	No Δ	No Δ	No Δ likely	Surgical risk	Facial lipoatrophy Buffalo hump	II

*For example, polylactic acid, calcium hydroxylapatite.

Q = quality of evidence: I = evidence from at least one randomized controlled trial; II = evidence from at least one randomized trial, dramatic results from uncontrolled trial, or cohort or case control trial; III = evidence from respected authorities or expert committee reports. ψ = values did not return to normal in the majority of cases; HDL = high density lipoprotein; LDL = low density lipoprotein; Δ = change; NRTI = nucleoside reverse-transcriptase inhibitor; tNRTI = thymidine analog NRTI; PI = protease inhibitor; NNRTI = non-nucleoside reverse-transcriptase inhibitor; P450 = hepatic cytochrome P450 enzyme system; GHRH = growth hormone releasing hormone.

used in HIV-infected patients on antiretroviral therapy, the drug improves insulin sensitivity but does not increase limb fat. Analysis of subcutaneous fat shows that rosiglitazone fails to stimulate PPAR-gamma expression in patients on NRTIs. Second, certain therapeutic agents improve some aspects of lipodystrophy while making other features worse. Examples include metformin and recombinant human growth hormone. Metformin improves insulin resistance but exacerbates lipoatrophy. Growth hormone, although reducing visceral fat accumulation, may worsen insulin resistance, an effect thought to be related to excess insulin-like growth factor 1 (IGF-1). Use of a synthetic growth hormone releasing hormone (GHRH) seems to be effective in reducing central obesity without the unwanted effects of excess IGF-1. Lastly, because many drugs are metabolized by similar pathways, care needs to be taken when using interventional strategies in the presence of antiretroviral therapy. Statins and PIs are metabolized through the cytochrome P450 3A4 enzyme complex, resulting in altered concentrations of both drug classes. Pravastatin, which is less reliant on CYP3A4 metabolism, is generally preferred in HIV-infected patients.

Encouraging results have arisen from a pilot study of supplementation with the nucleoside uridine. In a group of patients with lipodystrophy on antiretroviral therapy containing NRTIs, uridine supplementation for 3 months resulted in an increase of approximately 900mg in limb fat compared to placebo. However, it also decreased HDL cholesterol levels, which may adversely affect cardiovascular risk.

Switch strategies—that is, changing antiretroviral drugs suspected of contributing to lipodystrophy to ones with more metabolically friendly profiles—have been extensively investigated. Studies have involved switching from PI- to non-PI-based regimens to treat metabolic derangements and from NRTI-based to NRTI-sparing regimens to improve lipoatrophy. Overall, this strategy results in some improvement in metabolic and morphologic abnormalities, but, in regard to lipoatrophy, the change is very gradual and often incomplete.

An important initial step in managing hyperlipidemia is an assessment of the effect of all contributing factors on the patient's cardiovascular risk. For example, a 50% rise in cholesterol concentration may not have a significant impact on cardiovascular risk in a 30-year-old nonsmoking female. In contrast, in a 55-year-old, hypertensive male smoker, it would be important. Decisions on the use of therapeutic interventions for hyperlipidemia should be based on the patient's cardiovascular risk, the likely reduction in risk achievable with the intervention, and its associated risk.

There are several methods of calculating cardiovascular risk, using parameters such as age, cholesterol concentration, blood pressure, and smoking status. Examples of online risk calculators are listed at the end of this chapter. A guide to the assessment and treatment of hypercholesterolemia is contained in the third report of the National Cholesterol Education Program (NCEP), which offers target cholesterol concentrations depending on cardiovascular risk (Table 6-6).

Table 6-6.   Treatment of Hypercholesterolemia**

Risk Category	Baseline LDL Level	Decision to Use Lipid-Lowering Drug Therapy	Target LDL (mg/dL)
CHD or risk equivalent (10-year risk >20%)	≥130 <130	Yes Consider	<100
Multiple (≥2) risk factors (10-year risk ≤20%)	≥160 ≥130	Consider if 10-year risk <10% Consider if 10-year risk 10–20%	<130
0-1 risk factors (10-year risk <10%)		Consider if LDL ≥190 mg/dL	<160

*Summary of the Third National Cholesterol Education Program Report.
CHD = coronary heart disease; CHD risk equivalent is met when 10-year risk of CHD exceeds 20% or patient is diagnosed with diabetes mellitus. LDL = low density lipoprotein cholesterol.

Hepatotoxicity

Hepatotoxicity results in considerable morbidity and mortality, and management of this condition in HIV-infected patients has become increasingly important. Both disease and treatment-associated factors contribute to liver dysfunction in this setting (Box 6-2). Important disease-associated factors include coinfection with hepatitis B virus (HBV) or hepatitis C virus (HCV) and immune reconstitution disease. As for treatment-associated factors, all antiretroviral drugs and many other therapies have the potential for hepatotoxicity. The management of HBV and HCV infections in the context of HIV disease is discussed in Chapter 9.

Antiretroviral drug-related hepatotoxicity can be classified as early (1 to 6 weeks of starting therapy) or later (beyond 6 weeks) (Table 6-7). Early hepatotoxicity can occur either as a result of hypersensitivity to a drug or as a component of immune reconstitution disease. Hypersensitivity hepatotoxicity has been described with the use of several antiretroviral drugs, most notably nevirapine (NVP), a non-nucleoside reverse-transcriptase inhibitor (NNRTI). Depending on the group studied, between 6% and 17% of patients treated with NVP experience some evidence of hepatitis. The majority of cases are asymptomatic and resolve with continued treatment, although women with a low body mass index and CD4 count >250 cells/mm^3 may be at increased risk of severe hepatic damage if NVP is used as part of an initial antiretroviral regimen.

Box 6-2.   Factors Associated with Hepatotoxocity

Alcohol and substance abuse

Viral hepatitis co-infection (especially hepatitis B or C)

Opportunistic infections (CMV infection, MAC, varicella-zoster, tuberculosis)

Malignancy (lymphoma, metastatic carcinoma)

Immune reconstitution syndrome

Drug toxicity:

☐ ART
  • Hepatitis
  • Drug hypersensitivity
  • Lactic acidosis / acidemia

☐ Mycobacterial therapy
  • Necrosis and cholestasis

☐ Antifungal therapy (azoles)
  • Hepatitis and cholestasis

ART = antiretroviral therapy; CMV = cytomegalovirus; MAC = *Mycobacterium avium* complex.

Table 6-7. Mechanisms of Hepatic Dysfunction with Antiretroviral Therapy

	Lactic Acidemia	Hypersensitivity	Isolated Hepatitis	Immune Reconstitution
Antiretroviral class	NRTIs	NRTIs, abacavir	NNRTIs and PIs	All classes
Drug(s)	Stavudine, didanosine	Nevirapine	Ritonavir, nevirapine	Any
Onset	Late	Early	Early/late	Early
Risk factors (possible in italics)	*NRTI duration* / *Pregnancy* / *HCV treatment (ribavirin)*	*Female* / *HLA B57*01*	HCV/HBV coinfection / ↑ ALT pre-therapy	Pre-ART CD4+ <100 cells/μL or pre-ART OI / HCV/HBV co-infection
Clinical features:				
Fever	No	Common	Occasional	Yes
Jaundice	No	Occasional	Occasional	Common
Dyspnea	Common	No	No	No
Rash	No	Common	No	No
Fulminant hepatic failure*	Occasional	1%–2%	Unknown	Relatively common
Chronic liver failure	Rare	Not described	2° to HCV/HBV	Not described
Laboratory features:				
ALT >10 × ULN	Rare	Common	Common	Common
Lactate >2 mmol/L	Yes	No	No	No
Therapy	Cease NRTIs if lactate >5 mmol/L or symptomatic	Cease NNRTI if symptomatic	Cease drugs; treat HBV/HCV	Cease ARVs until underlying OI treated
Prognosis	Mortality 80% if lactate >10 mmol/L	Good	Good	Good if OI treated effectively

* Features of acute liver failure are peripheral edema, ascites, encephalopathy, hypoalbuminemia, and prolonged clotting times.
ALT = alanine aminotransferase; ART = antiretroviral therapy; HBV = hepatitis B virus infection; HCV = hepatitis C virus infection; NNRTI = non-nucleoside reverse-transcriptase inhibitor; NRTI = nucleoside reverse-transcriptase inhibitor; OI = opportunistic infection; PI = protease inhibitor; ULN = upper limit of normal.

Immune reconstitution disease can result in episodes of symptomatic hepatitis from pre-existing subclinical infections with HBV, HCV, cytomegalovirus (CMV), or *Mycobacterium avium complex* (MAC), especially in patients with advanced HIV disease who were recently started on antiretroviral therapy. Hepatitis from immune reconstitution disease can sometimes be severe, but it is usually self-limited.

Late hepatotoxicity is more commonly associated with long-term exposure to antiretroviral drugs than immune-related effects. The predominant histopathologic lesions are steatosis and cirrhosis rather than hepatitis. ZDV, d4T, and some PIs have been associated with late hepatotoxicity. NRTIs are thought to affect liver function through mitochondrial toxicity, which leads to hepatic steatosis. PI-induced hyperlipidemia and insulin resistance can also result in hepatic steatosis. Although late hepatotoxicity is often reversible, liver failure and death have been reported, in some cases, several years after drug cessation.

HIV/HCV coinfection is increasing worldwide, especially in parts of Asia and eastern Europe, and is associated with a higher risk of drug-related hepatotoxicity. Treatment of HIV and HCV concurrently can be complicated from both drug and infection burdens on the liver.

In patients coinfected with HBV, antiretroviral therapy with drugs active against HBV, such as the NRTIs 3TC, emtracitabine (FTC), or tenofovir (TDF), can provide added benefit. It is currently recommended that treatment of HIV/HBV coinfected patients should include TDF along with either 3TC or FTC. Rebound hepatitis has been reported in HIV/HBV coinfected patients in whom an NRTI with HBV activity was withdrawn.

Management of hepatotoxicity in the setting of HIV infection should include 1) cessation of the responsible drugs when necessary, 2) treatment of concurrent viral hepatitis, 3) immunizations against hepatitis A virus and HBV in seronegative patients, and 4) avoidance of alcohol.

Renal Toxicity

Of recent interest has been the association between TDF, a nucleotide reverse-transcriptase inhibitor, and renal dysfunction. TDF undergoes renal excretion through glomerular filtration and active tubular excretion. Although prospective data have failed to show a consistent relationship between TDF use and renal failure, there are numerous case reports of a Fanconi-like syndrome (proximal tubular dysfunction) in HIV-infected patients treated with the drug. However, in the largest published randomized study, one which compared TDF with d4T with a background of EFV and 3TC, several renal parameters, including serum creatinine, calculated creatinine clearance (CCrCl), and rates of renal failure, did not change significantly over 144 weeks of follow-up. Another study identified subtle but statistically significant differences in CCrCl and anion gap in patients on

TDF-containing antiretroviral therapy compared with those on non-TDF-containing regimens. In most case reports, renal dysfunction associated with TDF occurred in the context of pre-existing kidney disease and improved upon withdrawal of the drug. Avoiding TDF in this setting and careful monitoring of renal function in patients on TDF are recommended.

Peripheral Neuropathy

Distal sensory polyneuropathy (DSP) is a common medium- to long-term toxicity of antiretroviral treatment. It can result in pain, reduced mobility, and psychological sequelae. DSP has been mainly described in patients treated with NRTIs, specifically ddI, d4T, and zalcitabine (ddC). In phase I trials of ddI and d4T, peripheral neuropathy was reported in 12% to 21% of patients. The first symptom is usually a distal symmetrical paraesthesia of the extremities associated with pain and numbness, which can be reversed if the antiretroviral drugs are stopped promptly. However, if continued, the process may become severe and permanent.

Risk factors for DSP include a low baseline CD4 cell count, high baseline HIV RNA, longer exposure to NRTIs, and regimens containing a greater number of drugs. The neuropathy is likely the result of NRTI-induced mitochondrial toxicity in peripheral nerves superimposed upon the direct cytotoxic effect of HIV. Histopathology of nerves from affected patients has revealed axonal degeneration with more than half the mitochondria exhibiting abnormal size and structure. Decreased levels of mitochondrial DNA within peripheral neurons have also been demonstrated.

Management of DSP has proven difficult. In cases of chronic DSP, many therapies have been tested, but few have shown conclusive benefit (Table 6-8). Drugs used to treat DSP include anticonvulsants, such as lamotrigine and gabapentin, and acetyl-l-carnitine, which promotes nerve regeneration. Management of chronic severe pain should be individualized, with involvement of a pain specialist as warranted.

Lactic Acidemia and Acidosis

In addition to inhibition of viral reverse transcriptase, use of NRTIs, particularly the synthetic thymidine analogs, is thought to result in inhibition of mitochondrial DNA pol-gamma. In vivo studies demonstrating decreased mtDNA content of tissues exposed to NRTIs support this hypothesis. Decreased mitochondrial function leads to disruption of intracellular oxidative capacity, which causes the cell to revert to anaerobic metabolism, the end product of which is lactate.

Table 6-8. Treatment of Distal Sensory Polyneuropathy

Intervention	N	Outcome	Limitations	Q
Lamotrigine	227	Faster rate of improvement in pain score with lamotrigine	Rash Improvement only in those on neurotoxic ART	I
Lidocaine gel	64	No Δ from placebo		I
Gabapentin	26	Improvements in pain score	Somnolence (reported in 80%)	II
Acetyl-l-carnitine	21	Nerve regeneration on biopsy	Improvements in grade of neuropathy	I
Nerve growth factor	270	Improvement in symptoms	Injection 39% unblinded due to injection site pain	I
Amytriptyline	145	No Δ from placebo	—	I
Mexiletine	145, 22	No Δ from placebo	Adverse effects in 39%	I
Acupuncture and/or amitriptyline	250	No Δ from placebo	—	I
Nimodipine	41	Trend towards improvement	No significant Δ from placebo	I
Peptide T	81	No Δ from placebo	—	I

Δ = change; ART = antiretroviral therapy; RCT = randomized controlled trial; Q = quality of evidence: I = evidence from at least one randomised controlled trial; II = evidence from at least one randomised trial, dramatic results from uncontrolled trial, or cohort or case control trial.

Hyperlactatemia (> 2 mmol/L) can be been classified as asymptomatic lactic acidemia, symptomatic lactic acidemia, and lactic acidosis. Lactic acidosis describes the condition where accumulation of serum lactate (generally > 5 mmol/L) leads to an uncompensated metabolic acidosis. Patients with mild-to-moderate lactic acidemia complain of fatigue, anorexia, weight loss, gastrointestinal symptoms, and often have liver function test abnormalities. Patients with lactic acidosis may present with a sepsis-like syndrome, myopathy, and/or peripheral neuropathy. Once metabolic decompensation occurs, widespread end-organ damage rapidly follows and is associated with high mortality.

Lactic acidemia is diagnosed by demonstration of a high venous lactate level associated with an increased anion gap. Falsely high lactate levels can occur through inappropriate sample collection and delay in sample transport to the laboratory. Therefore, it is appropriate to repeat the test when a high reading is obtained. If lactic acidosis is suspected, all antiretroviral drugs should be discontinued immediately. Mild-to-moderate lactic acidemia may permit continuation of drug therapy with modification of the regimen. Management of metabolic acidosis and organ failure generally requires hospitalization in an intensive care setting.

The usefulness of obtaining a serum lactate level in asymptomatic patients treated with NRTIs remains controversial. The incidence of chronic stable hyperlactatemia is relatively high ($>8\%$) in patients on ZDV or d4T, while lactic acidosis is rare (3.9 to 14.5 cases/1000 patient years). However, increased serum lactate levels may help identify a subset of persons who may be at risk of insulin resistance, lipoatrophy, peripheral neuropathy, and osteopenia. Monitoring lactate concentrations should also be considered in situations where there is a higher risk of acidosis, such as during pregnancy or in the context of ribavirin therapy for HCV infection.

Bone Abnormalities

HIV infection and its management have been associated with a variety of bone abnormalities. Osteopenia, osteoporosis, pathological fractures, and avascular necrosis have all been described. With the exception of avascular necrosis, these conditions appear to arise secondary to abnormalities in bone metabolism.

Osteopenia and Osteoporosis

The prevalence of osteopenia in cross-sectional cohorts of HIV-infected adults is between 20% and 50%. In this setting, there appears to be uncoupling of the equilibrium normally existing between bone formation by osteoblasts and bone resorption by osteoclasts. Similar to lipodystrophy, patient factors (age, gender, baseline weight, hypogonadism) and treatment factors (antiretroviral drugs, corticosteroid use) have been implicated in its pathogenesis.

Bone and lipid metabolism are closely linked, and PI effects on lipid tissues may have an indirect effect on bone. Although decreased, bone mineral density has been shown to be stable over time in persons on PI-containing regimens. Mitochondrial toxicity induced by NRTIs can also result in loss of bone mineral. One possible explanation is that the chronic lactic acidemia may result in mobilization of calcium. Lactic acidemia has been shown to be independently associated with osteopenia in HIV-infected patients on antiretroviral therapy.

Avascular Necrosis

Bilateral avascular necrosis (osteonecrosis) of the femoral and humeral heads has been described with increasing frequency in patients on anti-retroviral therapy, many of whom also have evidence of lipodystrophy. While diabetes mellitus, insulin resistance, and hypertriglyceridemia are recognized risk factors for avascular necrosis in the general population, their role in the HIV-infected population has not been established. Use of corticosteroids in the treatment of opportunistic infections such as *Pneumocystis jiroveci* pneumonia (formerly *Pneumocystis carinii* pneumonia [PCP]) is relatively common and may be a contributing factor in some instances.

Management

Case reports have described the use of bisphosphonates for the treatment of osteopenia or osteoporosis in HIV-infected patients; however, randomized controlled trials of their effectiveness and safety in this setting have not been performed. Other factors that may help to maintain bone density, such as diet, exercise, and replacement of calcium and vitamin D, have also not been studied in HIV disease. As is the case with lipodystrophy, the clinical significance of osteopenia in the HIV-infected population will probably not be known for some years to come.

Management of avascular necrosis of the hips is symptomatic. Severe cases may necessitate joint replacement surgery.

KEY POINTS

- HIV-infected patients are living longer on combination antiretroviral therapy, but complications associated with treatment present a concern. These include lipodystrophy, hepatotoxicity, renal toxicity, peripheral neuropathy, lactic acidemia, and bone abnormalities.
- Lipodystrophy consists of loss of peripheral subcutaneous fat, accumulation of central visceral fat, hyperlipidemia, and/or glucose

intolerance. Its pathophysiology is complex and incompletely understood, and its management is syndromic.

- HIV-infected patients may be at increased risk for atherosclerotic disease. Modifiable risk factors for coronary artery disease should be identified and addressed in this patient population. Management of metabolic abnormalities may not be as effective as in the general population.
- Hepatic dysfunction in HIV-infected patients may be caused by drug toxicity, coinfection with hepatitis viruses and opportunistic pathogens, and immune reconstitution syndrome.
- Renal dysfunction in HIV-infected patients has been reported with tenofovir, a nucleotide reverse-transcriptase inhibitor. Persons with underlying renal insufficiency appear to be at greatest risk.
- Distal sensory polyneuropathy, a frequent long-term complication of antiretroviral therapy, can be reversed when it is detected early.
- Lactic acidemia has been associated with NRTI therapy, and mild cases can be managed on an individual basis. If lactic acidosis is suspected, all antiretroviral drugs should be discontinued immediately. Routine monitoring of serum lactic acid levels in asymptomatic patients is not recommended.
- Patients receiving PIs appear to be at increased risk for osteopenia and osteoporosis. Use of NRTIs may also lead to premature bone loss. The optimal management of bone abnormalities in HIV-infected patients is unknown.
- Avascular necrosis of the hips has also been described in HIV-infected patients, and its management is usually symptomatic.

SUGGESTED WEB SITES
Framingham cardiovascular disease risk calculator (http://hp2010.nibihin.net/atpiii/calculator. asp?usertype=prof).
Lipodystrophy case definition calculator (http://www.med.unsw.edu.au/nchecr).
PROCAM cardiovascular disease risk equation (http://www.chd-taskforce.de/calculator/ calculator.htm).

SUGGESTED READINGS
Bastard JP, Caron M, Vidal H, Jan V, Auclair M, Vigouroux C, et al. Association between altered expression of adipogenic factor SREBP1 in lipoatrophic adipose tissue from HIV-1-infected patients and abnormal adipocyte differentiation and insulin resistance. Lancet. 2002;359:1026-31.

Caron M, Auclair M, Vigouroux C, Glorian M, Forest C, Capeau J. The HIV protease inhibitor indinavir impairs sterol regulatory element-binding protein-1 intranuclear localization, inhibits preadipocyte differentiation, and induces insulin resistance. Diabetes. 2001;50:1378-88.

Carr A, Samaras K, Burton S, Law M, Freund J, Chisholm DJ, et al. A syndrome of peripheral lipodystrophy, hyperlipidaemia and insulin resistance in patients receiving HIV protease inhibitors. AIDS. 1998;12:F51-8.

Data Collection on Adverse Events of Anti-HIV Drugs (DAD) Study Group. Combination antiretroviral therapy and the risk of myocardial infarction. N Engl J Med. 2003;349:1993-2003.

Foulkes AS, Wohl DA, Frank I, Puleo E, Restine S, Wolfe ML, et al. Associations among race/ethnicity, ApoC-III genotypes, and lipids in HIV-1-infected individuals on antiretroviral therapy. PLoS Med. 2006;3:e52.

Grinspoon S, Carr A. Cardiovascular risk and body-fat abnormalities in HIV-infected adults. N Engl J Med. 2005;352:48-62.

HIV Lipodystrophy Case Definition Study Group. An objective case definition of lipodystrophy in HIV-infected adults: a case-control study. Lancet. 2003;361:726-35.

Lewis W, Day BJ, Copeland WC. Mitochondrial toxicity of NRTI antiviral drugs: an integrated cellular perspective. Nat Rev Drug Discov. 2003;2:812-22.

Mallon PW, Ward H, Law M, et al. Buffalo hump seen in HIV-associated lipodystrophy is associated with hyperinsulinemia but not dyslipidemia. J Acquir Immune Defic Syndr. 2005;38:156-62.

Rosey Investigators. No effect of rosiglitazone for treatment of HIV-1 lipoatrophy: randomised, double-blind, placebo-controlled trial. Lancet. 2004;363:429-38.

Tebas P, Powderly WG, Claxton S, Marin D, Tantisiriwat W, Teitelbaum SL, et al. Accelerated bone mineral loss in HIV-infected patients receiving potent antiretroviral therapy. AIDS. 2000;14:F63-7.

Chapter 7

Prevention of Opportunistic Infections

MATTHEW R. LEIBOWITZ, MD
JUDITH S. CURRIER, MD, MSc

Prevention of opportunistic infections (OIs) is a major goal in the management of HIV disease. Rates of AIDS-related mortality and OIs have declined dramatically since the advent of effective combination antiretroviral therapy in 1996. The extent to which specific types of OI prophylaxis have contributed to this decline in infection rates is difficult to determine. This chapter addresses the risk for OIs, drugs for primary prophylaxis, and recommendations for their use. Secondary prophylaxis (maintenance therapy) for established OIs is addressed in Chapter 9. Prophylaxis recommendations stratified by CD4 cell count are summarized in Table 3-2 in Chapter 3.

The characteristics of immune recovery in patients with HIV disease who achieve a good response to antiretroviral therapy continue to be studied. Data suggest that after initiating antiretroviral therapy, CD4 cell reconstitution occurs in several phases. Initially, there is an expansion of existing memory T cells. This is followed by a reduction in T-cell activation with improved CD4 cell reactivity to recall antigens, and then a rise in naïve CD4 lymphocytes. Thus, it is possible that immune recovery for patients who begin antiretroviral therapy when their CD4 cell count is low may be incomplete or delayed.

As our understanding of the critical measures of protection against OIs has improved, published recommendations for the use of prophylactic drugs have been updated. A significant number of studies have now examined the safety of discontinuing prophylaxis against specific OIs in patients whose CD4 cell count has increased on antiretroviral therapy. Data now suggest that primary prophylaxis for *Pneumocystis jiroveci* pneumonia (formerly known as *Pneumocystis carinii* pneumonia [PCP]) and *Mycobacterium avium* complex (MAC) infection can be stopped in this setting. Unfortunately, some patients respond poorly to antiretroviral drugs or have difficulty tolerating them. In addition, some patients who initially respond to treatment may develop drug resistance and progressive immune dysfunction over time. For these groups, prophylactic therapies remain important in the effort to decrease mortality and improve quality of life.

Several factors should be considered when deciding to initiate specific types of OI prophylaxis. These include infection risks and consequences, prophylactic drug effectiveness (e.g., impact on disease severity, mortality), drug toxicities, drug interactions, regimen complexity, the likelihood of inducing drug resistance, and cost. Detailed guidelines about OI prevention, including primary prophylaxis, secondary prophylaxis, and prevention of exposure, have been published by the U.S. Public Health Service in conjunction with the Infectious Diseases Society of America. Primary prophylaxis is recommended in specific clinical settings for PCP, toxoplasmosis, MAC infection, and tuberculosis (TB). It is not routinely advocated for localized or systemic fungal disease or for cytomegalovirus (CMV), herpes simplex, or varicella-zoster infection.

Pneumocystis jiroveci (carinii) Pneumonia

Incidence

Prophylaxis for PCP is a cornerstone of effective management of patients with AIDS. Before the widespread use of antimicrobial prophylaxis and combination antiretroviral therapy, this infection was the most common OI. PCP affected 40% to 60% of patients with a CD4 cell count of less than $200/mm^3$. The introduction of prophylactic therapies in the late 1980s and early 1990s led to a significant decline in new cases of PCP and decreased mortality.

Drug Therapy

Four drugs have been demonstrated to reduce the incidence of PCP in patients at risk: trimethoprim-sulfamethoxazole (TMP-SMX), dapsone, aerosol pentamidine (AP), and atovaquone (Table 7-1). Of these, TMP-SMX is clearly the drug of choice because it is both effective and inexpensive. The failure rate of TMP-SMX in preventing PCP is negligible in patients who reliably take the drug. TMP-SMX also provides excellent prophylaxis against toxoplasmosis and reduces the incidence of conventional bacterial infections. Three dosage regimens of TMP-SMX have been shown to be effective in preventing PCP. These include one double-strength (DS) tablet per day, one single-strength (SS) tablet per day, and one DS tablet three times per week.

The incidence of side effects from TMP-SMX is between 25% and 50% in HIV-infected patients. Adverse drug reactions include fever, rash, liver function test abnormalities, and leukopenia. Lower-dose regimens seem to be somewhat better tolerated than one DS tablet per day. In addition, one study has suggested that the number of adverse effects of TMP-SMX therapy can be reduced by gradually increasing the dose of the drug during the first two weeks. Patients who have a history of a non–life-threatening

Table 7-1. *Pneumocystis jiroveci (carinii)* **Pneumonia Prophylaxis Regimens**

Drug	Recommended Dosage	Annual Cost*	Comments
TMP-SMX	1 DS PO qd *or* 1 SS PO qd *or* 1 DS PO 3 times/wk	$108	Prophylaxis of choice
Dapsone	100 mg/d PO	$130	Do not use in G6PD-deficient patient
Aerosol pentamidine	300 mg/mo via Respirgard II nebulizer	$1185	Less desirable than either TMP-SMX or dapsone
Atovaquone suspension	1500 mg/d PO	$13,140	High cost and limited clinical data to support use

DS = double-strength; G6PD = glucose-6-phosphate dehydrogenase; SS = single-strength; TMP-SMX = trimethoprim-sulfamethoxazole.

*Costs for aerosol pentamidine and atovaquone represent average wholesale prices; all other costs represent retail prices and were obtained from www.drugstore.com.

adverse reaction to TMP-SMX can often be "desensitized" to the drug. This process involves rechallenging the patient with gradually increasing doses of TMP-SMX over a period ranging from 1 day to 2 weeks. A variety of desensitization regimens have proven successful. One commonly used protocol is outlined in Table 7-2. Given the many advantages of TMP-SMX over alternative regimens, desensitization should be considered in patients who cannot tolerate the drug because of fever, rash, or other mild-to-moderate side effects. However, TMP-SMX should not be used in patients who had anaphylaxis or Stevens-Johnson syndrome when previously exposed to it.

Dapsone is considered the second choice for PCP prophylaxis. Like TMP-SMX, it provides systemic protection against *P. jiroveci* infection and is inexpensive. Pyrimethamine can be added to confer protection against toxoplasmosis. Failure of prophylaxis is more common in patients on dapsone than in those taking TMP-SMX. A dosage of 100 mg/d seems to be more effective than 50 mg/d. The incidence of side effects from dapsone is nearly as high as with TMP-SMX. These include rash, fever, liver function test abnormalities, anemia, and leukopenia. In addition, because dapsone can cause hemolysis in patients deficient in glucose-6-phosphate dehydrogenase (G6PD), a G6PD qualitative assay is recommended before starting the drug.

Patients who are unable to take TMP-SMX or dapsone generally should receive AP as prophylaxis against PCP. AP is usually well tolerated, although bronchospasm may sometimes occur. AP prophylaxis is less desirable than TMP-SMX or dapsone for a number of reasons. AP costs more than 10 times as much as either of the other two drugs and provides protection against

Table 7-2.   TMP-SMX Oral Desensitization Protocol*

Day	Dilution†		Serial Doses‡		➝
1	1:1,000,000	1 mL	2 mL	4 mL	8 mL
2	1:100,000	1 mL	2 mL	4 mL	8 mL
3	1:10,000	1 mL	2 mL	4 mL	8 mL
4	1:1000	1 mL	2 mL	4 mL	8 mL
5	1:100	1 mL	2 mL	4 mL	8 mL
6	1:10	1 mL	2 mL	4 mL	8 mL
7	1:1	1 mL	2 mL	4 mL	8 mL
8	Full strength	5 mL	10 mL	20 mL	1 DS tab

* "Treating through" mild-to-moderate symptoms should be attempted. Low-grade fevers and myalgias can be managed with acetaminophen, and mild rashes can be treated with an antihistamine.
† Dilutions are made by pharmacist from a standard oral suspension of trimethoprim-sulfamethoxazole (TMP-SMX), which contains 40 mg of TMP and 200 mg of SMX per 5 mL.
‡ Gradually increasing doses of each day's dilution should be taken 4 times per day.
Protocol developed by Marcus Conant, MD, San Francisco; used by permission.
DS = uble-strength.

only pulmonary infection because of its lack of systemic absorption. In addition, AP is less effective in preventing PCP than TMP-SMX or dapsone, especially in patients with a CD4 count of less than 100 cells/mm^3. The usual dosage of AP is 300 mg/month administered with a Respirgard II nebulizer. Active TB should be ruled out with a purified protein derivative (PPD) skin test, chest x-ray, and other studies as warranted before initiating AP.

Atovaquone is used infrequently for PCP prophylaxis because its cost is more than 100 times that of TMP-SMX and dapsone, and data supporting its efficacy are relatively few. One clinical trial demonstrated that atovaquone suspension at a dosage of 1500 mg/d is as effective as dapsone 100 mg/d in preventing PCP. The rate of adverse effects of the two regimens was similar.

The combination of clindamycin and primaquine, sometimes used for the treatment of PCP, has not been shown to provide adequate PCP prophylaxis when compared with the standard regimens described above and therefore is not recommended.

Recommendations

Prophylaxis for PCP should be given to HIV-infected patients with a CD4 count of less than 200 cells/mm^3 and to those who meet other diagnostic criteria for AIDS. HIV-infected patients with thrush or a more than two-week history of unexplained fever should also receive prophylaxis. TMP-SMX is the drug of choice, with alternative regimens outlined above (see Figure 3-1 in Chapter 3). Data indicate that primary prophylaxis for PCP can be discontinued safely in patients on antiretroviral therapy whose CD4 count rises to over 200 cells/mm^3 for at least 3 months.

Toxoplasmosis

Incidence

Toxoplasmic encephalitis is one of the most common neurologic complications of HIV disease. Nearly all cases result from reactivation of latent *Toxoplasma gondii* infection. Most patients who have had primary infection with *T. gondii* have detectable serum antibody (IgG) to the organism. The rate of seropositivity varies around the world; it has been estimated to be between 10% and 40% in the United States. Without effective antiretroviral therapy and toxoplasmosis prophylaxis, approximately one-third of patients with *Toxoplasma* antibodies eventually will develop encephalitis. Reactivation of this infection generally occurs in HIV-infected patients with a CD4 count of less than 100 cells/mm^3.

Drug Therapy

The two regimens commonly used to prevent toxoplasmosis are TMP-SMX and dapsone plus pyrimethamine. TMP-SMX is the prophylactic drug of choice. Although there have been no prospective randomized trials, data from numerous studies show that patients taking TMP-SMX for PCP prophylaxis are rarely diagnosed with toxoplasmosis. In an Australian retrospective study of 155 patients receiving secondary PCP prophylaxis, none of 60 patients on TMP-SMX developed toxoplasmic encephalitis during a 3-year period, whereas 13% of 95 patients on AP developed this complication. The doses of TMP-SMX typically used for PCP prophylaxis seem adequate for toxoplasmosis prophylaxis.

The combination of daily dapsone and pyrimethamine given once per week also is effective in preventing toxoplasmosis. In a French study comparing AP to the combination of dapsone (50 mg/d) plus pyrimethamine (50 mg/wk) and folinic acid (25 mg/wk), toxoplasmosis developed in 16% (28/176) of patients receiving AP compared with 3% (5/173) of patients receiving dapsone plus pyrimethamine.

A Spanish study compared TMP-SMX DS dosed twice daily three times each week with dapsone 100 mg and pyrimethamine 50 mg dosed twice weekly, and found low rates of *Toxoplasma* reactivation in both groups (4% vs. 7% at 24 months). Pyrimethamine alone does not seem as effective as the combination of dapsone plus pyrimethamine. Atovaquone as dosed for PCP prophylaxis also may protect against toxoplasmosis, but it is much more expensive than TMP-SMX.

Recommendations

HIV-infected patients should have their *Toxoplasma* IgG antibody level checked at baseline. Patients with a positive test result and a CD4 count of less than 100 cells/mm^3 should receive prophylaxis as outlined below. Patients without detectable antibody presumably have never been infected with the organism and therefore are not at risk of reactivation. However, they should be counseled about methods to avoid primary infection, including refraining from eating raw or undercooked red meat and avoiding contact with cat feces. Patients without *Toxoplasma* antibody on initial presentation should have a repeat test performed if their CD4 count drops below 100 cells/mm³ to determine if they have become infected in the interim.

The choice of prophylactic drug for toxoplasmosis depends on what is given for PCP prophylaxis. Patients who are already receiving TMP-SMX or atovaquone need no additional prophylaxis for toxoplasmosis. However, in patients receiving dapsone for PCP prophylaxis, pyrimethamine (50 mg/wk) and folinic acid (25 mg/wk) to prevent pyrimethamine-induced bone marrow suppression should be added if their CD4 count drops below 100 cells/mm³.

Data from observational studies and two randomized trials have shown that primary prophylaxis for toxoplasmosis can be discontinued safely in patients on antiretroviral therapy whose CD4 count rises to over 200 cells/mm³ for at least 3 months. The median CD4 count upon stopping prophylaxis was more than 300 cells/mm³, and follow-up time ranged from 7 to 22 months.

Mycobacterium avium Complex Infection

Incidence

The risk of disseminated MAC infection increases as the CD4 cell count falls and is highest when it is below 50/mm³. Earlier in the epidemic, 40% to 50% of patients with an AIDS diagnosis could be expected to develop MAC. In one study from 1993, 18% of patients with a CD4 cell count of less than 200/mm³ who did not take prophylaxis developed MAC after a median follow-up of 38 weeks. More recent data show an encouraging decline in the incidence of MAC. The proportion developing MAC in the Johns Hopkins cohort decreased from 16% before 1996 to 4% after 1996, with a current rate of less than 1% per year. This trial included some patients who were receiving MAC prophylaxis, so it is difficult to determine the relative contributions of antimicrobial prophylaxis and antiretroviral therapy. In the EuroSIDA cohort study of more than 7000 HIV-infected patients, the incidence of MAC infection decreased from 3.5 cases/100 person years of follow-up before September 1995 to 0.2 cases/100 person years of follow-up after March 1997. The rate of use of MAC prophylaxis among those patients with a CD4 count of less than 50 cells/mm³ was 8% in the precombination antiretroviral therapy era and 14% in the more recent study period.

Drug Therapy

Azithromycin, clarithromycin, and rifabutin are approved for use as prophylaxis against MAC (Table 7-3). Randomized trials have shown each of these drugs to be superior to placebo in preventing MAC bacteremia. In ad-

Table 7-3.   *Mycobacterium avium* Complex Prophylaxis Regimens

Drug	Recommended Dosage	Annual Cost*	Comments
Azithromycin	1200 mg/wk PO	$1386	Least expensive
Clarithromycin	500 mg PO twice daily	$2808	—
Rifabutin	300 mg/d PO	$4693	Less effective than macrolides; drug interactions are problematic

* All costs represent retail prices and were obtained from www.drugstore.com.

dition, clarithromycin prophylaxis has been shown to decrease mortality in a placebo-controlled trial.

The California Collaborative Treatment Group (CCTG) compared once-weekly azithromycin (1200 mg) to daily rifabutin (300 mg) and to the combination of these two drugs. In an intent-to-treat analysis, the 1-year cumulative incidence of disseminated MAC was 15.3% in the rifabutin group, 7.6% in the azithromycin group, and 2.8% in the combination therapy group. After adjustment for CD4 cell count, the risk of MAC was 72% lower with combination therapy than with rifabutin alone, and 47% lower than with azithromycin alone. The risk of MAC infection in patients taking azithromycin was 47% lower than in patients taking rifabutin. Azithromycin- and clarithromycin-resistant MAC was identified in 11% (2/18) of breakthrough isolates on azithromycin and in none on the combination arm. Dose-limiting toxicity was 21% in the combination arm, 16% in the azithromycin arm, and 13% in the rifabutin arm.

The ACTG 196/CPCRA 009 study compared clarithromycin (500 mg twice daily) to rifabutin (300 mg/d) and to the combination of these two drugs. The cumulative incidence of MAC infection at one year in an intent-to-treat analysis was 5% in the clarithromycin recipients, 10% in the rifabutin recipients, and 5% in the combination arm. Therefore, in contrast to the CCTG results, the addition of rifabutin added no further protection against MAC. Clarithromycin resistance was observed in 28% of breakthrough isolates.

No data exist comparing clarithromycin and azithromycin for the prevention of MAC. However, both drugs seem to be more effective than rifabutin. Azithromycin has the advantages of once-weekly dosing, fewer drug interactions, and lower cost. Their gastrointestinal side effects are comparable. The lowest effective dose of these drugs is not known.

An added benefit of both clarithromycin and azithromycin over rifabutin is protection conferred against conventional bacterial infections. In the CCTG study, there were more bacterial infections in the rifabutin arm compared with the azithromycin-containing arms (RR: 1.58; 95% CI: 1.10 to 2.30). The risk of sinusitis and bacterial pneumonia was reduced by 50% in azithromycin recipients compared with rifabutin recipients. Preliminary data also indicate that patients on macrolide prophylaxis for MAC infection have a lower incidence of PCP than those receiving rifabutin.

Recommendations

Prophylaxis against MAC infection using azithromycin (1200 mg/wk) or clarithromycin (500 mg twice daily) is recommended for HIV-infected patients with a CD4 count of less than 50 cells/mm^3. Rifabutin is less effective and difficult to coadminister with protease inhibitors and non-nucleoside reverse-transcriptase inhibitors. While some clinicians question the need for initiating MAC prophylaxis among patients with a low CD4 cell count who are initiating antiretroviral therapy, published recommendations continue to promote its use in this setting. Data suggest that primary prophylaxis for MAC infection can be discontinued safely in patients on antiretroviral therapy whose CD4 count rises to over 100 cells/mm^3 for at least 3 months.

MAC infection presenting as immune reconstitution disease with inflammatory lymphadenitis has been described shortly after initiating antiretroviral therapy. It is not known whether the use of MAC prophylaxis is effective at preventing this syndrome.

Tuberculosis

Incidence

HIV disease is the greatest known risk factor for the development of active TB. It has been estimated that an HIV-infected patient with a positive PPD has a 10% risk per year of developing active infection. This is in contrast to the 10% lifetime risk of active TB in an HIV-seronegative person. Active TB can affect patients with any CD4 cell count, but extrapulmonary disease is seen mainly in those with advanced immunodeficiency.

The PPD is the best method of assessing a patient's risk of developing active TB. Unfortunately, the test is less sensitive in HIV-infected patients, especially in those with a lower CD4 cell count. Based on this observation, the Centers for Disease Control and Prevention (CDC) has defined induration of 5 mm or greater to constitute a positive test in HIV-infected persons. Routine anergy testing is no longer recommended because of its lack of standardization.

Drug Therapy

Isoniazid (INH) significantly lowers the incidence of active TB in HIV-seropositive patients with evidence of previous infection. In a randomized trial in Haiti, 12 months of INH given to HIV-infected patients with a positive PPD reduced the risk of active TB by 83% during a 3-year period.

Another study demonstrated a 38% reduction in the incidence of TB with INH prophylaxis among HIV-infected South African men prior to the availability of combination antiretroviral therapy.

The recommended dosage of INH is 300 mg/d. The drug usually is given with pyridoxine (50 mg/d) to decrease the risk of peripheral neuropathy. Based on results of other studies, 9 months of therapy is now recommended in HIV-infected patients. INH, in a dosage of 900 mg twice per week, as directly observed therapy (DOT) in patients with a history of poor medication adherence, is also effective.

Data have shown that the combination of rifampin plus pyrazinamide given for 2 months is as effective as INH given for 12 months in reducing the incidence of active TB in HIV-infected patients with a positive PPD. However, because of reports of severe hepatotoxicity associated with the use of this short-course regimen, its use is strongly discouraged.

Recommendations

HIV-infected patients should have a PPD done at baseline and annually thereafter if the initial test was negative and there are historical risk factors for TB exposure. Induration of 5 mm or greater indicates previous infection with *Mycobacterium tuberculosis* and the need for prophylactic therapy. Active TB should be excluded by clinical assessment, chest x-ray, and other studies as warranted before prophylaxis is started. Prophylaxis is recommended for all HIV-infected patients with a history of a positive PPD regardless of age and should also be given if there has been recent contact with a person who has infectious TB.

Prophylaxis consists of INH and pyridoxine (300 mg and 50 mg/d, respectively, or 900 mg and 100 mg twice weekly [DOT], respectively) for 9 months. Few data exist to support the recommendation of a 4-month course of daily rifampin (10 mg/kg up to 600 mg) or rifabutin (5 mg/kg up to 300 mg) in HIV-infected patients, but this regimen is a possible alternative for those who cannot take INH. If the patient has been exposed to drug-resistant TB, other prophylactic regimens may be indicated. Consultation with an infectious disease specialist is advised.

Fungal Infections

Incidence

Fungal infections that occur in the context of HIV disease can be divided into superficial (oropharyngeal and vaginal candidiasis) and invasive (cryptococcal meningitis or fungemia, disseminated histoplasmosis, coccidioidomycosis, and esophageal candidiasis). Oropharyngeal candidiasis is extremely common, affecting more than 90% of people with AIDS. Before the advent of combination antiretroviral therapy, esophageal candidiasis was the most common invasive fungal infection, with a lifetime risk of 20% to 30% compared with 5% to 10% for cryptococcosis, and 2% to 5% for histoplasmosis (with higher rates in endemic areas).

The incidence of fungal infections has declined dramatically since the introduction of protease inhibitors. Data from the French Clinical Epidemiology Study demonstrated a 69% decline in the rate of *Candida* esophagitis from the first 6 months of 1996 through the first 6 months of 1997. In this database, the rates of cryptococcal meningitis fell 70% during the same time period. Similar significant decreases in esophageal candidiasis and cryptococcosis were described in the Adult and Adolescent Spectrum of Disease Project in the United States.

Drug Therapy

Preventive therapies for fungal infections include topical nystatin and clotrimazole and oral fluconazole and itraconazole. There are few data on newer azoles such as voriconazole and posaconazole. Randomized trials have demonstrated the benefit of prophylaxis for oropharyngeal candidiasis, vaginal candidiasis, and invasive fungal infections.

The largest study of fungal prophylaxis was ACTG 981, which compared daily fluconazole (200 mg) to clotrimazole troches five times daily in patients with a CD4 count of less than 200 cells/mm^3. The study demonstrated a significant reduction in the overall rate of invasive fungal infections from 11% in patients receiving clotrimazole troches to 4% in patients receiving fluconazole. This difference was primarily the result of a decrease in the rates of esophageal candidiasis and cryptococcal disease, and benefit was greatest among patients with a CD4 cell count of less than 50/mm^3. No survival advantage was demonstrated. This study also showed a significant reduction in the rate of oral candidiasis from 45% in the clotrimazole group to 15% in the fluconazole group. A recent metaanalysis of five randomized trials of fungal prophylaxis in HIV-infected patients (n=1316) found that the incidence of cryptococcal disease was decreased in those taking primary prophylaxis (RR, 0.21; 95% CI, 0.09 to 0.46) compared with those on placebo. However, there was no significant difference in overall mortality (RR, 1.01; 95% CI, 0.71 to 1.44).

Fluconazole (200 mg/wk) has also been compared with placebo for the prevention of vaginal candidiasis in HIV-infected women. This study found a 37% decrease in the rate of vaginal candidiasis in the fluconazole group and a decrease in the overall rate of mucosal candidiasis. Rates of resistance of isolates to fluconazole were similar in the study arms.

Itraconazole, an azole that is superior to fluconazole in treating histoplasmosis, has been studied for its ability to prevent fungal infections in patients residing in histoplasmosis-endemic areas. Results from a study of 295 patients randomized to receive itraconazole (200 mg/d) or placebo showed that after a median 16 months of follow-up, itraconazole prophylaxis reduced the risk of systemic fungal infections from 11.6% to 4.0%. This finding was the result of a decrease in the rate of histoplasmosis from 6.8% in placebo recipients to 2.7% in itraconazole recipients and a decrease in the rate of cryptococcosis from 5.5% to 0.7%. Surprisingly, there was no reduction in the rate of mucosal candidiasis.

Recommendations

Despite the proven efficacy of fluconazole in preventing both superficial and invasive fungal infections, the use of this drug for primary prophylaxis is not generally recommended. Long-term use of fluconazole may predispose to the development of azole-resistant *Candida* infections. In addition, fluconazole prophylaxis is not cost-effective because of the low incidence of invasive fungal disease. However, in settings where antiretroviral therapy is not available or tolerated, the use of fluconazole prophylaxis might be considered.

Itraconazole prophylaxis (200 mg/d) may be warranted to prevent histoplasmosis in patients with a CD4 count of less than 100 cells/mm³ who reside in endemic areas. Issues to consider when deciding about itraconazole prophylaxis include potential drug interactions, the risk of other fungal infections, and cost.

Cytomegalovirus Infection

Incidence

Between 95% and 98% of homosexual men and injection-drug users have CMV antibody, which indicates prior infection and places them at risk of reactivation in the context of advanced HIV disease. Before the advent of effective combination antiretroviral therapy, CMV disease was a common complication of HIV infection. One study found that 25% of men with a CD4 cell count of less than 100/mm³ developed CMV retinitis in 4 years of follow-up. Autopsy studies showed that up to 75% of patients who died of AIDS showed evidence of CMV infection in one or more organ systems. The use of antiretroviral therapy has led to a dramatic decline in the incidence of CMV disease.

Drug Therapy

The only drug proven effective in preventing CMV disease in advanced AIDS patients is oral ganciclovir. In 1996, Spector and coworkers published the results of a double-blind, placebo-controlled trial of oral ganciclovir (1000 mg tid) versus placebo in 725 AIDS patients who had a CD4 cell count of less than 50/mm³ or less than 100/mm³ combined with a history of an AIDS-defining OI. The incidence of CMV retinitis after 12 months was

24% in the placebo group compared with 12% in the patients who received ganciclovir. There was no significant difference in mortality between the groups. Anemia and neutropenia were common in patients who received ganciclovir; 14% of them required erythropoietin, and 24% required granulocyte colony-stimulating factor. Comparative data for the placebo group were 6% and 9%, respectively.

A second study performed by the Community Programs for Clinical Research on AIDS (CPCRA 023) did not confirm the efficacy of oral ganciclovir in preventing CMV disease. Nine-hundred ninety-four patients with a CD4 cell count of less than 100/mm^3 were randomly assigned to oral ganciclovir (1000 mg tid) or placebo. No difference in the incidence of CMV disease or death was seen between the groups. Similar to the previous trial, the patients on ganciclovir experienced significantly more neutropenia than those receiving placebo.

In a randomized trial, valganciclovir, the orally administered valine ester of ganciclovir, was shown to be as effective as intravenous ganciclovir for induction therapy of CMV retinitis in HIV-infected patients. The role of valganciclovir for CMV prophylaxis in patients with advanced HIV disease who do not respond to combination antiretroviral therapy is under investigation.

Recommendations

Primary prophylaxis for CMV disease generally is not recommended for a number of reasons, including conflicting data about its efficacy, large daily pill burden, potential for bone marrow suppression, and cost. In addition, many patients on ganciclovir require colony-stimulating factors to prevent anemia and neutropenia, which adds further to the expense of treatment. Studies are being performed to determine which AIDS patients are at the greatest risk of CMV disease so that prophylaxis can be better targeted.

HIV-infected patients who are not thought to be at high risk of having prior CMV infection may benefit from CMV antibody screening. HIV-seropositive patients who are CMV antibody–negative and require a blood transfusion should receive only leukocyte-depleted products to avoid transfusion-associated primary CMV infection.

KEY POINTS

- Despite the success of combination antiretroviral therapy, prophylactic treatment for OIs remains critically important.
- There are data to support the withdrawal of primary PCP, toxoplasmosis, and MAC infection prophylaxis in patients who have shown a significant rise in CD4 cell count in response to antiretroviral therapy.

- Patients with a CD4 count of less than 200 cells/mm^3 are at risk of PCP if they do not receive antibiotic prophylaxis; TMP-SMX is the drug of choice. Desensitization may be possible if there is a history of a non–life-threatening drug reaction. Dapsone, atovaquone, and aerosol pentamidine can be used as alternative agents if TMP-SMX is not tolerated.

- Prophylaxis against toxoplasmosis should be provided in patients with a CD4 count of less than 100 cells/mm^3 and serologic evidence of previous *Toxoplasma* infection. TMP-SMX is the drug of choice; dapsone with weekly pyrimethamine is an alternative treatment.

- Prophylaxis against MAC infection with azithromycin or clarithromycin should be initiated in patients with a CD4 count of less than 50 cells/mm^3. Rifabutin is less effective and may be problematic to administer because of drug interactions.

- HIV-infected patients with a positive PPD ($\geq$5 mm induration) should receive 9 months of INH therapy.

- The use of fluconazole as primary prophylaxis for fungal infections is not recommended in general because of its lack of effect on overall survival.

- The use of oral ganciclovir for CMV prophylaxis is not advised because of its high cost and potential hematologic toxicity.

SUGGESTED READINGS

American Thoracic Society. Targeted tuberculin testing and treatment of latent tuberculosis infection. MMWR. 2000;49(RR-6):1-51.

Currier JS, Williams PL, Koletar SL, Cohn SE, Murphy RL, Heald AE, et al. Discontinuation of Mycobacterium avium complex prophylaxis in patients with antiretroviral therapy-induced increases in CD4+ cell count. A randomized, double-blind, placebo-controlled trial. AIDS Clinical Trials Group 362 Study Team. Ann Intern Med. 2000;133:493-503.

Furrer H, Opravil M, Bernasconi E, Telenti A, Egger M. Stopping primary prophylaxis in HIV-1-infected patients at high risk of toxoplasma encephalitis. Swiss HIV Cohort Study [Letter]. Lancet. 2000;355:2217-8.

Gluckstein D, Ruskin J. Rapid oral desensitization to trimethoprim-sulfamethoxazole (TMP-SMZ): use in prophylaxis for *Pneumocystis carinii* pneumonia in patients with AIDS who were previously intolerant to TMP-SMZ. Clin Infect Dis. 1995;20:849-53.

Gordin F, Chaisson RE, Matts JP, Miller C, de Lourdes Garcia M, Hafner R, et al. Rifampin and pyrazinamide vs isoniazid for prevention of tuberculosis in HIV-infected persons: an international randomized trial. Terry Beirn Community Programs for Clinical Research on AIDS, the Adult AIDS Clinical Trials Group, the Pan American Health Organization, and the Centers for Disease Control and Prevention Study Group. JAMA. 2000;283:1445-50.

Grupo de Estudio del SIDA 04/98. A randomized trial of the discontinuation of primary and secondary prophylaxis against *Pneumocystis carinii* pneumonia after highly active antiretroviral therapy in patients with HIV infection. Grupo de Estudio del SIDA 04/98. N Engl J Med. 2001;344:159-67.

Kaplan JE, Hanson D, Dworkin MS, Frederick T, Bertolli J, Lindegren ML, et al. Epidemiology of human immunodeficiency virus-associated opportunistic infections in the United States in the era of highly active antiretroviral therapy. Clin Infect Dis. 2000;30 Suppl 1:S5-14.

Moore RD, Chaisson RE. Natural history of opportunistic disease in an HIV-infected urban clinical cohort. Ann Intern Med. 1996;124:633-42.

Palella FJ Jr., Delaney KM, Moorman AC, Loveless MO, Fuhrer J, Satten GA, et al. Declining morbidity and mortality among patients with advanced human immunodeficiency virus infection. HIV Outpatient Study Investigators. N Engl J Med. 1998;338:853-60.

United States Public Health Service/Infectious Disease Society of America guidelines for the prevention of opportunistic infections in persons infected with human immunodeficiency virus. Ann Intern Med. 2002;137:435-77. Available as a living document on AIDSinfo: Department of Health and Human Services website at http:www.aidsinfo.nih.gov.

Weverling GJ, Mocroft A, Ledergerber B, Kirk O, Gonzáles-Lahoz J, d'Arminio Monforte A, et al. Discontinuation of *Pneumocystis carinii* pneumonia prophylaxis after start of highly active antiretroviral therapy in HIV-1 infection. EuroSIDA Study Group. Lancet. 1999;353:1293-8.

Willemot P, Klein MB. Prevention of HIV-associated opportunistic infections and diseases in the age of highly active antiretroviral therapy. Exp Rev Anti Infect Ther. 2004;521-32.

Chapter 8

Diagnostic Approach to Common Clinical Syndromes

AMITA GUPTA, MD, MHS
LISA R. HIRSCHHORN, MD, MPH
PETER J. PILIERO, MD
JOEL E. GALLANT, MD, MPH

The incidence of HIV-related opportunistic infections (OIs) and malignancies has declined dramatically since the advent of effective combination antiretroviral therapy and improved antimicrobial prophylaxis. In the United States, OIs are now seen mainly among persons who initially present with advanced HIV disease, among those who do not seek care or adhere to therapy, and among those for whom treatment has failed. In patients with advanced HIV disease who are initiating antiretroviral therapy, OIs may also occur as a result of immune reconstitution. This chapter reviews the diagnostic approach to common HIV-related clinical syndromes encountered by the primary care practitioner. For details on the prevention and treatment of OIs, the reader is referred to Chapters 7 and 9, respectively, as well as to published guidelines.

Traditionally, the diagnostic approach to HIV-related conditions has been influenced by the patient's degree of immunodeficiency. For example, respiratory symptoms are evaluated differently in a patient with a normal CD4 count than in a patient with a CD4 count of <200 cells/mm^3 who is not on prophylaxis for *Pneumocystis jiroveci (carinii)* pneumonia (PCP). Data from a number of cohorts have shown that a high viral load, particularly in advanced HIV disease, is also an independent risk factor for OIs.

Effective antiretroviral therapy results in suppression of viral replication followed by a rapid increase in the CD4 count that is associated with enhanced immune function. This leads to a significant decline in the risk of OIs within 3 to 6 months. The risk of certain malignancies also decreases. For patients responding to antiretroviral therapy, a CD4 count above 200 cells/mm^3 is the most important predictor of OI-free survival. However, atypical presentations of OIs have been described as a manifestation of immune reconstitution in this setting.

As the frequency of OIs decreases and the risk of comorbid diseases increases in the aging HIV-infected population, non-HIV-related conditions may account for a greater proportion of new health problems. For example, chronic obstructive pulmonary disease (COPD) and congestive heart failure

(CHF) should be included in the differential diagnosis of dyspnea in an older patient. In addition, complications of antiretroviral therapy (e.g., lactic acidosis, avascular necrosis of the hips) should also be considered in the evaluation of symptoms.

The diagnostic approach to an HIV-infected patient who presents with a new complaint starts with a thorough history (Box 8-1). This information should be interpreted in the context of physical findings and immune status as assessed by the most recent CD4 count, as well as the degree and duration of virologic suppression if on antiretroviral therapy. Once these data are obtained, diagnostic tests guided by the patient's symptoms and signs may be warranted. If initial studies are not revealing, more extensive testing, empiric treatment, or both are then considered.

A number of technological advances in the past decade have added to our ability to identify complications in HIV-infected patients. They have decreased the need for invasive procedures and the time required for making a diagnosis. For example, the ability to diagnose infections caused by intracellular organisms such as mycobacteria and fungi has greatly improved with the use of more sensitive blood culture methods such as lysis-centrifugation and radiometric systems. These cultures become positive within a few days to weeks, reducing the need for liver and bone marrow biopsies.

The increasing use of polymerase chain reaction (PCR) technology for diagnostic purposes has also improved the care of HIV-infected patients. For example, the diagnosis of cytomegalovirus (CMV) central nervous system (CNS) infection has improved significantly with the introduction of

---

Box 8-1.   Diagnostic Approach to an HIV-Infected Patient Presenting with a New Complaint

History
- Current condition (duration, severity, associated symptoms, precipitating factors, prior history)
- Exposures (travel, occupational, food, pets, hobbies, similar illness in household and other close contacts)
- Sexual behaviors
- Drug and alcohol use
- Risk factors for or presence of cardiopulmonary disease and other comorbid conditions
- Medications (prescription, over-the-counter, and complementary; adherence to medical therapies)
- Degree of immunosuppression (lowest and current CD4 count, response to antiretroviral therapy)

Physical Examination
- Complete examination with attention to symptomatic regions

Laboratory Studies
- Choice of specific tests guided by symptoms and signs
- Chest radiograph, sputum examination, and culture if pulmonary symptoms are present
- Blood, urine, and other cultures if fever is present

CMV-PCR testing of spinal fluid. This technology is now also being used for the diagnosis of progressive multifocal leukoencephalopathy (PML), Epstein-Barr virus (EBV) infection, herpes simplex virus (HSV) infection, and the rapid differentiation of tuberculosis (TB) from atypical mycobacterial infection. Other new diagnostic techniques have facilitated detection of other viral pathogens, *Cryptococcus neoformans*, *Histoplasma capsulatum*, and *Legionella pneumophila*.

The final area in which great progress has been achieved is in radiologic evaluation. The use of magnetic resonance imaging (MRI), improved computed tomography (CT) scanning, and enhanced resolution ultrasound and nuclear medicine studies has facilitated the noninvasive diagnosis of many clinical conditions.

Fever

The approach to the HIV-infected patient with fever is determined mainly by the presence and nature of accompanying symptoms; the degree of immunodeficiency as measured by a recent CD4 count; and the duration and magnitude of the virologic response to antiretroviral therapy. This section focuses on fever without localizing symptoms or signs (Table 8-1).

Studies in the early 1990s examining fever of unknown origin (FUO) in HIV-infected patients reported high rates of mycobacterial disease, including, disseminated *Mycobacterium avium* complex (MAC) infection and TB, as well as lymphoma and drug fever. An increased risk for these conditions occurred as the CD4 count declined. However, results varied significantly

Table 8-1. Causes of Fever Without Localizing Symptoms or Signs

Etiology	Examples	Comments
Medications	TMP-SMX, dapsone, abacavir, penicillins, and many others	Increased rate of drug reactions in HIV disease
Infections Bacterial	Sinusitis, endocarditis, occult abscess, PID, TB, MAC salmonellosis, SA	Atypical manifestations of TB with low CD4 count; MAC with CD4 count < 50 cells/mm^3
Fungal	Histoplasmosis, coccidioido-mycosis, *Penicillium marneffei* infection, cryptococcosis	Diagnosis made by culture, biopsy, or antigen detection
Parasitic	Toxoplasmosis, PCP, malaria, babesiosis, leishmaniasis	Travel and animal exposures important
Viral	CMV	CD4 count < 50 cells/mm^3
Neoplasia	Lymphoma	Usually with adenopathy
Endocrine	Hypoadrenalism	Adrenal disease with CMV or mycobacterial infection

CMV = cytomegalovirus; MAC = *Mycobacterium avium* complex; PCP = *Pneumocystis jiroveci (carinii)* pneumonia; PID = pelvic inflammatory disease; SA = *Staphylococcal aureus*; TB = tuberculosis; TMP-SMX = trimethoprim-sulfamethoxazole.

based on the population. For example, one study of HIV-infected patients hospitalized with fever in a public hospital documented bacterial infections as a source in the majority of cases.

In HIV-infected patients who present with a fever but without localizing symptoms or signs, mycobacterial disease should be considered in the differential diagnosis. In patients with advanced HIV disease, extrapulmonary TB is relatively common. Manifestations consist of fever, lymphadenopathy, and/or nonspecific laboratory findings, such as anemia and an increased serum alkaline phosphatase level, in the absence of pulmonary symptoms. Disseminated MAC infection is unusual until the CD4 count falls below 50 cells/mm^3; patients present with fever, weight loss, diarrhea, and anemia. The organism can usually be isolated from blood, bone marrow, lymph nodes, and/or liver but may take up to 8 weeks to grow. Diagnosis is made in over 90% of cases by blood culture using a lysis-centrifugation or radiometric system.

CMV infection also occurs in patients with a CD4 count less than 50 cells/mm^3. It typically presents as retinitis, or less commonly, as gastrointestinal tract disease, both of which may initially present with fever alone. A dilated funduscopic examination will confirm the presence of CMV retinitis, whereas endoscopic esophageal, gastric, or intestinal biopsy is needed to diagnose gastrointestinal involvement.

Other infections, including cryptococcosis, histoplasmosis, and *Toxoplasma* encephalitis, may present with fever in patients with advanced HIV disease. Finally, both community-acquired (e.g., *Streptococcus pneumoniae*) and nosocomial (e.g., *Pseudomonas aeruginosa*) pneumonia with or without bacteremia should also be considered in the differential diagnosis in all HIV-infected patients.

Limited information exists about the epidemiology of FUO in the context of antiretroviral therapy and OI prophylaxis. Standard diagnostic approaches for FUO should be used in HIV-infected patients with higher CD4 counts (>200 cells/mm^3), with the proviso that increased rates of TB, bacterial pneumonia with bacteremia, and bacterial sinusitis have been reported. With the exception of TB and recurrent bacterial pneumonia, HIV-related OIs generally do not occur until the CD4 count has fallen below 200 cells/mm^3. In such patients, the differential diagnosis broadens to include the OIs described above and lymphoma.

The clinician evaluating a patient with fever should begin with a history of the present illness (including duration, degree, and pattern of the fever), an evaluation of potential pathogen exposures (e.g., occupational, geographic region of origin and travel history, animal exposure, sexual practices, food history, sick contacts, injection drug use), and a review of systems. Both recent and past travel history are important in assessing patients with fever. For example, a patient from Southeast Asia with fever may have disseminated *Penicillium marneffei* infection, whereas a traveler to or former resident of Southern California may have acute coccidioidomycosis.

A history of past medical conditions, including TB, bacterial infections, OIs, malignancies, and the presence of other potential sources of infection (e.g., intravascular catheter, surgery, trauma), should be reviewed. Fever associated with immune reconstitution has been described in advanced HIV disease. A drug history, including any recent changes, should be obtained. For patients presenting with fever after starting a new medication, drug fever should be considered. For example, abacavir induces a hypersensitivity reaction in 2% to 8% of patients, with over 93% of cases occurring within 6 weeks of initiation of treatment. The reaction is characterized by fever and "flu-like" symptoms, which are accompanied by a rash in 70% of cases.

Physical examination should emphasize the skin, lymph nodes, fundi, oral cavity, sinuses, heart, lungs, abdomen, and pelvis. Initial laboratory studies, in addition to reviewing a recent CD4 cell count and viral load, should include a complete blood count (CBC) with differential count, urinalysis, and liver function tests (LFTs). Additional studies to consider include a TB skin test (PPD), chest x-ray, conventional blood cultures, syphilis and viral hepatitis serologies, and lysis-centrifugation blood culture and serum cryptococcal antigen in patients with a CD4 count of less than 100 cells/mm^3.

Further evaluation is based on the results of the initial laboratory tests. For example, LFT abnormalities may prompt abdominal imaging with CT or ultrasound, whereas an abnormal chest x-ray may be further investigated with sputum induction, CT, or bronchoscopy with bronchoalveolar lavage (BAL), and/or biopsy as indicated. Other diagnostic studies to consider in patients with normal initial tests include thoracic, abdominal, and pelvic CT scans looking for lymphadenopathy, malignancy, or occult abscess; an MRI or CT scan of the brain; and an examination of the cerebrospinal fluid (CSF). Gallium scanning for occult infection and malignancy is highly nonspecific. Bone marrow biopsy may be useful in patients with fever accompanied by neutropenia and/or anemia, with a 25% diagnostic yield for disseminated mycobacterial and fungal infections in this setting. Liver biopsy should be considered in patients with advanced HIV disease who have unexplained hepatomegaly or an increased serum alkaline phosphatase level.

HIV-infected patients with a fever are generally evaluated on an outpatient basis. The need for hospitalization and empiric antimicrobial therapy is determined by the severity of presentation and the probability of a bacterial or fungal infection for which treatment delay may have an adverse effect on clinical outcome.

Pulmonary Symptoms

The risk of several infectious and noninfectious pulmonary conditions is increased in HIV-infected patients (Table 8-2). Key considerations in the evaluation of respiratory symptoms are the acuity and nature of presentation,

Table 8-2.   Causes of Pulmonary Symptoms in HIV Disease

	Characteristics
Bacterial Infections	
Streptococcus pneumoniae, Haemophilus influenzae	Occur at all stages of HIV disease; acute presentation with fever and purulent sputum production
Gram-negative bacteria	Acute presentation; generally in hospitalized patients
Legionella pneumophila	Acute presentation with constitutional symptoms and variable sputum production
Rhodococcus equii	Subacute presentation with minimal sputum production
Staphylococcus aureus	Acute, subacute, or chronic presentation with purulent sputum production
Mycobacterium tuberculosis	Acute or subacute presentation, usually with constitutional symptoms
Viral Infections	
Influenza	Acute presentation with variable sputum production, winter season
CMV, HSV, VZV	Usually seen with involvement of other organ systems
Fungal Infections	
Pneumocystis jiroveci (formerly *carinii*)	Acute or subacute presentation; dry cough, fever and dyspnea common
Cryptococcus neoformans	May be associated with meningitis
Histoplasma capsulatum	Acute to subacute presentation, often with systemic involvement
Coccidioides immitis	Often with meningitis and skin lesions
Malignancies/Other	
Kaposi's sarcoma	Subacute to chronic presentation with chest pain, dyspnea, and hemoptysis
Lymphocytic interstitial pneumonitis	Chronic progressive dyspnea, usually associated with nonproductive cough; hepatosplenomegaly and parotid enlargement may be present
Lymphoma	Subacute to chronic presentation with constitutional symptoms and adenopathy
Lung cancer	Constitutional and/or pulmonary symptoms
Other Diseases	
Congestive heart failure	Acute or subacute in presentation; dyspnea often with signs including S3 gallop and rales
Asthma and COPD	Acute or chronic in presentation; cough often associated with wheezing

AFB = acid-fast bacillus; BAL = bronchoalveolar lavage; CMV = cytomegalovirus; COPD = chronic obstructive pulmonary disease; DLCO = carbon monoxide diffusion in the lungs; ECG = electrocardiogram; HSV = herpes simplex virus; PFTs = pulmonary function tests; VZV = varicella-zoster virus.

Diagnostic Findings	Comments
Lobar or bronchopneumonia; diagnosis by sputum Gram stain and culture or blood culture	Pneumococcal vaccine indicated for HIV-infected patients with CD4 count $\geq$ 200/mm^3
Lobar or bronchopneumonia; diagnosis by sputum gram stain and culture or blood culture	*Pseudomonas aeruginosa* seen in patients with neutropenia or low CD4 count
Gram stain is nondiagnostic; urinary antigen test may be useful	Uncommon cause of pneumonia in HIV patients
Cavitary lesions common	—
Septic emboli, cavitary lesions, lobar and/or pleural effusion; diagnosis by sputum gram stain and culture or blood culture	Usually seen as septic emboli from endo-carditis; less common after viral pneumonia
Lobar pneumonia, cavitary lesions, hilar adenopathy; miliary pattern diagnosis by AFB stain and culture of sputum or isolator blood culture; bronchoscopy with BAL and biopsy may be necessary in some cases	May present with extrapulmonary disease in patients with advanced HIV disease
Interstitial infiltrates; nasopharyngeal washings for viral antigen may be useful	—
Reticulonodular or diffuse infiltrates; transbronchial biopsy is necessary for definitive diagnosis	Uncommon, but may be seen in patients with advanced HIV disease (CMV), in intubated patients (HSV), or in pregnant women (VZV) presence of CMV or HSV by PCR may not reflect disease need tissue diagnosis
Interstitial infiltrates; examination may be normal, but oxygen saturation is usually decreased; induced sputum examination or BAL by monoclonal antibodies is very sensitive	Desaturation with exercise common; decreased DLCO on PFTs
Focal or diffuse infiltrates; diagnosis by sputum or BAL culture; less commonly cavitary; positive serum cryptococcal antigen	Often indistinguishable from other causes of atypical pneumonia with fever, dry cough
Focal or nodular infiltrates, hilar adenopathy, and effusions; diagnosis by bronchoscopy, isolator blood culture, or bone marrow biopsy; serum or urinary antigen test may be useful	Seen in patients from or visiting endemic areas including Ohio and Mississippi valleys, parts of Caribbean and South and Central America, Southeast Asia, and Africa
Reticular nodular or focal infiltrates; diagnosis by bronchoscopy, isolator blood culture, or bone marrow biopsy; complement fixation antibody usually positive	Seen in patients from or visiting endemic areas in southwestern U.S. and parts of South and Central America
Nodular or interstitial infiltrates; diagnosis by biopsy of other sites or bronchoscopy	May present with fever due to involvement of internal organs
Interstitial infiltrates; diagnosis by bronchoscopy	Responds to prednisone; may flare with initiation of antiretroviral drugs
Nodular or interstitial infiltrates; diagnosis by biopsy of involved sites	—
Nodule or mass; diagnosis by biopsy	Some reports of increased risk in HIV disease
ECG and echocardiographic abnormalities	May be HIV-related or due to underlying cardiac risk factors
Chest radiograph may show hyperinflation and other characteristic changes; peak flow measurements and PFTs useful	—

the radiographic findings, the degree of immunodeficiency as measured by a recent CD4 count, the OI prophylaxis and immunization status, and whether there is active injection-drug use.

Acute bronchitis, pneumococcal pneumonia, TB, influenza (during the winter), and *Staphylococcal aureus* pneumonia (in injection drug users) are the most common causes of pulmonary symptoms in patients with a CD4 count greater than 200 cells/mm³. Opportunistic infections, such as PCP, cryptococcal pneumonia, *Toxoplasma* pneumonia, *Mycobacterium kansasii* infection, *P. aeruginosa* infection, aspergillosis, and pulmonary Kaposi's sarcoma (KS), are included in the differential diagnosis at lower CD4 counts. Fungal infections such as histoplasmosis (endemic in midwestern United States, Mexico, and Central America) and coccidioidomycosis (endemic in southwestern United States) may be considered if the patient has relevant geographic exposure history. *Nocardia asteroides* and *Rhodococcus equi* should be considered in the setting of cavitary lung disease. Atypical pneumonia caused by *Mycoplasma pneumoniae*, *Chlamydia trachomatis*, and *L. pneumophila* are relatively uncommon in HIV-infected patients. Invasive disease caused by *Aspergillus* species has been described in patients with advanced HIV disease and coexisting risk factors, including neutropenia and exposure to antibiotics, corticosteroids, or marijuana. MAC and CMV systemic infections in patients with advanced HIV disease are not generally associated with lung disease. Non-HIV-related conditions, including asthma, COPD, CHF, and respiratory manifestations of drug toxicity (e.g., abacavir hypersensitivity, lactic acidosis), also need to be considered in the differential diagnosis of pulmonary symptoms.

The most common AIDS-defining OI in the United States is PCP, which usually presents subacutely with fever, nonproductive cough, dyspnea, and interstitial infiltrates on chest x-ray. The radiographic findings of PCP may be atypical, especially in patients receiving aerosol pentamidine prophylaxis, who may present with upper lobe disease or spontaneous pneumothorax. In 10% to 20% of patients, the chest x-ray may be normal, but high resolution chest CT will show ground glass opacities.

Although the differential diagnosis of pulmonary symptoms in HIV-infected patients is broad, history, physical examination, and selective laboratory and radiographic studies can narrow the possibilities and provide guidance in management. History should include duration and nature of symptoms, presence of other complaints, history of TB exposure, travel history, underlying pulmonary or cardiac disease, and current medications. If the patient is receiving antiretroviral therapy and OI prophylaxis, the risk of PCP, TB, and, in some instances, conventional bacterial infections will be decreased. Physical examination should focus on the oropharynx, sinuses, heart, lungs, and extremities. Measurement of oxygen saturation is often helpful as a screening tool and in assessing the severity of the condition. Desaturation with exercise increases the likelihood of PCP or another interstitial process.

The diagnostic evaluation of an HIV-infected patient with pulmonary symptoms is based on the results of history and physical examination and measurement of oxygen saturation. Laboratory studies, in addition to reviewing a recent CD4 count and viral load, should include a CBC with differential count, sputum for Gram stain and culture, and usually a chest x-ray. If dyspnea is present or PCP is suspected clinically, an arterial blood gas should be performed to measure the partial pressure of oxygen and the alveolar-arterial oxygen gradient. Both are used to assess severity and to determine the need for adjunctive corticosteroids.

Chest radiography is often helpful in narrowing the differential diagnosis. Diffuse infiltrates are suggestive of PCP, TB (in patients with a low CD4 count), pulmonary KS, cryptococcal pneumonia, histoplasmosis, viral pneumonitis (e.g., influenza, adenovirus), and lymphocytic interstitial pneumonitis (LIP). Focal infiltrates are more common with *S. pneumoniae*, *Hemophilus influenzae*, *L. pneumophila*, *M. pneumoniae*, and TB (in patients with a normal CD4 count). Cavitary lesions should raise the possibility of TB, septic pulmonary emboli from endocarditis with *S. aureus* or other pathogens, aspergillosis, cryptococcosis, or other disseminated fungal infections (histoplasmosis or coccidioidomycosis), infection with *P. aeruginosa*, *N. asteroides, M. kansasii*, or *R. equi*, or aspiration pneumonia. A normal chest x-ray may represent early pneumonia, sinusitis, or bronchitis. In addition, it may represent a noninfectious process such as asthma, COPD, pulmonary hypertension, or lactic acidosis.

If PCP is suspected clinically, an induced sputum for examination has a sensitivity ranging from 50% to 90%, with the lower figure reported in patients receiving aerosol pentamidine for PCP prophylaxis and in facilities with limited experience with the test. Bronchoscopy with BAL is usually needed to establish the diagnosis in patients with a negative induced sputum. Continuing empiric treatment for PCP without a microbiologic diagnosis is generally discouraged because of the prolonged course of therapy required and its potential toxicity, the broad differential diagnosis, and the potential for exacerbation of other undiagnosed OIs in patients requiring adjunctive corticosteroids.

The HIV-infected patient with suspected active TB should be evaluated with a PPD (induration of ≥5 mm is positive) and examination of three expectorated sputum samples for acid-fast bacilli (AFB) stain and culture. False-negative PPD results are possible in patients with a low CD4 count. If there is no sputum production, induced sputum or bronchoscopy should be considered. Although the AFB smear may be negative in up to 70% of patients with advanced immunodeficiency or chest x-ray findings suggestive of primary TB, cultures are positive in over 93% of cases, and lysis-centrifugation blood cultures are positive in up to 20% of cases.

Other diagnostic tests that may be useful in selected clinical instances include *Legionella* urinary antigen, rapid viral culture for influenza and other respiratory viruses, serum cryptococcal antigen, and serum or urine *Histoplasma* antigen. Pulmonary function tests, echocardiography, and exercise tolerance test may be warranted in other settings in which noninfectious causes are considered likely.

The decision about the need for hospitalization may be difficult. If upper airway infection is suspected, symptomatic management for viral infection or an empiric trial of antibiotic therapy for sinusitis as an outpatient is reasonable. If mild bacterial pneumonia or PCP is suspected, an adherent patient may also be managed as an outpatient with close follow-up. However, pneumonia manifesting with high fever, increased respiratory rate, or hypoxemia warrants hospitalization, with rapid collection of sputum for bacterial pathogens and prompt initiation of antibacterial therapy, as well as consideration of empiric PCP coverage if the CD4 count is less than 200 cells/mm^3.

For patients in whom initial evaluation is nondiagnostic, bronchoscopy with BAL and transbronchial biopsy should be considered. Transbronchial biopsy is required for the diagnosis of lymphoma, LIP, and usually for pulmonary KS, although bronchoscopic visualization of typical endobronchial lesions may be diagnostic for KS. Open-lung biopsy in patients with HIV disease is generally reserved for instances in which empiric treatment is ineffective and the transbronchial biopsy is nondiagnostic.

An algorithmic approach to pulmonary symptoms in the HIV-infected patient is presented in Figure 8-1.

Gastrointestinal Symptoms

Diarrhea

Diarrhea may be the most frequently reported HIV-related symptom, especially in patients with advanced disease (Table 8-3). In patients with a normal CD4 count, diarrhea related to medications or non-HIV-related disorders, such as viral gastroenteritis and lactose intolerance, is most common. However, in patients with a CD4 count of less than 100 cells/mm^3, opportunistic pathogens, such as *Cryptosporidium* species and microsporidia, CMV infection, and disseminated MAC infection need to be considered in the differential diagnosis. *Clostridium difficile* colitis, which is associated with recent antibiotic use, can occur at any CD4 count. Salmonellosis and isosporiasis are now unusual because of the widespread use of trimethoprim-sulfamethoxazole (TMP-SMX) for PCP prophylaxis.

The evaluation of diarrhea in an HIV-infected patient is greatly influenced by history. The characteristics of diarrhea to consider include volume (small vs. large), frequency, consistency, duration (acute vs. chronic), and associated symptoms such as tenesmus and blood or mucus in the

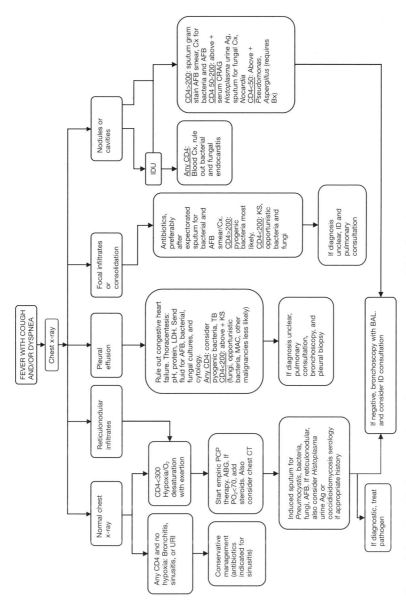

Figure 8-1. Algorithmic approach to pulmonary symptoms in the HIV-infected patient.

Table 8-3.   Causes of Diarrhea in HIV Disease

	Characteristics	Diagnostic Findings	Comments
Infections			
Cryptosporidium	Subacute course; may be associated with wasting	Stool for Cryptosporidium; small bowel biopsy may be necessary	CD4 count < 200 cells/mm³
Microsporida	Subacute course; may be associated with wasting, cholangiopathy	Stool for microsporida; small bowel biopsy may be necessary	CD4 count < 200 cells/mm³
Giardia lamblia	Acute or chronic course; upper and/or lower GI symptoms	Stool for ova and parasite (may require more than one specimen) or duodenal aspirate; Giardia antigen	Any CD4 count; risks include oral–anal sex, travel, and well/fresh water exposure
Cytomegalovirus	Acute to subacute course; may be associated with fever or evidence of retinitis	Colonoscopy with biopsy	CD4 count < 50 cells/mm³
Enteroviruses	Acute, self-limited course	Diagnosed presumptively	—
Bacterial enteritis	Acute course; watery and/or bloody diarrhea	Stool for enteric pathogens; blood cultures if fever present	Increased risk of bacteremia; food history and local epidemiology, sexual history
Clostridium difficile	Acute course; associated with fever	Stool for toxin	Recent antibiotic therapy or hospitalization
Mycobacterium avium complex	Chronic course; fever and constitutional symptoms; may be associated with wasting	Isolator blood or bone marrow culture; colonoscopy with biopsy sometimes necessary	CD4 count < 50 cells/mm³
Drugs	Usually occurs within 4 weeks of initiation of therapy	May require discontinuation of suspected drug, followed by rechallenge (except abacavir); consider anti-diarrheal drug or calcium carbonate	More common with lower CD4 counts and on initiation of treatment

Acute course = ≥3 loose stools for 3–10 days; GI = gastrointestinal.

stool. The patient's degree of immunodeficiency should be considered, as well as the food and travel history, sick contacts, sexual activity, and family history of colitis. In addition, current medications should be reviewed. If a drug likely to cause diarrhea has been recently started and the patient has no constitutional symptoms or blood in the stool, interruption of the drug or the use of an antimotility agent is appropriate.

Physical examination should evaluate for abdominal tenderness, mass, organomegaly, or ascites; the anorectal area should be examined for external lesions, occult blood, or mucus in the stool. Laboratory studies, in addition to reviewing a recent CD4 count and viral load, should include a CBC with differential count, serum electrolytes, serum amylase and lipase if abdominal pain is present, and blood cultures if fever is present. For acute diarrhea, a stool culture for bacterial pathogens and an assay for *C. difficile* toxin are indicated. Evaluation of chronic diarrhea should also include stool ova and parasite examinations (up to three collected at different times), *Giardia* antigen, and, in patients with a CD4 count less than 100 cells/mm^3, a modified AFB stain for *Cryptosporidium* species and microsporidia. If this approach is nondiagnostic, referral to a gastroenterologist for colonoscopy is warranted. An algorithmic approach to diarrhea in the HIV-infected patient is presented in Figure 8-2.

Abdominal Pain

The physical examination and laboratory evaluation of abdominal pain in the HIV-infected patient is guided by the clinical presentation and the degree of immunodeficiency.

One of the most serious causes, usually associated with nausea and vomiting, is acute pancreatitis. Its etiologies include drugs such as pentamidine and didanosine (ddI), hypertriglyceridemia (which can be caused or exacerbated by antiretroviral therapy), excessive alcohol use, OIs, and non–HIV-related conditions such as cholelithiasis and abdominal trauma. Physical examination generally shows periumbilical tenderness. Laboratory studies are noteworthy for increased serum amylase and lipase levels. OIs, such as CMV, and less commonly, cryptosporidiosis, MAC infection, TB, and microsporidiosis, should be considered in the differential diagnosis of pancreatitis in patients with a CD4 count of less than 100 cells/mm^3.

Increasingly recognized in recent years is the syndrome of lactic acidemia related to mitochondrial toxicity from nucleoside reverse-transcriptase inhibitors (NRTIs). In studies to date, lactic acidemia has been most often associated with the combination of ddI and stavudine (d4T), which is no longer recommended, followed by d4T, zidovudine (ZDV), and ddI. Other risk factors for lactic acidemia include female sex, pregnancy, obesity, and use of ribavirin or hydroxyurea. Symptoms may include anorexia, fatigue, nausea, abdominal pain, and diarrhea. Detailed discussion of this topic is presented in Chapter 6.

Another important cause of abdominal pain in patients with a CD4 count of less than 100 cells/mm^3 is lymphoma, which is often accompanied by constitutional symptoms and weight loss. CT scan and tissue biopsy are necessary to establish the diagnosis. Other causes of abdominal pain in persons with advanced immunodeficiency include CMV colitis, MAC infection with mesenteric lymphadenopathy, and TB and MAC immune reconstitution syndromes.

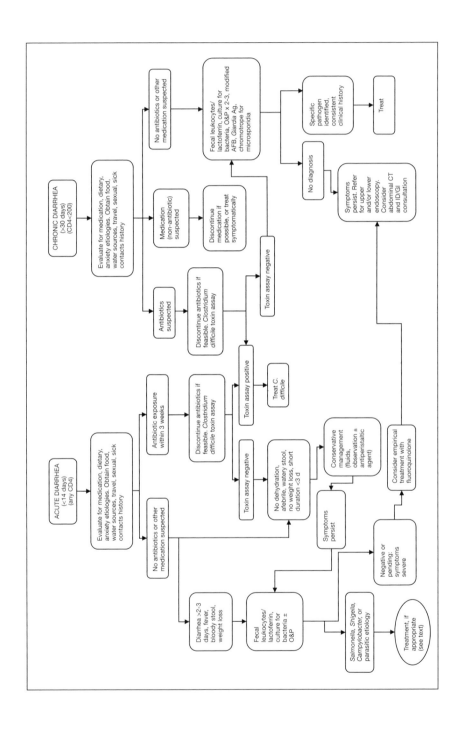

Hepatitis

Hepatitis, both drug-induced and viral, is an important problem in HIV disease (Table 8-4) (see Chapters 6 and 9). Unfortunately, many patients have components of each, which can complicate diagnosis and management of this condition.

Drug-induced hepatitis is defined as increased serum transaminase levels in conjunction with the use of a known hepatotoxin. NRTIs, especially d4T, ZDV, and ddI, have been associated with hepatic steatosis, usually in the setting of lactic acidemia. Drug-induced hepatitis has also been reported with non-nucleoside reverse-transcriptase inhibitors (NNRTIs) and protease inhibitors (PIs). Nevirapine (NVP), an NNRTI, has been associated with severe hypersensitivity-mediated hepatotoxicity, especially in women who initiate NVP with a CD4 count above 250 cells/mm^3. The risk of NVP hypersensitivity reaction is greatest within the first 6 weeks of initiating therapy. When used at full dose, ritonavir (RTV) is the PI most associated with hepatotoxicity. However, RTV is rarely prescribed for its antiretroviral effect anymore; it is now given at much lower doses to inhibit the hepatic metabolism of other PIs. All PIs, whether combined with RTV or not, have the potential for hepatotoxicity. Other medications, including rifabutin, rifampin, isoniazid, and anabolic corticosteroids, can also cause hepatotoxicity.

Hepatitis A virus (HAV), hepatitis B virus (HBV), and hepatitis C virus (HCV) infections occur frequently in the context of HIV disease. In addition, increases in chronic HBV and HCV-related morbidity and mortality have been described in this setting. Initial assessment of an HIV-infected patient with increased serum transaminase levels should include serologic tests for these pathogens. In general, antibody to HAV (anti-HAV), hepatitis B surface antigen (HBsAg), hepatitis B core antibody (HBcAb), and antibody to HCV (anti-HCV) should be obtained. If these tests are negative but HBV or HCV infection is still suspected clinically, quantitative PCR studies should be done.

Figure 8-2. Algorithmic approach to diarrhea in the HIV-infected patient. Antimicrobials should be avoided for EHEC (*E. coli* O157:H7). Antibiotic therapy is not required in many cases of acute bacterial diarrhea because the illness is usually self-limited. Empiric antibiotic therapy is typically given in the following situations: 1) patients with moderate-to-severe travelers' diarrhea as characterized by more than four unformed stools daily, fever, blood, pus, or mucus in the stool; 2) patients with more than eight stools per day, volume depletion, and symptoms for more than one week; 3) patients in whom hospitalization is being considered; and 4) patients with immunocompromised hosts (CD4 < 200 cells/mm^3). Treatment is indicated for *Salmonella typhi, Entamoaba histolytica, Cyclospora cayetanensis, Isospora belli,* and *Giardia lamblia.* Some also advocate treatment for *Shigella* given its high rates of transmission. Seafood exposure: consider *Vibrio* sp. Traveler's diarrhea: treat with empiric fluoroquinolone or TMP-SMX. Proctitis in men who have sex with men: consider sigmoidoscopy.

Table 8-4.   Causes of Abnormal Liver Function in HIV Disease

	Characteristics	Diagnostic Findings	Comments
Viral Infections			
Hepatitis A	Acute onset of fever, constitutional symptoms, jaundice; self-limited >99%; no chronic form	Positive HAV IgM	Fecal-oral transmission
Hepatitis B	Acute or chronic (10%)	Acute: Positive HBsAg anti HBc IgM Chronic: HBsAg > 6 mo	Sexual or bloodborne transmission
Hepatitis C	Acute or chronic (80%); most have progressive disease; may be asymptomatic until cirrhotic	Positive HCV antibody test with confirmatory HCV RNA	Injection-drug users at highest risk
Cholangiopathy	Subacute onset of jaundice; RUQ pain	Increased serum bilirubin and alkaline phosphatase levels; diagnosis by MRCP or ERCP	CD4 count < 200 cells/mm³ etiologies include *Cryptosporidium* (most common); microsporidia, CMV. 20–40% idiopathic
Drugs	Acute or subacute onset; nevirapine-induced hepatitis can be acute and fulminant	Usually mildly to moderately increased serum transaminases	Any CD4 count
Opportunistic Diseases			
Cytomegalovirus	Subacute onset; usually associated with retinitis or GI tract involvement	Liver biopsy may be necessary	CD4 count < 50 cells/mm³
MAC infection	Subacute; associated with fever, GI symptoms, wasting, and/or pancytopenia	Positive isolator blood or bone marrow culture	CD4 count < 50 cells/mm³
Pneumocystis jiroveci (formerly carinii) infection	Subacute; often associated with pulmonary involvement	Liver biopsy	CD4 count < 200 cells/mm³
Bacillary angiomatosis	Subacute; associated with characteristic skin lesions	Liver biopsy	CD4 count < 100 cells/mm³
Lymphoma	Subacute; associated with fever, adenopathy, and/or hepatomegaly	Liver biopsy	CD4 count < 200 cells/mm³

CMV = cytomegalovirus; ERCP = endoscopic retrograde cholangiopancreatography; GI = gastrointestinal; HAV = hepatitis A virus; HBsAg = hepatitis B surface antigen; HCV = hepatitis C virus; IgM = immunoglobulin M; MRCP = magnetic resonance cholangiopancreatography; RIBA = recombinant immunoblot assay.

The pattern, duration, and degree of LFT abnormalities will help define the most likely diagnoses. In an asymptomatic patient, mildly increased transaminases with a normal bilirubin level are often caused by drug toxicity, alcohol use, or chronic HBV or HCV infection. A patient presenting with a febrile illness, moderately to severely increased transaminases, and an increased bilirubin level will most likely have acute HAV or HBV infection. The majority of patients with acute HCV infection will be asymptomatic and have generally lower transaminase levels. Patients with chronic HBV or HCV infection can have acute and usually self-limited increased transaminase levels soon after starting antiretroviral therapy related to immune reconstitution. A cholestatic profile (high serum alkaline phosphatase and bilirubin levels with mildly or modestly increased transaminases) raises the possibility of biliary tract obstruction from gallstones or malignancy, lactic acidemia with hepatic steatosis (see above), or cholangiopathy from cryptosporidiosis, microsporidiosis, CMV, MAC, or HIV infection itself (if the CD4 count is less than 100 cells/mm^3). A very high serum alkaline phosphatase level with mildly or modestly increased transaminases may indicate the presence of infiltrative liver disease. Abdominal ultrasonography or CT or MRI scanning may be useful in this setting.

Upper Gastrointestinal Symptoms

Upper gastrointestinal tract symptoms associated with HIV infection is a common problem. Important causes of anorexia, nausea, and vomiting include medications (antiretroviral and antimicrobial drugs, opiates), lactic acidemia, gastroenteritis, peptic ulcer disease, gastroparesis, hepatobiliary disease, pancreatitis, and OIs. Evaluation is guided by the history and physical examination and may include a CBC with differential count, LFTs, serum amylase, *Helicobacter pylori* antibody test, viral hepatitis serologies, and lactic acid level. Severe or persistent symptoms warrant radiologic imaging and/or endoscopic evaluation. Depression should be considered in the differential diagnosis of patients with persistent unexplained anorexia.

Mouth lesions, which may be exudative or ulcerative, are common in HIV disease. Oropharyngeal candidiasis is seen in patients with a CD4 count of less than 300 cells/mm^3. Candidiasis is sometimes asymptomatic but more often associated with a "bad taste" in the mouth, oral discomfort, or "cut" lips. Physical examination reveals white curd-like exudates (thrush), which can be easily scraped off with a tongue blade, on the buccal mucosa, palate, tongue, or posterior pharynx. Alternative presentations include angular cheilitis (fissured lip margins) and atrophic candidiasis (erythema involving the palate). The diagnosis of candidiasis is suspected clinically and confirmed with a potassium hydroxide (KOH) preparation that reveals budding yeast and pseudohyphae. Fungal cultures are not useful, because *Candida* species can be found in the pharynx of patients without evidence of infection.

Oropharyngeal candidiasis is sometimes confused with oral hairy leukoplakia (OHL). In contrast to thrush, OHL is found on the lateral margins of the tongue and appears as vertically oriented, white, linear plaques that cannot be scraped off with a tongue blade. The causative agent is EBV, and the diagnosis is made clinically. Ulcerative oral lesions usually present with

Table 8-5.   Common Causes of Oral Ulcers in HIV Disease

	Characteristics	Diagnostic Findings	Comments
Herpes simplex virus	Multiple shallow ulcers < 1 cm on buccal mucosa, labia, and/or tongue	Positive Tzanck smear, PCR, or culture	Any CD4 count
Cytomegalovirus	Several shallow ulcers < 1 cm, usually on buccal mucosa	Positive PCR, culture, or biopsy	CD4 count < 50 cells/mm^3
Aphthous ulcers	Multiple punched-out ulcers < 0.5 cm with surrounding erythema; on buccal mucosa and/or labia	Diagnosis of exclusion	Any CD4 count

PCR = polymerase chain reaction.

pain. Common etiologies include aphthous stomatitis, HSV infection, adenovirus infection, and CMV infection (Table 8-5). Oral ulcers are less often associated with syphilis, lymphoma, and medications (e.g., zalcitabine [ddC]).

Candida esophagitis is the most common cause of odynophagia in patients with advanced HIV disease. The likelihood of esophageal candidiasis is increased when thrush is present, but its absence does not exclude the diagnosis. In patients who present with esophageal symptoms without thrush or who do not respond to empiric therapy with fluconazole or another systemic azole, alternative etiologies (e.g., aphthous esophagitis, CMV or HSV infection, or azole-resistant candidiasis) should be considered. Upper endoscopy with biopsy and cultures is required to establish these diagnoses. Biopsies of ulcers caused by CMV or HSV infection show characteristic viral inclusions, whereas no such abnormalities are seen with aphthous esophagitis, which presents with large, sometimes solitary ulcers. In patients with a CD4 count greater than 200 cells/mm^3 who present with odynophagia, esophageal reflux disease or spasm, and other non-HIV-related conditions should be considered in the differential diagnosis.

Weight Loss and Change in Body Habitus

Wasting syndrome—defined as loss of greater than 10% of baseline body weight with chronic diarrhea, weakness, or fever in the absence of a known cause—was one of the earliest recognized manifestations of AIDS. However, lesser degrees of weight loss are clinically significant, and it has now been shown that a 5% reduction is associated with increased risk of OIs and death. In addition to wasting syndrome, other causes of weight loss include: hypogonadism or other endocrine abnormalities; decreased oral

Table 8-6.   Factors Contributing to Weight Loss in HIV Disease

	Etiology	*Management*
Inaccessible food or preparation difficulties	Social or health issues	Social service, homemaker, dietary supplements
Anorexia	Intercurrent illness HIV infection Depression	Treat Megestrol acetate, dronabinol Antidepressant therapy
Nausea, vomiting	Medications HIV gastroparesis	Discontinue, anti-emetic therapy Metoclopramide
Mouth pain, dysphagia, odynophagia	Gingivitis, periodontitis Opportunistic diseases	Dental referral Specific therapy
Diarrhea, malabsorption	Opportunistic diseases HIV infection	Specific therapy Antiretroviral therapy

Adapted from Libman H, Witzburg RA, eds. HIV Infection: A Primary Care Manual. Boston: Little Brown; 1996.

intake because of limited access to food, upper gastrointestinal symptoms, or depression; and loss of nutrients from diarrhea or malabsorption. Weight loss in advanced HIV disease can also be caused by OIs that limit oral intake or nutrient absorption.

When a patient presents with weight loss, the history can elucidate possible causes and the appropriate evaluation and management (Table 8-6). Weight change over time, diet, the presence of diarrhea or symptoms of hypogonadism or depression, medications, and illicit drug use should be elicited. Laboratory studies should include CBC with differential count, serum albumin, thyroid stimulating hormone (TSH), serum testosterone level, PPD, and other studies as warranted by history or physical findings.

Lipodystrophy is a recognized complication of long-term antiretroviral therapy. This condition is characterized by abnormal visceral fat accumulation (abdomen, cervicodorsal fat pad, breasts, lipomas), loss of subcutaneous fat (face, extremities, buttocks), and metabolic derangements (hyperlipidemia, glucose intolerance). More recent data indicate that its pathophysiology is complex. For example, fat accumulation may be secondary to the metabolic complications of PI therapy, whereas lipoatrophy appears to be the result of mitochondrial toxicity from NRTIs. Detailed discussion of this topic is presented in Chapter 6.

Neurologic Symptoms

Neurologic disorders in HIV-infected patients can affect both the central and peripheral nervous systems. Some conditions such as headache, lower extremity pain from drug-induced neuropathy, or weakness from an inflammatory demyelinating polyneuropathy (e.g., Guillain-Barré syndrome),

---

Box 8-2.   Differential Diagnoses of Neurologic Syndromes in HIV Disease

Headache
- Acute/chronic sinusitis
- Cryptococcal meningitis
- Lymphoma
- Toxoplasmosis
- TB meningitis
- Bacterial meningitis
- Syphilis
- Medication-related

Altered Mental Status
- Toxoplasmosis
- Cryptococcal meningitis
- HIV encephalopathy
- Progressive multifocal leukoencephalopathy
- CMV encephalitis
- Syphilis
- Medication-related

Painful Extremities
- Distal sensory polyneuropathy
- CMV polyradiculopathy
- HIV infection
- Syphilis
- Polymyositis
- Diabetes mellitus
- B_{12} deficiency
- Alcohol
- Isoniazid

Focal Deficits
- Toxoplasmosis
- CNS lymphoma
- CNS tuberculosis
- Brain abscess
- Neurosyphilis

CMV = cytomegalovirus; CNS = central nervous system; TB = tuberculosis.

---

can occur at any CD4 cell count, but most other complications are associated with advanced HIV disease (Box 8-2).

Headache, Seizure Activity, and Focal Neurologic Symptoms

In patients with a CD4 count over 200 cells/mm^3, headache is usually caused by muscle tension, migraine, or sinusitis. In patients with a lower CD4 count, OIs should also be considered in the differential diagnosis. The three most common opportunistic diseases that produce headache are cryptococcal meningitis, toxoplasmic encephalitis, and primary CNS lymphoma; less frequent causes include coccidioidomycosis, histoplasmosis, TB, nocardiosis, and pyogenic brain abscess.

The history should include duration, location, and precipitants of headache; associated neurologic and other symptoms; and potential exposures (e.g., travel, TB, drug use). Physical examination should focus on the head, neck, and the central and peripheral nervous systems. For the patient with a CD4 count of less than 200 cells/mm^3 and significant or persistent headache, or headache associated with seizure activity or focal neurologic symptoms, imaging with a contrast-enhanced MRI or CT scan of the brain should be performed to rule out a localized infection or mass lesion. If this study is normal, lumbar puncture with CSF analysis, including cell count, chemistries, cryptococcal antigen, syphilis serology, cytology, and stains and cultures for specific pathogens are indicated. PCR testing may identify CMV, HSV, JC virus (progressive multifocal leukoencephalopathy [PML]), and EBV (primary CNS lymphoma). The serum cryptococcal antigen is a highly sensitive test for diagnosing cryptococcal meningitis.

When enhancing mass lesion(s) are present on CT or MRI, the most likely diagnosis is toxoplasmosis or primary CNS lymphoma. Toxoplasmosis generally appears as multiple ring-enhancing lesions within the gray matter, whereas lymphoma lesions are more likely to be solitary, periventricular, and have substantial surrounding edema and mass effect. The serum IgG antibody to *Toxoplasma* is positive in most patients with toxoplasmic encephalitis because it represents reactivation of a latent infection; a negative serology increases the likelihood of other conditions. In patients with a mass lesion who are seropositive for *Toxoplasma*, empiric antimicrobial therapy is warranted. If a clinical and radiologic response is not seen within 10 to 14 days, SPECT scan with early thallium uptake and CSF-EBV-PCR (sensitivity, 50% to 80%; specificity, >94%) should be considered, but brain biopsy may be necessary to establish a definitive diagnosis of lymphoma. Other less common causes of CNS mass lesions include PML, TB, cryptococcosis, nocardiosis, and pyogenic brain abscess.

Seizure activity and focal neurologic symptoms can be manifestations of CNS disorders in advanced HIV disease. Opportunistic diseases associated with seizures include toxoplasmosis (seizures in 30% of patients), CNS lymphoma (15% of patients), and cryptococcal meningitis (10% of patients). Less commonly, neurosyphilis, TB, and other CNS infections present with seizure activity.

An algorithmic approach to headache in the HIV-infected patient is shown in Figure 8-3.

Altered Mental Status

The evaluation of altered mental status in an HIV-infected patient should follow the same approach as in the general population, with recognition of an increased risk of infectious and neoplastic causes (Table 8-7). History should include the course, nature, and pattern of cognitive change; presence of associated symptoms (e.g., fever, headache, seizure activity, focal neurologic symptoms); medications; and trauma, alcohol, and drug use. All of the CNS processes discussed previously can present with altered mental status, and several other diagnoses should be considered in patients with advanced HIV disease. These include HIV encephalopathy (also known as HIV-associated dementia [HAD]), PML, and CMV encephalitis (Table 8-8).

A slowly progressive decline in cognitive function is the chief characteristic of HAD. In early stages, patients present with short-term memory and concentration loss and slowing of motor function. They may also experience subtle behavioral changes. As HAD progresses over months, pa-

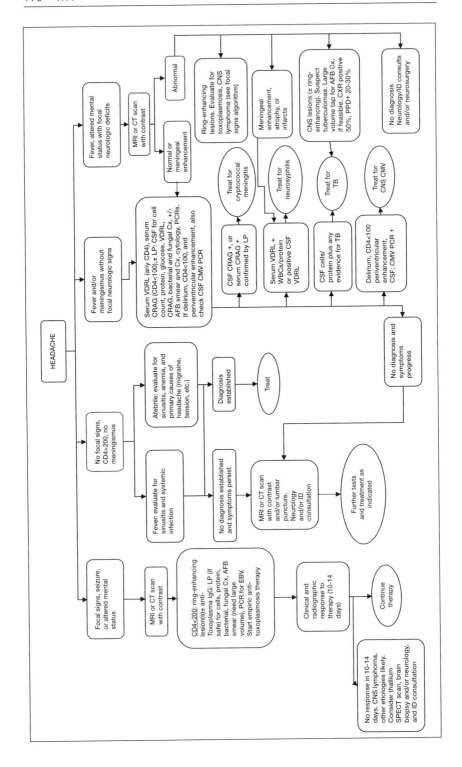

Table 8-7.   Differential Diagnosis of Altered Mental Status ("MEND A MIND")

Etiology	Examples	Comments
Metabolic	Renal or hepatic dysfunction, electrolyte imbalances	Increased risk of chronic liver disease from HBV and HCV
Endocrine	Hyperglycemia, hypoadrenalism	Glucose intolerance and diabetes mellitus have been described with antiretroviral therapy
Neoplasia	Lymphomatous meningitis or primary CNS lymphoma	—
Drugs	Prescribed, complementary, or illicit	Medication levels can be affected by drug interactions
Autoimmune	Systemic lupus erythematosus	—
Mechanical	Subdural hematoma, brain abscess	History or trauma, alcoholism, or injection-drug use
Infections	Toxoplasmosis or CMV encephalitis, bacterial or fungal meningitis, sepsis	Requires prompt and aggressive evaluation
Neuropsychiatric	CVA, seizures, psychosis, schizophrenia	—
Dementia	HIV encephalopathy	Diagnosis of exclusion; may improve with antiretroviral therapy

CMV = cytomegalovirus; CNS = central nervous system; CVA = cerebrovascular accident; HBV = hepatitis B virus; HCV = hepatitis C virus.

tients can develop global dementia. A combination of history, physical examination, and neuropsychologic testing is used to establish the diagnosis. MRI or CT scan of the brain shows diffuse atrophy, and CSF analysis reveals mild pleocytosis and increased protein.

PML commonly manifests with focal neurologic deficits, seizure activity, altered mental status, or a combination of these features. Diffuse nonenhancing white matter abnormalities on radiologic imaging should prompt either lumbar puncture to obtain CSF for JC virus by PCR assay or brain biopsy, which remains the gold standard for diagnosis. A negative PCR for JC virus does not rule out PML, because of its low sensitivity.

CMV encephalitis is the least common of these disorders and presents with rapid evolution of fever, delirium, disorientation, and meningismus in a patient with established systemic CMV disease. Radiologic imaging shows periventricular confluent lesions with enhancement. A positive CSF-CMV-DNA by PCR assay confirms the diagnosis.

Figure 8-3.   Algorithmic approach to headache in the HIV-infected patient.

Table 8-8.   Characteristics of HIV-Associated Dementia, Progressive Multifocal Leukoencephalopathy, and Cytomegalovirus Encephalitis

Diagnosis	Radiologic Imaging	CSF Profile
HAD	Multifocal periventricular white-matter abnormalities	Mild lymphocytic pleocytosis; mildly increased protein
PML	Diffuse nonenhancing white-matter abnormalities	Mild lymphocytic pleocytosis; mildly increased protein; positive JC virus DNA
CMV encephalitis	Diffuse periventricular white-matter enhancement	Moderate lymphocytic pleo-cytosis and increased protein; positive CMV DNA

Painful Extremities

The most frequent cause of painful extremities in HIV-infected patients is distal sensory polyneuropathy, which presents with symmetric numbness, tingling, burning, and/or pain in the feet or hands. Motor weakness is not present. This condition is often the result of drug toxicity (e.g., ddI, d4T) and/or HIV infection itself. Other causes or contributing factors may include alcoholism, thyroid disease, vitamin B_{12} deficiency, syphilis, and diabetes mellitus. In drug-induced neuropathy, early interruption of the offending medication usually leads to resolution of the symptoms. Dose reduction is no longer recommended. Effective antiretroviral therapy may result in improvement in HIV-related neuropathy. Detailed discussion of this topic is presented in Chapter 6.

CMV myelitis and polyradiculitis cause rapidly progressive weakness and numbness in the upper and lower extremities. These syndromes generally occur in patients with a CD4 count of less than 50 cells/mm^3. Myopathy, related to HIV itself or drugs (e.g., ZDV, statins), presents with pain in the muscles, usually in the thighs and shoulders, proximal weakness, and an increased serum creatine phosphokinase (CPK) level.

The history should include the nature, duration, and progression of symptoms, medications, and occupational exposures. Physical examination consists of a neurologic and musculoskeletal assessment. Laboratory studies should include fasting glucose, TSH, CPK, vitamin B_{12} level, and syphilis serology. MRI or CT imaging of the spine should be performed if significant weakness is present. If CMV infection is suspected, lumbar puncture with examination of the CSF for CMV-DNA by PCR assay is necessary. Depending on the clinical presentation, electromyography, nerve conduction studies, and muscle biopsy may also be warranted.

HIV-associated neuromuscular disease is an uncommon cause of weakness related to mitochondrial toxicity from NRTIs. It manifests with ascending paresis and areflexia and can sometimes involve the cranial nerves. Serum CPK and lactic acid levels are increased.

Gynecologic Symptoms

Gynecologic complaints may be the initial manifestation of HIV infection in women. Vulvovaginal candidiasis, cervical dysplasia/cancer, and pelvic inflammatory disease (PID) are more frequent and sometimes more difficult to treat.

Vaginal Discharge and Pelvic Pain

One of the most common complaints in HIV-infected women is vaginal discharge. This symptom can be caused by vaginitis, or it can be the initial manifestation of a more significant problem such as PID. A common problem is recurrent vaginal candidiasis, which is characterized by pruritis and a thick white discharge. Genital HSV infection, which may be recurrent, manifests as painful vesicles.

Pelvic pain can be a manifestation of PID, ectopic pregnancy, HSV infection, or other gynecologic abnormalities, including uterine fibroids, ovarian cysts, and endometriosis. HIV-infected women with PID may have fewer signs of infection and be at increased risk of complications. HIV-infected women are also at increased risk for cervical dysplasia and cancer, both of which are related to human papillomavirus (HPV) infection.

Evaluation of HIV-infected women presenting with vaginal discharge or pelvic pain requires a history and careful abdominal and pelvic examinations. History should focus on the location and nature of symptoms, characteristics of any discharge, and the presence of fever or other associated complaints. Testing for gonorrhea and *Chlamydia* should be performed. Discharge should be examined with KOH preparation for yeast and with normal saline for trichomoniasis and evidence of bacterial vaginosis ("clue cells"). A urine pregnancy test should be done if indicated. Other studies, including pelvic or abdominal ultrasound, and the need for empiric antimicrobial therapy, are determined by the clinical presentation and results of the initial investigation.

Menstrual Abnormalities

HIV-infected women experience menstrual abnormalities at no greater frequency than the general population. Evaluation of menstrual symptoms may include screening for pregnancy, uterine fibroids, and endocrinologic abnormalities. Referral to a gynecologist is appropriate if the patient has persistent dysfunctional bleeding and diagnostic studies are not revealing.

Dermatologic Symptoms

Over 90% of HIV-infected patients have dermatologic symptoms at some time (Table 8-9). Certain skin conditions are unique to HIV disease. These include eosinophilic folliculitis (EF) and dermatologic manifestations of

Table 8-9. Causes of Dermatologic Conditions in HIV Disease

	Clinical Manifestations
Viral Infections	
HIV exanthem (acute retroviral syndrome)	Fever, myalgias, urticaria; truncal, palmar, plantar maculopapules
Herpes simplex	May be relapsing with persistent erosions (*see* Fig. 9-6)
Varicella-zoster	May be recurrent; usually dermatomal (*see* Fig. 9-12)
Molluscum contagiosum	Clusters of white umbilicated papules
Oral hairy leukoplakia	Whitish, nonremovable verrucous plaques on sides of tongue
Warts (HPV)	Increased number and size of verrucous lesions
Fungal Infections	
Candida albicans	Oral mucosal white plaques, sore throat, dysphagia, angular cheilitis, deep tongue erosions (*see* Fig. 9-2); intractable vaginal infection; nail infection
Tinea versicolor	Thick, scaly hypopigmented or light-brown plaques on trunk
Dermatophytes (tinea corporis, pedis, cruris)	Extensive involvement, especially groin and feet
Bacterial Infections	
Staphylococcal	Superficial and subcutaneous infections; impetigo
Syphilis	Primary: painless chancre; secondary: generalized plaques and papulosquamous lesions (*see* Fig. 9-9)
Bacillary angiomatosis	Dome-shaped pedunculated solitary or multiple papules and nodules (4 mm–2 cm) (*see* Fig. 9-1); visceral involvement
Arthropod Infestations	
Scabies	Generalized crusted papules and eczematous lesions
Miscellaneous Disorders	
Seborrheic dermatitis	Red scaling plaques with yellow greasy scales and distinct margins on the face and scalp
Psoriasis	Activation of prior disease or no previous history
Xeroderma	Severe dry skin, possible erythroderma
Papular eruption	2–5-mm skin-colored papules on head, neck, upper trunk; pruritic, chronic
Eosinophilic and bacterial folliculitis	Groups of small vesicles and pustules that can become confluent
Thrombocytopenic purpura	Petechiae
Darkened nails	Dark blue appearance at bases of fingernails
Premature hair graying, long eyelashes	Usually with advanced HIV disease
Drug reactions	*See* Table 8-10
Kaposi's sarcoma	Pale-to-deep violaceous oval plaques and papules; oral lesions; visceral lesions (*see* Fig. 10-1)

Adapted from Libman H, Witzburg RA, eds. HIV Infection: A Primary Care Manual. Boston, Little Brown; 1996.

Diagnosis	Treatment
HIV antibodies usually within 12 weeks of infection; leukopenia, thrombocytopenia, hypergammaglobulinemia	Symptomatic treatment; initiation of antiretroviral therapy
HSV culture, DFA, Tzanck smear for multinucleated giant cells	Acyclovir or famciclovir
VZV culture, DFA, Tzanck smear for multinucleated giant cells	Acyclovir or famciclovir
Biopsy or KOH preparations of soft central material show large viral inclusions	Cryosurgery
Clinical appearance	None generally necessary
Clinical appearance	Topical agents, cryosurgery, surgical excision
KOH slide preparation	Topical: nystatin suspension, clotrimazole troche Systemic: fluconazole
KOH slide shows numerous short hyphae and spores	Topical: selenium sulfide, micronazole, clotrimazole, sodium thiosulfate
KOH slide shows branched, septated hyphae	Topical: miconazole Oral: fluconazole
Culture	Dicloxacillin or cephalexin; TMP-SMX or clindamycin for community-acquired MRSA
Positive VDRL or RPR *and* FTA-abs or MHA-TP	Penicillin
Biopsy	Macrolide or quinolone antibiotic; chronic suppressive therapy may be necessary
KOH or oil preparation shows mites	Permethrin cream; ivermectin for extensive involvement
Biopsy; KOH preparation to rule out tinea	Ketoconazole cream; low-potency topical steroids
Biopsy	Treatment-resistant cases may respond to etretinate
Clinical presentation	Lactic acid emollients
Biopsy shows lymphocytic perivascular infiltrate	Low-potency topical steroids; antipruritic lotions; antihistamines
Biopsy; negative culture for atypical organisms	Ultraviolet B phototherapy for EF; topical and/or systemic antibiotics for bacterial folliculitis
Complete blood count	Antiretroviral therapy
Recent history of zidovudine treatment	None
Physical examination	None
Clinical examination	Alternative drugs
Biopsy	Antiretroviral therapy Localized disease: intralesional chemotherapy, radiation therapy Systemic disease: chemotherapy, interferon

DFA = direct fluorescent antibody; EF = eosinophilic folliculitis; FTA-abs = fluorescent treponemal antibody, absorbed test; HSV = herpes simplex virus; HPV = human papillomavirus; KOH = potassium hydroxide; MHA-TP = microhemagglutination–*Treponema pallidum;* MRSA = methicillin-resistant *Staphylococcus aureus;* RPR = rapid plasma reagin test; TMP-SMX = trimethoprim-sulfamethoxazole; VDRL = Venereal Disease Research Laboratory test for syphilis; VZV = varicella-zoster virus.

primary HIV syndrome, OIs, and certain malignancies. Other conditions, which are seen in the general population as well, are more frequent (e.g., drug eruptions) or more severe or resistant to therapy (e.g., seborrheic dermatitis, psoriasis, xerotic eczema). Some dermatologic conditions may have atypical manifestations resulting in delay in diagnosis and treatment. Examples include ecthymatous varicella-zoster virus (VZV) infection, which presents as "heaped-up" hyperkeratotic lesions, and cryptococcosis manifesting as skin lesions resembling those of molluscum contagiosum. The use of antiretroviral therapy has affected the presentation and course of a number of conditions, with the worsening or precipitation of some of them shortly after initiation of treatment (e.g., EF, VZV), but improvement of others (e.g., KS, molluscum contagiosum, psoriasis). As HIV-infected patients live longer, age-related dermatologic conditions, such as squamous and basal cell cancers, are being reported more frequently.

The diagnosis of skin conditions relies on a history, including duration and distribution of lesions, associated local and systemic symptoms, and potential new exposures (e.g., drugs, travel, occupation, pets, soaps, lotions). Physical examination should focus on skin, mucous membranes, abdomen for organomegaly, and lymph nodes for enlargement. Laboratory studies, in addition to reviewing a recent CD4 count and viral load, should include a CBC with differential count, LFTs, serologies, and other studies as warranted by clinical presentation. Scaling lesions should be scraped and examined for fungal hyphae. If the diagnosis remains obscure, a skin biopsy is indicated. Specimens should be examined using appropriate stains and should be cultured for bacteria, fungi, and mycobacteria.

Infectious Disorders

A wide range of infections, including OIs and other conditions that occur more frequently with HIV disease, can present with skin manifestations. These include cryptococcosis (papular lesions resembling molluscum contagiosum), histoplasmosis (ulcerations or other nonspecific lesions), candidiasis (thrush, angular chelitis, paronychia), syphilis (maculopapular rash), bacterial infection (*S. aureus* folliculitis, abscesses, or pyomyositis), bacillary angiomatosis (cutaneous papular, nodular, or pedunculated lesions sometimes associated with constitutional symptoms), HSV, HPV (warts, dysplasia/cancer), VZV (shingles), and molluscum contagiosum poxvirus (umbilicated papules). Although parasitic cutaneous infestations are unusual in the developed world, scabies can present as a severe crusting disseminated eruption (crusted or "Norwegian" scabies), with the scraping or biopsy showing large numbers of mites. Disseminated cutaneous *Acanthamoeba* infection has also been described in HIV-infected patients.

Noninfectious Disorders

Drug Reactions

Drug reactions are common in HIV-infected patients and may limit the treatment of the virus and its complications (Table 8-10). The most frequent reactions are to sulfonamides, notably TMP-SMX, and to dapsone, which is a sulfone used in the treatment and prophylaxis of PCP and toxoplasmosis. Other agents that often cause rash include abacavir (in the setting of a systemic hypersensitivity reaction), NNRTIs (especially NVP), and the PI fosamprenavir. Drug reactions typically present as pruritic maculopapular, morbilliform, or urticarial eruptions, but they may also appear as erythema multiforme, erythema nodosum, or exfoliative dermatitis (toxic epidermal necrolysis, Stevens-Johnson syndrome). Manifestations of systemic involvement may include fever, increased serum transaminase levels, and interstitial

Table 8-10.   Manifestations of Drug Reactions

Drug	Manifestations	Comments
TMP-SMX	Exanthemous eruption, erythema multiforme, fixed drug eruption, toxic epidermal necrolysis, Stevens–Johnson syndrome	Increased frequency in HIV disease; eruption usually pruritic and associated with fever
Dapsone	Exanthemous eruption, Stevens–Johnson syndrome	May present as sulfone syndrome (fever, rash, hemolytic anemia, and fulminant hepatitis)
Zidovudine (ZDV)	Nail hyperpigmentation with mucous membranes and skin less commonly involved	—
Zalcitabine (ddC)	Oral ulcers	Less commonly associated with ddI
Abacavir	Rash accompanies hypersensitivity reaction in ~60% of cases	Usually associated with fever and worsening constitutional symptoms; drug rechallenge contraindicated
Nevirapine	Exanthemous eruption, Stevens–Johnson syndrome	Risk significantly decreased by dose escalation on initiation of therapy and CD4 count < 250 cells/mm³ in women and CD4 count < 400 cells/mm³ in men
Protease inhibitors	Acute exacerbation of chronic conditions (e.g., eosinophilic folliculitis); erythematous macular rash described with amprenavir	—
Foscarnet	Penile ulcers	Related to direct toxicity of drug on mucous membranes

ddI = didanosine; TMP-SMX = trimethoprim-sulfamethoxazole.

nephritis. Management consists of symptomatic treatment and/or drug discontinuation with careful observation for resolution.

Malignancies
The incidence of KS and anogenital squamous cancer is increased in HIV-infected patients. KS typically presents as reddish-purple macules, papules, nodules, or tumors on the skin or mucous membranes. Early lesions may resemble nevi or bruises, and diagnosis is established with biopsy. HPV-related squamous cell cancer may be asymptomatic or present as a nonhealing lesion or mass. This malignancy may be suspected by physical examination of the cervix or anus/rectum or by abnormal cervical or anal Pap smear results.

Other Conditions
A number of common dermatologic conditions may be more severe or resistant to treatment in the context of HIV disease. Seborrheic dermatitis occurs in up to 80% of HIV-infected patients. It is characterized by scaly erythematous plaques primarily involving the eyebrows, scalp, and nasolabial folds. Other such conditions include xerotic eczema, psoriasis, and Reiter's syndrome (palmoplantar pustules associated with arthritis, urethritis, and/or conjunctivitis).

Eosinophilic folliculitis, which is seen in patients with advanced HIV disease, presents as pruritic pustular lesions involving the chest above the nipples, the face, and the upper extremities. This condition often responds to ultraviolet light therapy. Another HIV-related condition, prurigo nodularis (sometimes referred to as "itchy red bump disease") is characterized by pruritic papular lesions that usually begin on the trunk but can involve any part of the body. This condition is difficult to treat and can result in the development of lichen simplex chronicum or secondary infection from persistent scratching.

KEY POINTS

- Since the introduction of combination antiretroviral therapy, the incidence of OIs has declined, and other infectious and non-infectious disorders now account for an increasing proportion of the complications seen in HIV-infected patients.
- For the assessment of fever in patients with a CD4 count of less than 200 cells/mm^3, the differential diagnosis expands to include HIV-related opportunistic diseases. The risk of OIs is greatest at the lowest CD4 counts.
- *Pneumocystis jiroveci (carinii)* pneumonia (PCP) remains the most common OI responsible for pulmonary symptoms in HIV-infected patients in developed countries.

- Diarrhea is a frequently reported HIV-related symptom. Acute diarrhea is often related to drug toxicity or gastroenteritis; chronic diarrhea, especially in patients with advanced HIV disease, may be a manifestation of a localized or systemic opportunistic disease.

- Neurologic complications, including peripheral neuropathy and central nervous system disorders, are seen in patients with advanced HIV disease. They may present with painful extremities, weakness, altered mental status, or seizure activity.

- In women, recurrent vulvovaginal candidiasis may be the initial manifestation of HIV infection.

- Dermatologic conditions affect more than 90% of HIV-infected patients. Common dermatoses in this setting may be more frequent, severe, and/or resistant to therapy.

SUGGESTED READINGS

Armstrong WS, Katz JT, Kazanjian PH. Human immunodeficiency virus-associated fever of unknown origin: a study of 70 patients in the United States and review. Clin Infect Dis. 1999;28:341-5.

Benson CA, Kaplan JE, Masur H, Pau A, Holmes KK; CDC; National Institutes of Health; Infectious Diseases Society of America. Treating opportunistic infections among HIV-exposed and infected children: recommendations from CDC, the National Institutes of Health, and the Infectious Diseases Society of America. MMWR Recomm Rep. 2004 Dec 17;53(RR-15):1-112. Erratum in: MMWR Morb Mortal Wkly Rep. 2005 Apr 1;54(12):311.

Cengiz C, Park JS, Saraf N, Dieterich DT. HIV and liver diseases: recent clinical advances. Clin Liver Dis. 2005;9:647-66, vii.

Currier JS, Havlir DV. Complications of HIV disease and antiretroviral therapy. Top HIV Med. 2005;13:16-23.

Feldman C. Pneumonia associated with HIV infection. Curr Opin Infect Dis. 2005;18:165-70.

Havlir DV, Barnes PF. Tuberculosis in patients with human immunodeficiency virus infection. N Engl J Med. 1999;340:367-73.

Kaplan JE, Masur H, Holmes KK. Guidelines for preventing opportunistic infections among HIV-infected persons—2002. Recommendations of the U.S. Public Health Service and the Infectious Diseases Society of America. MMWR Recomm Rep. 2002;51(RR-8):1-52.

Kotler DP. HIV infection and the gastrointestinal tract [Editorial]. AIDS. 2005;19:107-17.

Levine AM. Evaluation and management of HIV-infected women. Ann Intern Med. 2002;136: 228-42.

Maurer TA. Dermatologic manifestations of HIV infection. Top HIV Med. 2005;13:149-54.

Ogedegbe AE, Thomas DL, Diehl AM. Hyperlactataemia syndromes associated with HIV therapy. Lancet Infect Dis. 2003;3:329-37.

Shelburne SA, Visnegarwala F, Darcourt J, Graviss EA, Giordano TP, White AC Jr., et al. Incidence and risk factors for immune reconstitution inflammatory syndrome during highly active antiretroviral therapy. AIDS. 2005;19:399-406.

Skiest DJ. Focal neurological disease in patients with acquired immunodeficiency syndrome. Clin Infect Dis. 2002;34:103-15.

Thomas CF Jr., Limper AH. Pneumocystis pneumonia. N Engl J Med. 2004;350:2487-98.

Chapter 9

Diagnosis and Management of Opportunistic Infections

SONIA NAGY CHIMIENTI, MD
LORI A. PANTHER, MD, MPH
CAMILLA S. GRAHAM, MD, MPH

This chapter reviews the epidemiology, microbiology, pathogenesis, clinical manifestations, diagnosis, and management of opportunistic infections (OIs). Essential to the control of many OIs is reconstitution of the immune system. However, controversy exists regarding the appropriate timing of antiretroviral therapy (ART) in relation to treatment of active OIs. For patients who are on ART at the time of development of an OI, continuation of ART and optimizing it as necessary are recommended. For patients who are not taking ART at the time of development of an OI, it is unclear whether the benefits of immediate ART outweigh the risks of increased inflammation from immune reconstitution and toxicity from drug interactions. For cryptosporidiosis, microsporidiosis, progressive multifocal leukoencephalopathy, and Kaposi's sarcoma (KS), it is generally accepted that early ART is important. For tuberculosis (TB), *Mycobacterium avium* complex (MAC) infection, *Pneumocystis jiroveci* (formerly *carinii*) pneumonia (PCP), and cryptococcal meningitis, most experts recommend delaying ART until an initial response is seen from treatment of the OI.

The recommendations presented in this chapter are based on guidelines issued by the Centers for Disease Control and Prevention (CDC), the Department of Health and Human Services, and the HIV Medicine Association of the Infectious Diseases Society of America. The latest federal guidelines for the treatment of OIs are available at http://www.hivatis.org/guidelines.

Bartonellosis

Microbiology

Sophisticated molecular diagnostic techniques have resulted in better characterization and increased detection of *Bartonella* species. Bartonellosis in an AIDS patient was first described in 1983 presenting as subcutaneous nodules with bacterial forms on Warthin-Starry stain. Cat scratch disease (CSD) and its systemic equivalent, bacillary angiomatosis (BA), are caused by *B. henselae* or *B. quintana*. *B. henselae* infection has been linked to cat or flea exposure, whereas *B. quintana* infection has been associated with body or head lice infestation.

Pathogenesis

Inoculation with *Bartonella* species via a lick or bite from a cat or kitten evokes an inflammatory response and endothelial proliferation presenting as a nodule at the site of inoculation (CSD). In HIV-infected patients, the organism may disseminate because of compromised immune function. Bacteremia is associated with foci of vascular and endothelial cell proliferation manifesting as nodules or cysts within the skin, lymph nodes, bones, or viscera (BA).

Clinical Manifestations

In immunocompetent patients, CSD presents as an ulcerated nodule at the site of inoculation associated with fever and regional lymphadenopathy. CSD usually resolves in 1 to 2 months without treatment in healthy people and is rarely associated with systemic symptoms. The risk for BA is highest in HIV-infected patients with a CD4 count of less than 50 cells/mm^3. BA manifests as rapidly proliferating papules or ulcerated nodules that easily bleed and can be confused with KS (Table 9-1 and Figure 9-1). With systemic dissemination, fever is almost universal. Abdominal pain and increased serum transaminase and alkaline phosphatase levels are common with liver involvement ("peliosis hepatis"). *Bartonella* species has also been reported to cause "culture-negative" endocarditis, large vessel vasculitis, and neuroretinitis in HIV-infected patients.

Table 9-1.   Features of Bacillary Angiomatosis and Kaposi's Sarcoma

	Bacillary Angiomatosis	*Kaposi's Sarcoma*
Lesion appearance	Red papule/nodule, plaque rare; blanching; bleeds easily; painful	Purple papule/nodule/plaque; nonblanching; does not bleed easily; not painful
Progression in size and number of lesions	Often very rapid	Usually slow; occasionally rapid
Bone lesions	Sometimes	No
Systemic symptoms	Often	Rare
Histology	Round vascular space; plump endothelial cells; WBC infiltrate; stromal edema	Slit-like vascular space; spindled endothelial cells; no WBC infiltrate; no stromal edema

WBC = white blood cell.

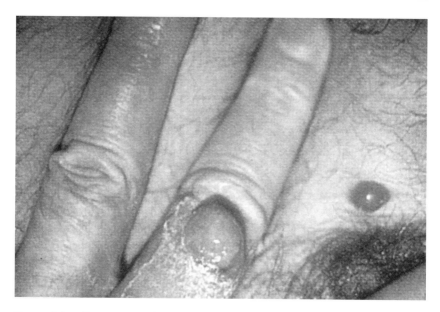

Figure 9-1. Characteristic skin lesions of bacillary angiomatosis. (From Koehler JE, LeBoit PE, Egbert BM, Berger TG. Cutaneous vascular lesions and disseminated cat-scratch disease in patients with acquired immunodeficiency syndrome (AIDS) and AIDS-related complex. Ann Intern Med. 1988;109:449-55; with permission.)

Diagnosis

Diagnosis of BA is problematic because of the low sensitivity (culture and Warthin-Starry silver stain) and low specificity (cytology, histopathology) of generally available tests. Hematoxylin and eosin stain of infected tissue shows lobular proliferation of small blood vessels with plump endothelial cells, stromal edema, inflammation, and granular clumps of eosinophilic material, which prove to be the trilaminar-walled bacilli on electron microscopy. Warthin-Starry silver stain is more specific for demonstrating *Bartonella* species. Culture of blood or involved tissues is recommended despite its low sensitivity for the purposes of speciation and public health reporting. The yield of blood cultures has improved with the use of enriched lysis-centrifugation tubes.

An IgG immunoflourescent antibody (IFA) test for *B. henselae* and *B. quintana* has a sensitivity of 82% to 95% and a specificity of 93% to 96% for the diagnosis of CSD. An IFA titer of greater than 1:256 strongly suggests active infection. The prevalence of a positive IFA in afebrile persons is 4% to 7%. An enzyme immunoassay (EIA) for IgM and IgG has been reported to have a sensitivity of 75% for IgG alone, 48% for IgM alone, and 85% overall when used for the diagnosis of CSD; its specificity is 98% to 100%. Whereas IFA cannot reliably distinguish between the various

Bartonella species, DNA detection by polymerase chain reaction (PCR) allows for speciation of the organism.

Management

Because *Bartonella* infection is unusual, treatment recommendations for HIV-infected patients are based on clinical experience. Standard doses of erythromycin, doxycycline, clarithromycin, and azithromycin have all been used with success. The length of therapy is determined by the severity of illness: two months is recommended for isolated cutaneous disease, three months for bacteremia or suspected bacteremia, and four months for deep organ infection, osteomyelitis, or endocarditis. Clinical response to treatment is generally seen within two to three days. A Jarisch-Herxheimer reaction has been described on initiation of therapy. A single episode of BA does not require maintenance therapy, but chronic suppression with erythromycin or doxycycline should be considered for recurrent disease, especially in patients with a CD4 count below 100 cells/mm^3.

Primary prevention is focused on the education of HIV-infected patients regarding cat ownership. They should avoid licks, scratches, or bites from cats and contact with kittens, and they should use flea-control measures. Declawing is not necessary. There is no evidence that routine laboratory screening of cats is useful in prevention.

Candidiasis

Epidemiology and Pathogenesis

Mucosal infections with *Candida* species, most commonly *C. albicans*, occur in the majority of HIV-infected patients. Esophageal candidiasis is an AIDS-defining diagnosis. In HIV-infected women, recurrent vulvovaginal candidiasis is a common initial complaint and usually presents before oral infection. Other factors that predispose to candidal infection include diabetes mellitus, antibiotic therapy, and nasal, inhaled, and systemic corticosteroid therapy. *Candida* species live as commensal organisms in the oral cavity and the female genital tract. Decreased lymphocyte proliferative response to *Candida* antigen and decreased specific mucosal antibodies may predispose to mucous membrane infection in the context of HIV disease.

Clinical Manifestations

Oral candidiasis, the pseudomembranous form of which is called "thrush," typically occurs in patients with a CD4 count between 200 and 500 cells/mm^3. Symptoms may include mouth discomfort and altered taste sensation, and physical examination shows "cottage cheese-like" white plaques on the oral mucosa. Esophageal candidiasis presents in patients with a CD4 count of less than 200 cells/mm³. Symptoms include dysphagia, odynophagia, and retrosternal pain with swallowing. Although 30% of patients with esophageal candidiasis do not have oral manifestations, esophageal symptoms occurring with thrush usually indicate contiguous spread of the infection.

Recurrent vulvovaginal candidiasis is common in HIV-infected women with a normal CD4 cell count, as well as in the general population. Symptoms of vulvovaginal candidiasis include vaginal itching, dysuria, vulvar pain, and dyspareunia. Physical examination shows a thick, adherent, white vaginal discharge with a pH of 4 to 4.5.

Despite the frequent occurrence of mucosal candidiasis, candidemia and deep tissue involvement are unusual. Disseminated infection, when it occurs, is associated with traditional risk factors, such as neutropenia, intravascular line infection, or chronic corticosteroid therapy.

Diagnosis

Diagnoses of thrush (Figure 9-2, *A*) and vulvovaginal candidiasis are suspected clinically and confirmed by potassium hydroxide (KOH) preparation. Invasive forms, which exhibit pseudohyphae, can be distinguished from commensal organisms, which exist as oval yeast. Other forms of oral candidiasis include atrophic candidiasis, manifested by erythema of the tongue or oral mucosa without white plaques (Figure 9-2, *B*), and angular cheilitis, manifested by crusting and fissures at the corners of the mouth. Differential diagnosis of oral candidiasis includes oral hairy leukoplakia, which presents as white plaques on the lateral aspect of the tongue or buccal mucosa. In esophageal candidiasis, upper endoscopy shows a white exudate overlying friable mucosa; biopsy and culture are necessary for confirmation. Differential diagnosis of esophageal symptoms in HIV-infected patients includes cytomegalovirus (CMV) and herpes simplex virus (HSV) infections, lymphoma, and KS.

Management

Treatment for candidiasis is presented in Table 9-2. For oral candidiasis, recommended topical therapy consists of 10-mg troches of clotrimazole or 5 mL of nystatin suspension taken orally up to 5 times daily for 7 to 10 days; systemic therapy with oral fluconazole 100 mg/d is reserved for refractory cases. If the clinical suspicion for esophagitis is high, empiric antifungal therapy is initiated with fluconazole 200 mg/d. If there is no response within 7 days, upper endoscopy with biopsy is recommended. For vulvovaginal candidiasis, topical cream or ointment containing clotrimazole, miconazole, butoconazole, tioconazole or terconazole, nystatin vaginal tablets (100,000 U/tab), or boric acid vaginal capsules (600 mg/cap) is usually successful. Oral fluconazole (150 mg given once) can be used as an alternative.

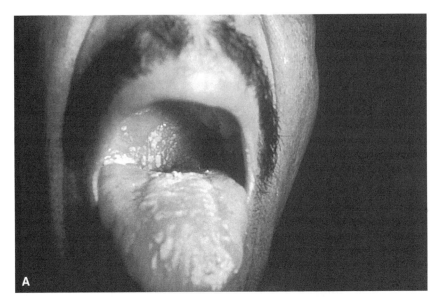

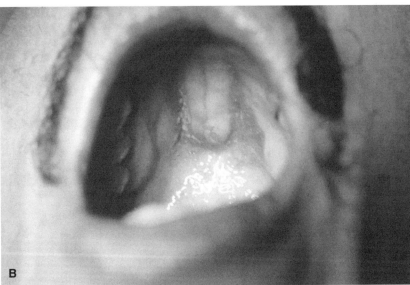

Figure 9-2. Pseudomembranous **(A)** and atrophic **(B)** variants of oral candidiasis. (For color reproduction, see Plates 1 and 2 at back of book.)

In fluconazole-refractory cases, higher doses of fluconazole (400 to 800 mg/d), oral itraconazole suspension (200 mg/d on an empty stomach), oral voriconazole (200 mg bid), oral posaconazole (400 mg bid), oral amphotericin B suspension (100 mg/mL, 1-5 mL qid), intravenous amphotericin B (0.3 to 0.6 mg/d), or intravenous caspofungin (50 mg/d) may be

Table 9-2.   Treatment of Candidiasis

Condition	Therapy
Oral infection (thrush)	Nystatin suspension swish-and-swallow 5 mL five times daily or clotrimazole troche 10 mg five times daily × 7–10 d
Cutaneous infection	Clotrimazole 2% or other antifungal cream*
Vulvovaginitis	Clotrimazole 2% or other antifungal cream or troches† or fluconazole 150 mg orally given once
Oral, cutaneous, or vulvovaginal infection; refractory to topical therapy or frequently recurrent	Fluconazole 100 mg/d orally × 7–14 d
Esophagitis	Fluconazole 200 mg/d orally × 14–21 d
Esophagitis; refractory to fluconazole	Voriconazole 200 mg twice daily or itraconazole suspension 200 mg/d orally or fluconazole 400–800 mg/d orally × 14–21 d
Fungemia or disseminated infection	Amphotericin B 0.3–0.6 mg/kg/d IV or caspofungin 50 mg/d IV after single loading dose of 70 mg IV or voriconazole 200 mg twice daily after two loading doses of 400 mg given the first day

* Miconazole, butoconazole, tioconazole, terconazole.
† Nystatin vaginal troches 100,000 U/tab or clotrimazole troches 10 mg.

necessary. The duration of treatment of *Candida* esophagitis is 14 to 21 days.

Maintenance antifungal therapy is generally not recommended for mucosal candidiasis in HIV-infected patients because of the potential for side effects, drug interactions, and the emergence of resistant nonalbicans *Candida* species. However, in patients with a CD4 count less than 50 cells/mm^3, prophylaxis reduces the frequency of recurrent infection without an impact on mortality. In this setting, oral fluconazole 50 to 200 mg/d is usually effective.

Coccidioidomycosis

Epidemiology

Coccidioides immitis is a dimorphic fungus that is endemic in the Southwestern United States and parts of Central and South America. Most disease is thought to result from reactivation infection from prior exposure, so a patient who has lived in an endemic area at any time should be considered at risk. The incidence of disease in HIV-infected patients from endemic areas has been estimated to be as high as 2% to 5%. Asians (especially Filipinos), African-Americans, and Hispanics are at increased risk for dissemination, as are women in the third trimester of pregnancy.

Pathogenesis

Primary infection is thought to occur via inhalation of *C. immitis* spores (arthroconidia), followed by subclinical or symptomatic pneumonia. The arthroconidia transform into spherules in pulmonary tissue. Persons who have had extensive exposure to disrupted soil harboring the organism are at greatest risk of acquiring the infection. Outbreaks have been reported after dust storms, earthquakes, and soil excavation.

Clinical Manifestations

Primary infection manifests as fever, respiratory complaints, arthritis, and/or rash (erythema multiforme, erythema nodosum). The most common presentation of coccidioidomycosis in AIDS is disseminated disease, with constitutional symptoms, generalized lymphadenopathy, nodular skin lesions, and involvement of the bones, joints, and liver. Approximately 25% of patients with disseminated disease have meningitis, which can be complicated by hydrocephalus and other neurologic sequelae.

Diagnosis

The diagnosis of coccidioidomycosis is made by culture of the organism from clinical specimens. Laboratory personnel should be alerted when specimens are sent for culture of this highly infectious pathogen so that appropriate safety measures can be taken. Direct examination of specimens using 10% KOH may reveal the typical thick-walled spherule containing endospores, which are released when it ruptures. Histopathology demonstrates both acute suppurative and granulomatous inflammation. The fungus may also be seen as hyphae in pulmonary cavities or in meningeal tissue. Blood cultures are generally negative. Serologic studies include IgM and IgG antibody tests. The IgM test is positive in 75% of patients with acute infection, appearing within 1 to 3 weeks and persisting for up to 3 to 4 months. Occasionally, it can become positive again in the setting of reactivation. The IgG test is helpful in determining the extent and progression of disease. For example, titers are greater than 1:32 in patients with disseminated disease or untreated extrapulmonary disease. For patients with meningeal involvement, cerebrospinal fluid (CSF) IgG serology is usually positive as well, and serum and CSF titers can be monitored to assess the response to treatment.

Management

Expert consultation is recommended for clinicians with limited experience in the treatment of coccidioidomycosis. The mainstay of therapy has been intravenous amphotericin B for pulmonary and disseminated disease without meningeal involvement. Data regarding dosing of this drug are limited;

patients are maintained on therapy until clinical improvement is demonstrated, usually following a total dose of 500 to 1000 mg. Oral fluconazole or itraconazole may be given as alternative therapy for mild disease, but the relapse rate approaches 50%. The role of azoles, given in conjunction or sequentially with amphotericin B, is unclear. In meningeal disease, fluconazole has been shown to be up to 80% effective. Intrathecal amphotericin B may be given as alternative or adjunctive therapy, but toxicity may limit its use.

Serum titers should be followed at monthly intervals until there has been consistent clinical improvement. CSF titers and other abnormalities may persist despite appropriate therapy. Lifelong preventive therapy with fluconazole (400 mg/d) or itraconazole (200 mg/bid) is recommended after treatment is completed.

Community-Acquired Pneumonia

Epidemiology

Community-acquired pneumonia (CAP) is common in HIV-infected patients, with the highest risk in injection-drug users. The most frequent bacterial pathogens are the same as those in immunocompetent hosts and include *Streptococcus pneumoniae*, *Staphylococcus aureus*, *Haemophilus influenzae*, and *Klebsiella pneumoniae*. *Nocardia*, *Bordatella*, *Legionella*, and *Rhodococcus* species, although less common, have also been described. Two-thirds of HIV-infected patients presenting with CAP have a CD4 count of less than 200 cells/mm^3. Since the advent of effective combination antiretroviral therapy, the incidence of bacteremic pneumococcal pneumonia has decreased by 50%. While there is no evidence that influenza is more common in HIV-infected patients, it may be more severe.

Pathogenesis

The increased risk of bacterial CAP in HIV disease appears related to impaired immune function rather than increased exposure or colonization. Decreased B-cell lymphocyte activation, IgA and IgG production, opsonizing ability, alveolar macrophage function, and antibody-dependent cytotoxicity all likely contribute.

Clinical Manifestations

Symptoms of CAP in HIV-infected patients are similar to those of the general population, with acute onset of fever, productive cough, pleuritic chest pain, and dyspnea. Atypical pneumonia with *Legionella* species, *Mycoplasma pneumoniae*, and respiratory viruses should be considered in patients with a nonproductive cough. In patients with advanced HIV disease who present with pneumonia, it is necessary to consider the possibility of concurrent PCP, TB, and other OIs.

Diagnosis

Sputum should be sent for gram stain, bacterial culture, and mycobacterial stain and culture. Sputum examination establishes a presumptive diagnosis in 50% of patients with pneumococcal pneumonia. As with the general population, sputum cultures are less helpful for microbiologic diagnosis because of overgrowth of oropharyngeal flora. In patients with suspected concurrent PCP, induced sputum for immunofluorescent antibody stain should also be obtained. Ninety percent of patients with bacterial pneumonia have a unilateral infiltrate on chest x-ray; pleural effusions and cavitary lesions are less common. In patients with diffuse infiltrates, atypical pathogens or PCP should be considered in the differential diagnosis. Common laboratory abnormalities associated with CAP include leukocytosis (although less so in patients with advanced immunodeficiency) and hypoxemia.

Management

The response of CAP to a 10- to 14-day course of antibiotic therapy is similar to that in HIV-seronegative patients. Initial therapy, either with ceftriaxone or cefotaxime (with or without erythromycin) or with levofloxacin is recommended. Critically ill patients with a gram stain suggestive of *S. aureus* infection should be empirically started on vancomycin. More than one active pulmonary infection should be considered if the patient does not show rapid improvement to initial treatment. The rate of recurrent pneumococcal disease in HIV-infected patients is twice that of the general population. Penicillin-resistant *S. pneumoniae* does not seem to occur with greater frequency.

Although the immunogenicity of the 23-valent polysaccharide pneumococcal vaccine is decreased in HIV-infected patients, it is recommended if the CD4 count is greater than 200 cells/mm^3 (see Table 3-3 in Chapter 3). *H. influenzae* type B vaccine is not advised in HIV-infected adults because the strains covered by this preparation comprise only a minority of invasive infections. It is noteworthy that the frequency of bacterial pneumonia is decreased by more than 40% in HIV-infected patients taking trimethoprim-sulfamethoxazole (TMP-SMX) for PCP prophylaxis. Similar benefits may be associated with the use of macrolides for prophylaxis of MAC infection. Nevertheless, these antibiotics should not be prescribed solely for the primary prevention of bacterial pneumonia.

Cryptococcosis

Epidemiology

Earlier in the AIDS epidemic, 5% to 10% of HIV-infected patients, most of whom had advanced immunodeficiency, were diagnosed with cryptococcosis. Meningoencephalitis is the most common presentation, but pulmonary and cutaneous involvement has also been described. The incidence of cryptococcosis is highest in injection-drug users, Africans, African-Americans, and Haitians. The mortality rate of cryptococcal meningitis is approximately 20%.

Pathogenesis

The majority of cryptococcal disease in AIDS is caused by *Cryptococcus neoformans*. The organism is an encapsulated yeast that is ubiquitous in soil. Its primary mode of acquisition is via the respiratory route, with secondary spread hematogenously to the brain, lungs, bone marrow, liver, and spleen. HIV-related abnormalities in opsonization, cell-mediated immunity, and humoral immunity permit its growth and dissemination. The polysaccharide capsule of *Cryptococcus* is poorly immunogenic, and minimal inflammation is observed in pathologic specimens.

Clinical Manifestations

Pulmonary cryptococcosis may be asymptomatic, or it may present similarly to other atypical pneumonias with fever and a nonproductive cough. Occasionally skin lesions mimicking molluscum contagiosum have been described in patients with disseminated disease.

Symptoms and signs of cryptococcal meningitis are often indolent and nonspecific. Fever is present in 60% to 80% of cases, headache in over 70%, altered mental status in 25%, meningismus in 25% to 30%, seizure in 5%, and focal neurologic deficits in 6% to 11%. Extraneural cryptococcal disease occurs in 50% of patients. Clinical features on presentation that portend a poor prognosis include concomitant extraneural disease, altered mental status, hyponatremia, cerebrospinal fluid (CSF) cryptococcal antigen (CrAg) titer greater than 1:1024, CSF white blood cell count (WBC) of less than 20 cells/mm^3, and CSF opening pressure greater than 30 cm H$_2$O.

Diagnosis

When pulmonary or systemic cryptococcosis is suspected, sputum and blood fungal cultures, as well as a serum CrAg, should be performed, and cryptococcal meningitis should be ruled out with a lumbar puncture (LP). A positive CSF CrAg is diagnostic of cryptococcal meningitis. In general, the CSF WBC shows a mild lymphocytosis, the glucose is normal or slightly low, and the protein is mildly increased. AIDS patients with cryptococcal meningitis usually have a lower cell count and higher organism load in the CSF compared with others with the disease. India ink examination is positive in 75% to 80% of cases. The organisms are 4 to 6 μM narrow-based, budding, round yeast cells with a distinct capsule (Figure 9-3). Culture of the CSF remains the "gold standard" for diagnosis, although rarely it may

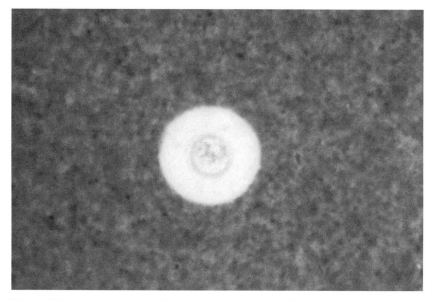

Figure 9-3. *Cryptococcus neoformans* on India ink stain of cerebrospinal fluid.

be negative. The serum CrAg is positive in over 99% of HIV-infected patients with cryptococcal meningitis. Rare false-positive tests occur with poorly encapsulated strains and from cross-reactivity with rheumatoid factor or systemic infection with *Trichosporon*. Blood cultures are positive in 75% of cases.

Brain imaging with computed tomography (CT) or magnetic resonance imaging (MRI) should be performed in all cases of suspected cryptococcal meningitis to rule out a space-occupying lesion. Differential diagnosis includes other subacute meningitides, partially treated bacterial meningitis (if the patient is on chronic antibiotic therapy), viral meningoencephalitis, syphilis, toxoplasmosis, and lymphoma.

Management

Expert consultation is recommended for clinicians with limited experience in the treatment of cryptococcal infection. Isolated pulmonary disease, urinary tract infection, or fungemia can be treated with oral fluconazole 200 to 400 mg/d with or without flucytosine 100 to 150 mg/kg/d or oral itraconazole 200 to 400 mg/d for 10 weeks (Table 9-3).

For patients with severe cryptococcal meningitis manifested by altered mental status, cranial nerve palsy, high opening CSF pressure, or CSF CrAg titer greater than 1:64, a 2-week induction with intravenous amphotericin B at 0.7 to 1.0 mg/kg/d plus flucytosine 100 mg/kg/d, followed by oral fluconazole 400 mg/d for 8 additional weeks is recommended. Amphotericin B

Table 9-3.   Treatment of Cryptococcosis

Condition	Initial Therapy	Maintenance Therapy
Nonmeningeal disease	Fluconazole 200-400 mg/d orally × 10 wk *or* Itraconazole 200-400 mg/d orally × 10 wk	None
Meningitis	Amphotericin B 0.7-1.0 mg/kg/d IV *plus* Flucytosine 25 mg/kg 4 times daily orally × 14 days *followed by* Fluconazole 400 mg/d orally × 8 wk *or* until CSF culture is sterile	Fluconazole 200 mg/d orally

is administered until a total dose of 15 mg/kg is reached and/or symptoms resolve. The clinical response rate is approximately 70% using this approach, and the mortality rate is under 10%. Toxicities of amphotericin B include phlebitis, fever, rigors, nausea, vomiting, anemia, hypokalemia, hypomagnesemia, and renal tubular acidosis. The addition of flucytosine to amphotericin B has been demonstrated to decrease the rate of relapse, but it may not be well tolerated in HIV-infected patients because of hematologic and renal toxicity. Liposomal amphotericin B is associated with less nephrotoxicity and can be used as an alternative agent in patients with significant renal dysfunction. Its optimal dose has not been determined, but treatment success has been reported with 4 mg/kg daily. Flucytosine should not be used in conjunction with liposomal amphotericin because of an increased risk of renal toxicity. Intrathecal amphotericin B is sometimes given for refractory cases of cryptococcal meningitis.

Compared with amphotericin B, fluconazole as initial therapy is associated with a higher early mortality, slower CSF organism clearance, and a lower response rate to treatment. An induction regimen of oral fluconazole 400 to 800 mg/d plus flucytosine 100 to 150 mg/kg/d for 6 weeks should be considered only in patients with mild cryptococcal meningitis (normal mental status, nonfocal examination, normal opening pressure, CSF CrAg < 1:64) and intolerance to standard therapy. Flucytosine monotherapy should never be used in the treatment of cryptococcosis because of the rapid emergence of resistance.

Since the prognosis of cryptococcal meningitis associated with a high CSF opening pressure is worse, it is recommended that patients with CSF opening pressures of 25 cm H_2O or greater have large-volume CSF drainage after an intracerebral mass lesion has been ruled out. Frequent, repeated LPs are indicated early to remove CSF and decrease intracranial pressure (ICP). There is no indication that high-dose corticosteroids or acetazolamide are of benefit in this setting. The importance of normalization of ICP cannot be overstated. Approximately 93% of deaths in the initial two weeks of treatment and 40% of deaths in weeks 3 to 10 are associated with a high ICP. CSF shunting may be necessary for patients who cannot tolerate daily LPs and for those whose symptoms and signs do not improve with this approach.

Initial treatment regimens should be changed to secondary prophylaxis after 10 weeks. Generally, oral fluconazole 200 mg/d is recommended for maintenance therapy. If a clinical response is obvious, it is not necessary to repeat the LP at the end of treatment to document clearance of the organism. However, if symptoms or signs of cryptococcal meningitis recur, a repeat LP must be performed. Relapse of cryptococcal meningitis on maintenance therapy may indicate persistent infection in sequestered sites such as the prostate gland and is associated with increased mortality. Retrospective data provide support for discontinuing secondary prophylaxis in patients who are asymptomatic, have completed their initial antimicrobial therapy, and have an increase in their CD4 count to over 100 to 200 cells/mm^3 for at least 6 months on ART.

Cytomegalovirus Infection

Epidemiology

Before the advent of effective combination ART, CMV disease was reported in 20% to 40% of HIV-infected patients, most of whom had a CD4 count of less than 50 cells/mm^3. However, in recent years, there has been a dramatic decrease in new cases. CMV disease is usually the result of reactivation of chronic latent infection and has ocular, gastrointestinal, and nervous system manifestations.

Clinical Manifestations

Retinitis represents 75% to 85% of CMV disease in AIDS. It may be asymptomatic or present with painless blurring of vision, blind spots, "floaters," or scotomata; retinal detachment may result in acute loss of vision. There have been reports of spontaneously resolving CMV retinitis during immune reconstitution with ART, as well as atypical presentations consisting of anterior chamber or vitreous inflammation.

CMV disease may also involve the gastrointestinal tract. The most common manifestations are esophagitis and colitis. Patients with esophagitis present with dysphagia, odynophagia, or retrosternal pain with swallowing; those with colitis present with abdominal pain, diarrhea, and hematochezia. Papillary sclerosis and sclerosing cholangitis also have been associated with CMV infection.

Many neurologic disorders attributable to CMV infection have been described. Polyradiculopathy presents as flaccid paralysis and urinary retention similar to the Guillan-Barré syndrome. Myelitis manifests as bilateral leg weakness and hyperreflexia. Encephalitis presents as neurocognitive impairment that is difficult to distinguish from AIDS dementia. Ventriculo-encephalitis manifests as a rapidly progressive delirium, cranial nerve palsies, nystagmus, and ataxia.

Other less common CMV-related syndromes include interstitial pneumonitis, adrenal disease, and viremia associated with constitutional symptoms.

Diagnosis

The diagnosis of CMV retinitis is made clinically. On ophthalmoscopic examination, there are fluffy, yellow-white, full-thickness retinal infiltrates in a vascular distribution. This "focal necrotizing retinitis" is often associated with intraretinal hemorrhage (Figure 9-4). Vitreal inflammation is minimal, except in the presence of immune reconstitution syndrome. Gastrointestinal tract disease is diagnosed by tissue biopsy revealing characteristic ulcerations and intranuclear and intracytoplasmic inclusions. CMV culture of the gastrointestinal mucosa is neither sensitive nor specific.

CMV polyradiculopathy is suspected if nerve root thickening is evident on imaging studies and is confirmed by LP results. The CSF typically shows a neutrophilic pleocytosis, an increased protein level, and a decreased glucose level. A positive CSF PCR for CMV is diagnostic of this condition. Myelitis may be associated with spinal cord enhancement on CT or MRI,

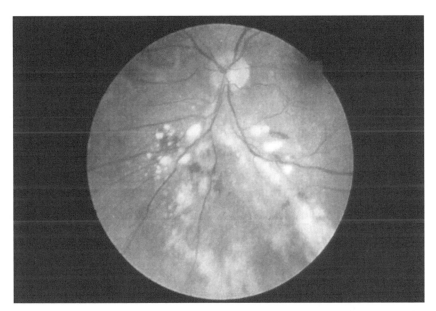

Figure 9-4. Retinal photograph of patient with cytomegalovirus retinitis. (For color reproduction, see Plate 3 at back of book.) (From Ann Intern Med. 1988;109:963-9; with permission.)

and, in contrast to polyradiculopathy, the CSF may be normal. Neuroimaging studies in patients with CMV encephalitis may show periventricular or meningeal enhancement, but these findings are nonspecific. The diagnosis of ventriculoencephalitis is supported by MRI showing periventricular enhancement on the T2-weighted signal and ventricular enlargement and is confirmed by CSF PCR for CMV. The CSF typically shows a mononuclear pleocytosis, an increased protein level, and a low or normal glucose level. CSF viral culture is not useful in the diagnosis of CNS CMV infection.

CMV viremia can be demonstrated using an antigen assay, PCR assay, or blood culture. Patients with CMV end-organ disease are usually viremic. CMV antigen tests are based on monoclonal antibodies directed against the CMV-specific 65-kD matrix protein in CMV-infected polymorphonuclear leukocytes. The assay is quantitative and reported as the number of infected cells per 200,000 neutrophils. It is more sensitive and rapid than CMV culture. While the assay can be positive in asymptomatic patients, studies suggest that a high number of infected cells predicts the development of clinical disease within three months. This assay is also useful for predicting relapse in patients on treatment for CMV infection. PCR testing of plasma and whole blood shows a quantitative correlation with the risk for CMV disease. The sensitivity, specificity, and positive predictive value of CMV PCR are 35%, 100%, and 100%, respectively, if the cutoff is greater than 1000 copies/mL, and 73%, 90%, and 73% if the cutoff is greater than 100 copies/mL. One study demonstrated a greater than three-fold increase in risk for CMV disease for each $\log_{10}$ increase in CMV PCR. Serologic tests are generally not helpful in diagnosing CMV disease.

Management

Expert consultation is recommended for clinicians with limited experience in the treatment of CMV infection. Several antiviral drugs, including ganciclovir (IV, oral, and intravitreal), foscarnet, valganciclovir, and cidofovir have been used. Ganciclovir is associated with hematologic toxicity, including neutropenia and thrombocytopenia; granulocyte colony-stimulating factor (GCSF) is sometimes required to treat these complications. Foscarnet is an effective alternative intravenous treatment for CMV retinitis but is associated with significant toxicities as well. These include nausea, neurologic symptoms, electrolyte disturbances (decreased calcium, phosphate, and magnesium), and renal dysfunction. The infusion takes two hours and requires a pump. Oral ganciclovir is not well absorbed and is not commonly used. The valine ester prodrug of ganciclovir, valganciclovir, is an oral agent that produces blood levels of ganciclovir similar to intravenously administered drug. A study of valganciclovir (900 mg orally bid for three weeks, then 900 mg/d) compared with intravenous ganciclovir as induction therapy for newly diagnosed CMV retinitis showed it to be as effective. Cidofovir has been associated with proximal tubular necrosis, proteinuria,

Table 9-4.   Treatment of Cytomegalovirus Retinitis

Drug	Route	Dose	Toxicity
Ganciclovir			
Initial therapy	Intravenous	5 mg/kg every 12 hours × 14–21 d	Neutropenia, anemia, nausea/diarrhea
Maintenance therapy	Intravenous	5 mg/kg/d 5–7 d/wk	
	Intravitreal implant*	Every 6 months	Blurred vision, iritis, vitreitis
Foscarnet			
Initial	Intravenous	90 mg/kg every 12 hours × 14–21 d	Nephrotoxicity, hypocalcemia, hypophosphatemia, hypomagnesemia, anemia, nausea, seizure
Maintenance	Intravenous	90–120 mg/kg/d	
Valganciclovir**			
Initial	Oral	900 mg twice daily × 14–21 d	Neutropenia, anemia
Maintenance	Oral	900 mg/d	
Cidofovir			
Initial	Intravenous	5 mg/kg/wk for 2 weeks with probenecid 2 g orally 3 hours before each dose and 1 g orally 2 and 8 hours after dose	Nephrotoxicity, neutropenia
Maintenance	Intravenous	5 mg/kg every other week with probenecid as above	
Fomivirsen			
Initial	Intravitreal	330 μg every other week × 2	Blurred vision, iritis, vitreitis
Maintenance	Intravitreal	330 μg every 4 weeks	

* May be used as initial or maintenance therapy; co-administration of a systemic agent is essential to prevent infection at other sites.

** Preferred for initial and maintenance therapies (together with a ganciclovir intravitreal implant if sight-threatening disease is present) if the patient is reliable and adherent. Otherwise intravenous therapy and hospitalization are necessary.

and renal dysfunction. Probenecid and intravenous hydration are necessary to reduce the risk of these toxicities.

Therapy for CMV retinitis is summarized in Table 9-4. Management depends upon whether the disease is sight-threatening (involving the macular or optic nerve) or not (involving the peripheral retina). Initial treatment for non-sight-threatening disease is valganciclovir 900 mg bid for 14 to 21 days, which is followed by maintenance therapy at 900 mg/d. For sight-threatening disease, a ganciclovir intraocular implant is placed surgically by an ophthalmologist, and valganciclovir is given at 900 mg/d to prevent occurrence of retinitis in the other eye and disease at other body sites. The ganciclovir implant provides intravitreal drug levels four times those obtained with systemic therapy. Surgical risks associated with this procedure include blurred vision lasting several weeks, retinal detachment, hemorrhage, and endophthalmitis. The implant is generally effective for 6 to 8 months, at which time active drug is depleted and a new implant is required. Alternatives for treatment of CMV retinitis include intravenous ganciclovir, foscarnet, cidofovir, or repeated intravitreal injections with fomivirsen (for relapses of disease, not for treatment of initial infection). Alternative maintenance regimens include foscarnet 90 to 120 mg/kg intravenously qd; cidofovir 5 mg/kg intravenously every other week (with probenecid 2 g orally 3 hours before and 1 g orally 2 hours after dosing, and again 8 hours after dosing); and fomivirsen (for retinal disease) injected intravitreally every 2 to 4 weeks.

Patients with severe gastrointestinal disease should be treated with intravenous ganciclovir or foscarnet; those with mild-to-moderate disease can be treated with valganciclovir. Unlike CMV retinitis, maintenance therapy has not extended the time to relapse and is generally not recommended. Treatment of CNS CMV disease consists of intravenous ganciclovir *and* foscarnet because of their association with improved survival, followed by maintenance therapy. Pulmonary disease should be treated if tissue histology is suggestive of CMV infection, and other pathogens have been excluded. Patients should be given induction therapy for 3 weeks or until clinical improvement occurs.

Patients with relapsing CMV disease should receive another course of induction therapy followed by maintenance therapy. Reinduction with the previously used drug is advised if the recurrence is not sight-threatening. Repeat induction with another drug or combination therapy is recommended if the recurrence is sight-threatening or rapidly progressing and there is a concern for resistance or if there is toxicity to the initial regimen. Dilated ophthalmologic examinations are essential for monitoring CMV retinitis and should be performed at the time of diagnosis, after the completion of induction therapy, and regularly thereafter while on maintenance therapy.

Initiation of ART should not be significantly delayed in the setting of newly diagnosed CMV disease. However, for patients with sight-threatening retinitis, CMV treatment should be started before ART. Immune recovery uveitis, an inflammatory reaction in the anterior chamber or vitreous, generally develops between 4 and 12 weeks after the initiation of ART. The inflammation can be complicated by macular edema, epiretinal membranes, and loss of vision. Treatment consists of periocular or systemic corticosteroids, but the response rate is only 50%.

Resistance to anti-CMV drugs has been described. Rates increase from 10% during the first 3 months of treatment to as high as 25% to 30% by 9 months. Low-level resistance to ganciclovir develops as a result of mutations at UL97 in the CMV phosphotransferase gene. High-level resistance is conferred by mutations at UL97 and UL54 (DNA polymerase gene), and cross-resistance to foscarnet and cidofovir occurs as a result of mutations at UL54. Resistance testing should be considered in the appropriate clinical setting. Patients with low-level resistance and CMV retinitis can be effectively treated with a ganciclovir implant; however, those with high-level resistance should be managed with fomivirsen injections.

Retrospective data provide support for discontinuing secondary prophylaxis in patients who are asymptomatic, have completed their initial antimicrobial therapy, and have an increase in their CD4 count to over 100 cells/mm³ for at least 3 to 6 months on ART. Primary prophylaxis of CMV infection is discussed in Chapter 7.

Gastrointestinal Parasite Infection

Pathogenesis and Clinical Manifestations

Diarrheal illness secondary to intestinal parasites is more common in HIV-infected patients living in or traveling to developing countries. The major pathogens are *Cryptosporidia*, microsporidia, *Isospora*, *Cyclospora*, and *Giardia*. All of these organisms affect the mucosa of the small intestine.

Cryptosporidiosis is acquired from fecally contaminated food or water. Oocysts are ingested, then excystate and release sporozoites that attach to the intestinal epithelium, causing profuse secretory diarrhea with low-grade fever, abdominal cramps, nausea, and vomiting. Patients with a CD4 count of less than 50 cells/mm³ are at increased risk for biliary tract disease and death. Microsporidiosis often coexists with cryptosporidiosis in HIV-infected patients.

Microsporidiosis is responsible for at least one-third of the chronic diarrhea in AIDS and is a frequent cause of cholangiopathy. *Enterocytozoon bieneusi* and *Encephalitozoon intestinalis* are the two clinically important species. Microsporidia are acquired via the oral or pulmonary route. The organism injects its nucleus into lumenal enterocytes and ultimately destroys them, distorting the mucosal architecture and causing malabsorption. Symptoms of microsporidiosis include chronic nonbloody diarrhea associated with abdominal cramping, anorexia, bloating, and weight loss.

Isospora species causes a malabsorptive diarrhea by disrupting mucosal architecture and causing inflammation in the lamina propria.

Symptoms of isosporiasis develop within one week of oocyst ingestion and consist of low-grade fever, anorexia, profuse watery diarrhea, and abdominal cramping, which may lead to dehydration and weight loss. Colitis, acalculous cholecystitis, and extraintestinal manifestations have also been described.

Cyclosporiasis is a coccidian infection linked to contaminated water or food. The organism invades and destroys the epithelium. Infection from *Cyclospora* species manifests as a prodrome of fever and malaise, followed by watery diarrhea, abdominal cramps, bloating, and flatulence that may wax and wane over weeks to months.

Giardiasis presents as nonbloody diarrhea associated with bloating and early satiety. Infection occurs by ingestion of as few as 10 cysts, which excystate into trophozoites that attach to luminal enterocytes and cause malabsorption.

Diagnosis

Examination of stool samples should be the initial strategy for diagnosing gastrointestinal parasites. *Cryptosporidia* and *Giardia* can be rapidly detected by a direct fluorescent antibody assay that is both sensitive and specific for these organisms. Modified acid-fast stains are used to identify *Isospora* and *Cyclospora*. Microsporidial spores are best identified with a modified trichrome stain. If species identification of microsporidia is important, electron microscopy should be performed. For diagnosis of

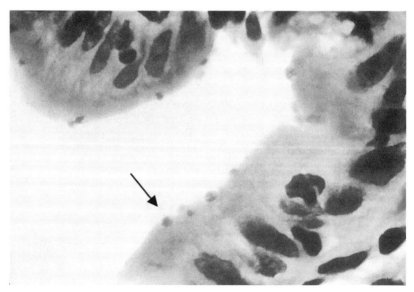

Figure 9-5. *Cryptosporidium* cysts on small bowel biopsy. (Courtesy of Centers for Disease Control and Prevention, Atlanta.)

Isospora, Cyclospora, and microsporidia, it is recommended that stool first be screened with a nonspecific chemofluorescent stain and, if positive, the diagnosis confirmed by a modified acid-fast or modified trichrome stain. In patients with persistent diarrhea and nondiagnostic stool samples, colonoscopy/endoscopy with biopsy should be considered (Figure 9-5).

Management

The diagnosis and treatment of gastrointestinal parasites in HIV disease are summarized in Table 9-5. Parasitic diarrhea in HIV-infected patients is generally associated with a poor clinical response, especially if the CD4 count

Table 9-5.   Diagnosis and Treatment of Gastrointestinal Parasites

Organism	Diagnostic Studies	Therapy	Alternatives	Comments
Cryptosporidiosis	DFA of stool; oocysts 4–5 μm	Nitazoxanide 500 mg orally twice daily until CD4 count > 100 cells/mm³	Paromomycin 25–35 mg/kg/d orally in 2–4 divided doses	Loperamide or octreotide for control of symptoms
Microsporidiosis				
Enterocytozoon bieneusi	Chemifluorescent screen, and, if positive, modified trichrome stain of stool for species identification	Fumagillin 60 mg orally once daily	—	Treatment response poor
Encephalitozoon intestinalis	As with *E. bieneusi* above for species identification	Albendazole 400 mg orally twice daily until CD4 count > 200 cells/mm³	—	Albendazole can eradicate infection
Isosporiasis	Chemifluorescent screen, and, if positive, modified acid-fast stain of stool; oocysts 30 × 12 μm	TMP-SMX DS orally four times daily for 10–14 days	Pyrimethamine 75 mg/d + leucovorin 5–10 mg orally once daily	—
Cyclospora infection	Chemifluorescent screen, and, if positive, modified acid-fast stain of stool; oocysts 8–10 μm	TMP-SMX DS orally twice daily for 10 days	Ciprofloxacin 500 mg orally twice daily	—
Blastocystis hominis	Stool ova and parasites	Metronidazole 750 mg orally three times daily for 10–20 days	TMP-SMX; iodoquinol	Pathogenicity uncertain

(cont'd)

Table 9-5.   Diagnosis and Treatment of Gastrointestinal Parasites (cont'd)

Organism	Diagnostic Studies	Therapy	Alternatives	Comments
Giardia lamblia	Stool ova and DFA parasites, or *Giardia* antigen test	Metronidazole 250 mg orally three times daily for 5–10 days *or* albendazole 400 mg orally daily for 5 days	Tinidazole 2 g orally (one-time dose) Nitazoxanide 500 mg orally twice daily for 3 days	—
Entamoeba histolytica	Stool ova and parasites	Metronidazole 750 mg orally three times daily for 10 days *or* tinidazole 2 g/d orally for 3 days	—	Acute treatment is followed by iodoquinol 650 mg orally three times daily for 20 days *or* paromomycin 500 mg orally three times daily for 7 days
Strongyloides stercoralis	Stool ova and parasites	Ivermectin 200 µg/kg/d orally for 1–2 days	Thiabendazole 25 mg/kg orally twice daily for 2 days	—

DFA = direct fluorescent antibody; DS = double-strength; TMP-SMX = trimethoprim-sulfamethoxazole.

is very low. In many cases, antiretroviral therapy is more important than antimicrobial therapy in clearing the infection. Antimotility drugs such as loperamide can be used adjunctively.

Successful treatment of cryptosporidiosis has been disappointing. Long-term cure rates are generally less than 50% with most drugs, including paromomycin plus azithromycin, atovaquone, metronidazole, TMP-SMX, and nitazoxanide. In outbreak settings, either boiling drinking water for one minute or using submicron water filters decreases the chances of ingesting cryptosporidial oocysts.

Microsporidial infection treatment has also been problematic. *E. intestinalis* often responds to albendazole or fumagillin, but *E. bieneusi* has been more difficult to manage. Endoscopic retrograde cholangiopancreatography (ERCP) with sphincterotomy offers pain relief for papillary stenosis and sclerosing cholangitis, which is associated with cryptosporidiosis and microsporidiosis, but symptoms may recur.

Isosporiasis can be managed effectively with TMP-SMX. Pyrimethamine with folinic acid can be used in instances of sulfonamide intolerance. Ciprofloxacin is not as effective. Since relapse is common in patients with a CD4 count below 200 cells/mm^3, secondary prophylaxis with TMP-SMX is recommended in this setting.

Cyclospora can be treated with TMP-SMX, with ciprofloxacin as an alternative agent. Secondary prophylaxis is advised in patients with a low CD4 count. Giardiasis is managed in the same manner as in the general population.

Proper storage, preparation, and handling of foods, avoidance of untreated or contaminated water sources, and careful attention to personal hygiene can decrease the risk of contracting gastrointestinal parasite infections.

Herpes Simplex Virus Infection

Epidemiology and Microbiology

In the United States adult population, seropositivity rates to herpes simplex virus, types 1 (HSV-1) and 2 (HSV-2), are approximately 80% and 12%, respectively. HSV latently infects trigeminal or sacral sensory ganglia and reactivates periodically from stimuli such as trauma, ultraviolet light exposure, acute illness, and immunosuppression. HIV-infected patients with a CD4 count of less than 200 cells/mm^3 may have frequent or severe recurrences. In the setting of HSV lesions, the risk of HIV transmission and acquisition is increased from coactivation of local HIV production within the ulcer as well as cytokine-mediated recruitment of HIV target cells.

Clinical Manifestations

HSV begins as vesicles on an erythematous base that are often preceded by 1 to 2 days of pain and tingling at the site of the eruption, usually the genitals, buttocks, or mouth (Figure 9-6). Over several days they begin to form a crust. HSV can cause prolonged ulcerative lesions in HIV-infected patients. HSV esophagitis, encephalitis, and keratitis also have been described, although the incidence of meningoencephalitis does not appear to be increased in comparison with the general population. Symptomatic reactivation of HSV may transiently increase the HIV viral load.

Diagnosis

Classic orolabial and genital HSV reactivation is usually diagnosed on clinical grounds. It can be confirmed by direct immunofluorescence assay (DFA). DFA has a 90% diagnostic yield compared with 65% with culture, and results are usually available within 24 hours. To obtain material for either DFA or culture, a fresh vesicle should be unroofed and the base of the shallow ulcer gently scraped with a Dacron swab or a scalpel to obtain cells. The Tzanck smear, which is a Giemsa or Wright stain of vesicular fluid used to demonstrate multinucleated giant cells, is less sensitive and dependent on the skill of the operator. Serology is helpful only in primary infection where a 4-fold or greater rise in the IgG titer is observed between acute and

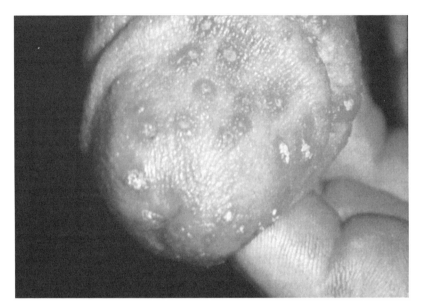

Figure 9-6. Herpes simplex virus infection involving penile glans.

convalescent sera. Diagnosis of acyclovir-resistant HSV is established by culture and sensitivity testing. HSV PCR testing of the CSF is useful in establishing the diagnosis of HSV meningoencephalitis.

Management

Treatment of orolabial or genital HSV infection consists of famciclovir or acyclovir given for 7 days (Table 9-6). Valacyclovir has been associated with hemolytic uremic syndrome in patients with advanced HIV disease and should be avoided in this setting. Severe cases of mucocutaneous HSV infection, meningoencephalitis, and involvement at other sites should be treated with intravenous acyclovir. Secondary prophylaxis should be considered in patients with advanced HIV disease who have frequent recurrences. Acyclovir-resistant HSV infection usually responds to a course of intravenous foscarnet or cidofovir.

Histoplasmosis

Epidemiology

Histoplasmosis is a relatively common diagnosis in HIV-infected patients from endemic areas (the Ohio and Mississippi River valleys, Haiti, Puerto Rico, South America, and Central America). Cases in patients who have not visited endemic areas for many years likely represent reactivation of latent infection.

Table 9-6.   Treatment of Herpes Simplex Virus and Varicella-Zoster Virus Infections

HSV Infection

Primary or recurrent mucocutaneous	Famciclovir 250–500 mg orally bid *or* Valacyclovir 1 g orally bid* *or* Acyclovir 400 mg orally tid
Extensive mucocutaneous	Acyclovir 5–7.5 mg/kg IV every 8 hours, then switch to oral therapy (as above) after lesions regress, total 7–14 d of rx
Visceral	Acyclovir 10 mg/kg IV every 8 hours for 14–21 days
Prevention of relapse	Acyclovir 400 mg orally bid *or* Famciclovir 250 mg orally bid *or* Valacyclovir 500 mg orally bid*
Acyclovir-resistant HSV strain	Foscarnet 60 mg/kg IV every 12 hours *or* Cidofovir 5 mg/kg IV once a week *or* Topical trifluridine 5%

VZV Infection

Localized (shingles)	Famciclovir 500 mg orally tid *or* Valacyclovir 1 g orally tid*
Primary or disseminated	Acyclovir 5 mg/kg IV every 8 hours, then switch to oral therapy (as above) for total 7–10 d
Prevention of relapse	No therapy indicated
Acyclovir-resistant VZV strain	Foscarnet 60 mg/kg IV every 12 hours
Visceral	Acyclovir 10 mg/kg IV every 8 hours until all cutaneous and visceral disease have resolved

*Avoid use in advanced HIV disease; see text for warning.
HSV = herpes simplex virus; VZV = varicella-zoster virus.

Pathogenesis

The dimorphic fungus *Histoplasma capsulatum* is found in soil. Primary histoplasmosis occurs when dust is stirred up and spores are aerosolized. Histoplasmosis is not transmitted from person to person, and infection in persons with normal immune function is asymptomatic or manifests as a self-limited respiratory illness. HIV-infected patients are at increased risk of disseminated infection, 90% of which occurs when the CD4 count is less than 150 cells/mm^3.

Clinical Manifestations

Disseminated histoplasmosis manifests subacutely with fever, weight loss, fatigue, malaise and respiratory complaints. Physical examination may reveal lymphadenopathy or splenomegaly. Chest x-ray often reveals bilateral diffuse nodular infiltrates with or without mediastinal/hilar lymphadenopathy. Involvement of the spleen, liver, lymph nodes, or bone marrow may occur in the absence of pulmonary involvement. Evidence of septic shock is present in up to 40% of patients with disseminated disease. Less common sites of involvement include the CNS, gastrointestinal tract, and skin.

Diagnosis

The sensitivity of sputum cultures for histoplasmosis ranges from 10% to 60% and increases with multiple specimens. The diagnostic yield of bronchoscopy is approximately 80% in the presence of pulmonary infiltrates. Bone marrow biopsy or blood culture has a sensitivity of approximately 50% in disseminated disease. Isolator blood cultures may require 2 to 4 weeks to become positive, limiting their utility in the acute setting. Serologic testing is not helpful in diagnosing reactivation histoplasmosis.

Detection of *Histoplasma* antigen in serum or urine is useful in establishing the diagnosis, although cross-reactivity with other fungal pathogens may occur. Antigen testing is positive in the urine in 95% and in the serum in 85% of patients with disseminated histoplasmosis, 40% of patients with cavitary pulmonary disease, and 20% with acute pulmonary disease. Antigen testing is also used to monitor the clinical response to therapy.

For the diagnosis of meningitis, a compatible clinical picture together with positive culture and/or antigen testing results are required. Fungal stains of the CSF are usually negative; cultures are positive in approximately 50% of patients, and antigen or anti-*Histoplasma* antibodies are positive in 70%.

Management

Expert consultation is recommended for clinicians with limited experience in the treatment of histoplasmosis. Intravenous amphotericin B (0.5 to 1.0 mg/kg/d for 3 to 10 days) is given as initial therapy for severe cases. Liposomal amphotericin has been demonstrated in a randomized controlled trial to be a reasonable alternative to amphotericin B and may be more effective. Patients who have completed the initial treatment for histoplasmosis should receive maintenance therapy with itraconazole 100 to 200 mg orally bid. Itraconazole (300 mg/bid orally for 3 days, then 200 mg/bid orally for 12 weeks) may be used for mild-to-moderate infections. For these patients, serum itraconazole levels can be monitored to ensure adequate therapeutic dosing. Patients with *Histoplasma* meningitis should receive amphotericin B or liposomal amphotericin for 12 to 16 weeks at the dosages noted above, followed by lifelong maintenance therapy with itraconazole.

HIV-infected patients with a CD4 count of less than 200 cells/mm³ should avoid activities associated with a risk for exposure to *H. capsulatum*, including caring for roosting birds, cleaning areas soiled with their droppings, and exploring caves. Itraconazole prophylaxis should be considered in patients with a CD4 count of less than 100/mm³ who live in endemic areas or engage in activities that put them at high risk for exposure.

Human Papillomavirus Infection

Epidemiology and Pathogenesis

Over 70% of sexually active adults will acquire genital human papillomavirus (HPV) infection during their lifetime. In the majority of cases, HPV infection is subclinical. HPV replication requires infection of the basal layer of the epithelium. As HPV-infected basal cells divide, mature, and migrate to the skin surface, new virions are formed. When the infected epithelial cells naturally slough, they carry millions of infectious viruses inside of them.

HPV infection causes warts and anogenital squamous intraepithelial dysplasia, which can progress to carcinoma (see Chapter 10). Most genital warts are associated with HPV types 6, 11, 42, 43, and 44, whereas the majority of cases of anogenital dysplasia and carcinoma are associated with types 16, 18, 31, 33, and 35. HPV-related dysplasia is more prevalent in HIV-infected patients, is more advanced at the time of diagnosis, and does not respond as well to standard therapies.

Clinical Manifestations

Anogenital warts (condylomata) can occur on any part of the external genitalia, vagina, cervix, or perianal region. They present as skin- or mucosa-colored papules that are rarely associated with pain, itching, burning, or bleeding. Anogenital dysplasia is generally asymptomatic. In patients who develop invasive squamous cell carcinoma, symptoms vary based upon the location and extent of tumor involvement. In vulvar cancer, local irritation and bleeding are usually present; in cervical cancer, postmenopausal or postcoital bleeding, menstrual irregularity, dysuria, and anemia may occur; and in anal cancer, rectal bleeding or pain and dyspareunia are often described.

Diagnosis

The diagnosis of anogenital warts is usually made on clinical grounds, but warts that are friable, ulcerated, or resistant to treatment should undergo biopsy to rule out dysplasia or carcinoma.

Cytologic testing by Pap smear is the most widely employed tool to screen for cervical dysplasia and carcinoma. Cervical Pap smear screening in HIV-infected women should be performed twice over 6 months and annually thereafter if the first two smears are negative. If the Pap smear shows atypical squamous cells (ASCUS) or dysplasia, colposcopic biopsy of the cervix is indicated.

Cytologic screening for anal cancer with anal Pap smears in HIV-infected men and women appears to have the same sensitivity and specificity as cervical Pap smears. Whether screening for and early treatment of anal dysplasia result in a survival benefit remains to be determined. Currently there are no formal recommendations for anal Pap smear screening in HIV-infected patients.

Management

In the absence of treatment, warts may regress, persist, or enlarge. Most therapies are topically applied, have equivalent success rates, and are administered on a repeated basis. Warts in moist intertriginous areas respond better to treatment than warts on dry skin surfaces.

Treatment modalities for external anogenital warts are listed in Box 9-1. Recurrences are common. Cervical and rectal warts should be managed by a specialist after dysplasia and carcinoma are ruled out. Treatment of external anogenital warts in men who have sex with men (MSM) should prompt investigation of whether there are coexisting internal lesions.

The management of high-grade cervical dysplasia is ablation, but recurrence in HIV-infected women is more common than in the general population. The optimal management of anal dysplasia is currently under investigation; ablation of high-grade lesions is usually recommended. Invasive anogenital carcinoma is managed with chemoradiation and radiation therapy.

Lymphogranuloma Venereum

Epidemiology and Microbiology

In 2003, an outbreak of *Chlamydia trachomatis* proctitis was reported among a group of mostly HIV-infected MSM in the Netherlands who were part of a sexual network. Further testing of serum samples revealed these

---

Box 9-1.   Treatment Modalities for Genital Warts

- Podofilox 0.5% solution or gel, available with prescription, applied twice daily to lesions for 3 consecutive days followed by 4 days without treatment

- Imiquimod 5% cream, available with prescription, applied to lesions at bedtime 3 nights a week, then washed with soap and water after 6-10 hours

- Cryotherapy with liquid nitrogen or cryoprobe applied to lesions and reapplied after eschar from the previous treatment has resolved

- Trichloroacetic acid (TCA) or bichloroacetic acid (BCA) 80-90% applied to lesions weekly. With this treatment, lesions will turn white as the acid reacts with the epithelial cells

- Surgical removal by electrocautery, laser, infrared coagulation, or cold-knife excision

infections to be related to the L serovars of *C. trachomatis*, the cause of lymphogranuloma venereum (LGV). Since that time, this infection has been reported throughout Europe and in the United States.

Clinical Manifestations

LGV classically begins with a shallow painless genital ulcer. Within days, bloody, purulent rectal discharge and tenesmus generally develop. Tender inguinal lymphadenopathy or bubos may accompany these symptoms.

Diagnosis

The diagnosis of LGV is suspected clinically and confirmed by serologic testing. Examination of the rectal mucosa shows edema with exudates and friable ulcerations. A complement fixation titer of greater than 1:64 or a microimmunofluorescence titer of greater than 1:128 suggests the diagnosis. Direct identification of *C. trachomatis* by culture of an ulcer or bubo aspirate can also be attempted, but the yield is limited. Although nucleic acid amplification testing is available for the detection of *C. trachomatis* in urine and urethral and cervical specimens, it has not been approved for rectal specimens. In patients diagnosed with LGV, testing for other sexually transmitted diseases should also be performed.

Management

The recommended treatment for LGV is doxycycline (100 mg/bid orally for 21 days). Erythromycin or azithromycin can be used as an alternative. Timely diagnosis and antibiotic therapy are important. If LGV goes untreated, involved lymph nodes may suppurate and form fistulae, and anal strictures may result from untreated proctitis.

Methicillin-Resistant *Staphylococcus aureus* (MRSA) Infection

Epidemiology and Microbiology

Since 2002, the incidence of community-acquired cellulitis and subcutaneous abscess caused by methicillin-resistant *S. aureus* (MRSA) has increased significantly. HIV-infected patients appear to be at particular risk. A history of shaving or clipping body hair in the affected region is present in 20% of cases. Methamphetamine use, multiple recent sexual contacts, and public hot tubs or saunas are also associated with increased risk for MRSA infection. Interestingly, patients who take TMP-SMX for PCP prophylaxis are somewhat protected from developing this infection.

Clinical Manifestations

Skin and soft tissue infections caused by MRSA appear in typical fashion. Cellulitis presents with the acute onset of localized erythema, swelling, and pain of the skin. Abscess manifests a tender subcutaneous nodule. The most commonly affected sites are the lower extremities and buttocks. Fever at the time of presentation is unusual, but, if the infection is left untreated, bacteremia associated with septic shock syndrome has been reported.

Diagnosis

The diagnosis of cellulitis and subcutaneous abscess is made clinically, and MRSA infection is suspected from the local epidemiology or lack of response to conventional antibiotic treatment. Radiologic imaging is sometimes useful in determining whether an abscess is present. Blood cultures should be obtained if the patient appears ill.

Management

Trimethoprim-sulfamethoxazole (TMP-SMX) is the treatment of choice for mild-to-moderate community-acquired MRSA infection. The dose is 1 to 2 double-strength tablets every 8 to 12 hours for at least 14 days. In patients with suspected bacteremia, intravenous vancomycin should be used. By definition, MRSA is resistant to beta-lactam antibiotics, including penicillins and cephalosporins. The majority of isolates are also resistant to ciprofloxacin and erythromycin, and resistance to tetracycline is common as well. Abscess collections should be incised and drained. If blood cultures are positive, the patient should be evaluated for endocarditis and other metastatic foci of infection.

Mycobacterium avium Complex (MAC) Infection

Epidemiology and Pathogenesis

Mycobacterium avium and M. *intracellulare*, referred to as *M. avium* complex, are atypical mycobacteria that cause systemic disease in HIV-infected patients with a CD4 count of less than 50 cells/mm^3. In the absence of antimicrobial prophylaxis, the incidence of disseminated MAC ranges from 20% to 40% in this setting. Ubiquitous in the environment, MAC is found particularly in water sources, including fresh and sea water, tap water, and steam heat. The portal of entry of the organism is inhalation or ingestion, and both respiratory and gastrointestinal colonization precede infection. However, routine surveillance cultures are not recommended in that 62% of patients with MAC infection have negative results. Additional factors associated with an increased risk for MAC infection include high HIV viral load (>100,000 copies/mL) and a history of other OIs, particularly CMV infection.

Clinical Manifestations

MAC infection commonly presents with fever, night sweats, fatigue, weight loss, abdominal pain, and diarrhea. On physical examination, patients may have lymphadenopathy, hepatosplenomegaly, and evidence of wasting. Unlike TB, MAC rarely causes pulmonary disease; cavitary and nodular pulmonary infiltrates occur in only 2.5% of patients.

MAC lymphadenitis has been reported after the institution of ART. Patients develop fever, lymphadenitis, necrotizing granulomata, and leukocytosis 1 to 3 weeks into therapy. This immune reconstitution syndrome is thought to represent an inflammatory response to previously subclinical infection.

Diagnosis

The diagnosis of MAC infection is suspected on the basis of symptoms and signs in the appropriate clinical setting and confirmed by isolation of the organism from blood or histopathologic evidence of it on a biopsy specimen. Laboratory examination may reveal anemia, leukopenia, thrombocytopenia, and/or an increased serum alkaline phosphatase level. Identification of MAC is best accomplished via lysis-centrifugation isolator blood cultures. These cultures, which are sensitive for intracellular organisms, are performed by lysing mononuclear cells and plating them to solid media on which colony counts can be quantified. Alternatively, blood can be inoculated into a Bactec system followed by radiometric growth detection. Once growth is noted, species can be identified using specific DNA probes, high-performance liquid chromatography (HPLC), or biochemical tests. Cultures may take several weeks to become positive. Occasionally, bone marrow or liver biopsy is necessary for the diagnosis of MAC infection. Pathology of infected sites shows distended histiocytes filled with acid-fast bacilli, minimal inflammatory response, and poorly formed granulomata (Figure 9-7). It is important to consider infection from TB and other nontuberculous mycobacteria in the differential diagnosis, as their clinical presentations may be similar.

Management

Expert consultation is recommended for clinicians with limited experience in the treatment of MAC infection. Medical regimens generally consist of three drugs, usually a macrolide, ethambutol, and rifabutin (Table 9-7). Clarithromycin is the best studied of the macrolides and clears cultures

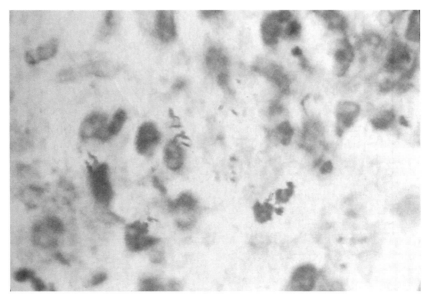

Figure 9-7. *Mycobacterium avium* complex infection diagnosed by liver biopsy. (From Hospital Physician. Turner-White Communications; April 1988; with permission.)

more rapidly than azithromycin. Azithromycin may be substituted, however, when drug interactions or intolerance is of concern. Randomized, controlled trials have demonstrated that the addition of rifabutin as a third agent results in improved survival and decreased development of resistance. Ciprofloxacin and amikacin may be used as alternative agents for rifabutin if necessary. Fluoroquinolones such as ciprofloxacin have activity against 20% to 30% of MAC isolates. Clofazimine, previously a component of MAC treatment regimens, has been associated with increased mortality and is no longer recommended for use.

Rifabutin interacts with many drugs. For example, concomitant use of clarithromycin and rifabutin increases rifabutin levels by 100% and decreases clarithromycin levels by 50%. Treatment with fluconazole also increases rifabutin levels. A dose reduction is necessary if rifabutin is given with most protease inhibitors (PIs), and a dose increase is necessary if it is given with efavirenz.

Resistance testing should be used to help guide therapy in patients who have developed disseminated MAC while on prophylactic therapy with macrolides and in those who are not responding to therapy. Suggested minimum inhibitory concentration (MIC) thresholds for resistance to clarithromycin and azithromycin are ≥ 32 and ≥ 256 mcg/mL, respectively.

Antiretroviral therapy should be initiated after 1 to 2 weeks of MAC treatment in patients not already receiving it. In patients being treated with ART at the time of development of MAC infection, therapy should be optimized whenever possible, with careful attention to drug interactions.

Table 9-7.   Drugs Used in the Treatment of Mycobacterial Infections

Drug	Usual Dose	Major Toxicities
Amikacin	7.5–15 mg/kg every 24 hours IV	Nephrotoxicity Ototoxicity
Azithromycin	600 mg/d orally	Gastrointestinal intolerance Hepatotoxicity Rash Headache Dizziness Reversible hearing loss
Ciprofloxacin	500–750 mg twice daily orally	Gastrointestinal intolerance Neurotoxicity Rash
Clarithromycin	500 mg twice daily orally	Gastrointestinal intolerance Hepatotoxicity Rash Headache Dizziness Reversible hearing loss
Ethambutol	15–25 mg/kg/d orally	Optic neuritis Rash Gastrointestinal intolerance Hepatotoxicity
Isoniazid	5 mg/kg/d orally (max dose 300 mg/d orally)	Hepatotoxicity Fever Rash Peripheral neuropathy
Pyrazinamide	25 mg/kg/d orally	Hepatotoxicity Hyperuricemia Rash
Rifabutin	300 mg/d orally; adjust dose based on interaction with other drug(s)	Gastrointestinal intolerance Hepatotoxicity Rash Orange discoloration of secretions Uveitis
Rifampin	10 mg/kg/d orally (max dose 600 mg/d orally)	Gastrointestinal intolerance Hepatotoxicity Rash Orange discoloration of secretions
Streptomycin	15 mg/kg/d IM	Ototoxicity Vestibular toxicity

Symptoms of reconstitution syndrome can be treated with nonsteroidal anti-inflammatory drugs or short-term corticosteroids (4 to 8 week course of prednisone 20 to 40 mg/d, followed by a gradual taper).

In some circumstances, three-drug regimens may eventually be consolidated to two-drug regimens, or treatment may be given three times per week rather than daily. These changes should only be made with guidance from an expert for reliable patients with mild disease who are at low risk for progression.

Response to treatment often takes several weeks. Surveillance blood cultures should be obtained 4 to 8 weeks after initiation of treatment to document clearance of bacteremia. Retrospective data provide support for discontinuing secondary prophylaxis in patients who are asymptomatic, have completed 12 months of antimicrobial therapy, and have an increase in their CD4 count to over 100 cells/mm^3 for at least 6 months on ART. Primary prophylaxis of MAC infection is discussed in Chapter 7.

Pneumocystis jiroveci (carinii) Pneumonia

Epidemiology

Historically, *P. carinii* had been classified as a protozoan, although ribosomal RNA sequencing has shown it to be more closely related to fungi, specifically *Saccharomyces* species. However, antifungal agents are not effective against *P. carinii* because its cyst wall sterols are unlike those of most fungi. The taxonomy was recently changed, such that *P. carinii* is now used to describe the species that causes infection in rodents and *P. jiroveci* is the preferred term used to describe the species that infects humans. For convention, the term *PCP* is still used to refer to the pneumonia in humans.

Before the availability of effective ART, approximately 70% to 80% of patients with AIDS developed PCP. However, the incidence of PCP in the United States and Europe has decreased in recent years, and the infection has always been relatively uncommon in developing countries. Mortality from PCP has also declined significantly, with survival rates increasing from 50% to 90%. Patients presenting with PCP generally have a CD4 count of less than 200 cells/mm^3. Other factors associated with PCP include AIDS wasting syndrome, thrush, a history of PCP or recurrent bacterial pneumonia, a CD4/total lymphocyte percentage of less than 15, and an HIV viral load above 100,000 copies/mL.

Pathogenesis

The organism is acquired via the respiratory route and not likely transmitted from person to person. Ninety-five percent of people are colonized with *P. jiroveci* by age 5, and it is believed that most cases in adults are a result of reactivation of latent cysts attached to alveolar epithelium. On reactivation, sporozoites form within the cyst and emerge as mature trophozoites, which cause inflammation and increased alveolar permeability.

Clinical Manifestations

Patients with PCP generally have fever, anorexia, fatigue, a nonproductive cough, and dyspnea on exertion for several days or weeks before presentation. Physical examination is often normal, but there may be dry rales on chest auscultation. Patients taking PCP prophylaxis may have an altered clinical presentation. The use of aerosol pentamidine (AP) has increased the risk of extrapulmonary pneumocystosis, which can involve the lymph nodes, bone marrow, spleen, liver, and other organs. Disseminated calcifications of lymph nodes and visceral organs should raise suspicion of this diagnosis.

Diagnosis

Chest x-ray classically reveals bilateral diffuse interstitial infiltrates in a central, butterfly-shaped pattern (Figure 9-8). However, while it is abnormal in 90% of patients on presentation, these findings are highly variable. Blebs, cysts, nodules, asymmetric infiltrates, and upper lobe disease have also been described; pleural effusions are rare. Patients receiving AP prophylaxis may present with upper lobe infiltrates, pneumothorax, or intraparenchymal cysts. The serum lactate dehydrogenase level, while nonspecific, is increased in over 90% of cases and may exceed 500 U/L. Patients with suspected PCP should have oximetry or a room-air arterial blood gas performed for the purpose of establishing the severity of disease.

Induced sputum using direct immunofluorescent antibody testing is the diagnostic test of choice. The yield of an induced sputum ranges between 50% and 90% and depends on the technical expertise in preparation of sample and the organism burden. Bronchoalveolar lavage (BAL) via bronchoscopy, with a sensitivity of 90% to 99%, is reserved for cases in which sputum induction is unavailable or when the test is negative but the index of suspicion for PCP remains high. It is acceptable to start empirical

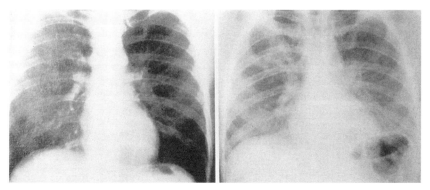

Figure 9-8.   Serial chest radiographs showing the development of *Pneumocystis jiroveci (carinii)* pneumonia. (From Western J Med. 1982;137:400-7; with permission.)

antimicrobial therapy before obtaining a definitive diagnosis because the yield of sputum examination does not decrease for several days into treatment. Transbronchial biopsy (TbBx), with a sensitivity of 95% to 100%, is reserved for cases in which BAL is nondiagnostic. The use of AP decreases the sensitivity of sputum induction and BAL, but the yield of TbBx is not affected. Open lung biopsy has a sensitivity of 95% to 100% but, given the operative risk involved, is reserved for situations in which all other testing is nondiagnostic.

The organism cysts and trophozoites can be demonstrated using cresyl violet, Giemsa, Diff-Quik, and Wright stains, while methenamine silver, Gram-Weigert, and toluidine blue stains show the cyst wall. Detection of cysts does not indicate whether they are viable. Nucleic acid amplification tests are in the process of development.

Management

Oral or intravenous TMP-SMX is the drug of choice for PCP, but other effective regimens are available (Box 9-2). Toxicities of TMP-SMX may include fever (30 to 40%), rash including Stevens-Johnson syndrome (30 to 55%), leukopenia (30 to 40%), thrombocytopenia (15%), and increased liver function tests (20%). If the drug rash is mild, it may be possible to "treat through" and manage it symptomatically. Oral desensitization to TMP-SMX is successful in the majority of patients who exhibit fever, rash, or liver

---

Box 9-2.   Treatment of *Pneumocystis jiroveci (carinii)* Pneumonia

Oral Regimens
- TMP-SMX 2 DS tablets orally every 8 hours for 21 days
- TMP 15 mg/kg/d *and* dapsone 100 mg/d orally for 21 days
- Clindamycin 300–450 mg orally four times daily *and* primaquine base 15 mg/d orally for 21 days
- Atovaquone suspension 750 mg orally twice daily for 21 days

Intravenous Regimens
- TMP-SMX (15–20 mg of TMP component per kilogram per day divided into 3–4 IV doses) for 21 days
- Pentamidine 3–4 mg/kg/d IV for 21 days
- Clindamycin 600–900 mg IV four times daily *and* primaquine base 15 mg/d orally for 21 days

Adjunctive Use of Corticosteroids*
- Prednisone 40 mg orally twice daily for 5 days, followed by 40 mg/d orally for 5 days, followed by 20 mg/d orally for 11 days

---

DS = double-strength; TMP-SMX = trimethoprim-sulfamethoxazole.
* Only if partial pressure of arterial blood (PaO$_2$) is less than 70 or alveolar-arterial gradient is greater than 35.

function test abnormalities (see Chapter 7). Patients who develop PCP while on TMP-SMX prophylaxis can usually be treated successfully with the drug. Intravenous pentamidine should be given to patients requiring parenteral therapy who cannot tolerate TMP-SMX. Toxicities of pentamidine may include hypotension, rash, hypoglycemia, neutropenia, and azotemia.

Adjunctive corticosteroid therapy is recommended in patients presenting with a room-air partial pressure of oxygen (PO_2) of less than 70 mmHg or an alveolar-arterial gradient of greater than 35 mmHg. Steroids act by decreasing inflammatory cytokines in the lung, stabilizing capillary permeability, and improving oxygenation.

Upon initiation of antimicrobial therapy, respiratory function occasionally worsens transiently as a result of cytokine release, but clinical improvement should occur within 5 days. Survival decreases to approximately 50% in patients who switch therapies because of drug failure and to 40% in patients requiring mechanical ventilation. Patients who do not improve or worsen after 5 days of TMP-SMX should be evaluated to rule out other OIs. If no other reason for clinical deterioration can be determined, alternative regimens, such as intravenous pentamidine, clindamycin/primaquine, or atovaquone (for mild disease) should be considered.

Immune reconstitution associated with ART may lead to deterioration in the respiratory status in patients with previously subclinical PCP. Because of this concern, as well as issues of overlapping toxicities from ART and PCP treatment, many clinicians defer initiation of ART until a response is seen from treatment of PCP.

Secondary prophylaxis is essential in patients following treatment for PCP who remain significantly immunosuppressed. Effective drugs include oral TMP-SMX 160/800 mg/d, dapsone 100 mg/d, AP 300 mg monthly, and atovaquone 1500 mg/d. Because the risk of prophylaxis failure is higher in patients taking AP prophylaxis, TMP-SMX or dapsone is preferred; AP is a useful alternative in those who are unable to tolerate systemic agents. Secondary PCP prophylaxis can be safely discontinued in patients whose CD4 count rises above 200 cells/mm³ for at least 3 months on ART. However, if a patient has a CD4 count above 200 cells/mm³ but a CD4/ total lymphocyte percentage of less than 15, maintenance of PCP prophylaxis should be considered. Primary prophylaxis of PCP is discussed in Chapter 7.

Salmonellosis

Epidemiology

Although *Salmonella* bacteremia accounts for less than 1% of OIs in HIV-infected persons in the United States, recurrent bacteremia (which meets the case definition for AIDS) occurs at 20-fold the rate in seronegative persons. Bacteremia is reported in about one-third of HIV-infected patients with enteritis. Whereas typhoidal *Salmonella* is mainly spread by person-to-person contact, transmission of nontyphoidal strains is generally from food or contact with birds or reptiles. Transmission from contaminated marijuana cigarettes has also been reported. The most frequent pathogenic strains in the United States are nontyphoidal and include *S. enteritidis*, serogroup D, and *S. typhimurium*, serogroup B.

Pathogenesis

HIV-induced defects in mucosal and systemic humoral and cell-mediated immunity lead to bloodstream invasion once *Salmonella* establishes an infection in the gastrointestinal mucosa. These same defects may be responsible for its persistence in macrophages and the resultant increased risk of recurrent bacteremia.

Clinical Manifestations

Patients with salmonellosis present with fever, chills, night sweats, anorexia, and weight loss, often in association with gastrointestinal complaints. Coexistence of CMV infection, parasitic infection, or KS may cause intestinal inflammation that predisposes to bacteremia. Focal suppurative complications of salmonellosis include splenic abscess, meningitis, septic arthritis, pneumonia, osteomyelitis, cholangitis, and endovascular infections (e.g., aortitis). The risk for recurrence is higher in patients who present with bacteremia and in those who do not receive quinolone therapy for their initial infection. In a study of *Salmonella* bacteremia in Spain, 17% of 172 patients experienced a relapse following treatment, and 60% of those who relapsed were HIV-infected.

Diagnosis

Blood cultures provide the highest yield for the diagnosis of salmonellosis in HIV-infected patients who have significant constitutional or gastrointestinal symptoms. Stool cultures should be performed as well. Laboratory studies may show leukocytosis and increased serum transaminase levels. If focal suppurative complications of salmonellosis are suspected, appropriate additional imaging studies and cultures should be obtained.

Management

Whereas antibiotics are usually not recommended for nonbacteremic salmonellosis in the general population, they are indicated in the HIV-infected patient. A 2-week course of therapy is advised if metastatic or endovascular infection is not clinically suspected. Initial therapy consists of a fluoroquinolone, usually ciprofloxacin (500 to 750 mg/bid). For systemic disease, a third-generation cephalosporin such as ceftriaxone should be added until sensitivity test results are available. Ceftriaxone has excellent tissue availability, which may be beneficial for focal metastatic infections. Treatment should continue for at least 6 weeks in patients with endovascular disease; surgical intervention is often necessary as well.

Long-term suppressive oral antibiotic therapy is recommended if salmonellosis recurs. Patient education regarding food handling, travel, and the health risks of keeping reptiles as pets is important. Household contacts of patients with the infection should be evaluated for asymptomatic carriage of the bacterium. Secondary prophylaxis can sometimes be discontinued following immune reconstitution from antiretroviral therapy.

Syphilis

Epidemiology and Pathogenesis

After declines in the late 1980s and the 1990s, the incidence of primary and secondary syphilis has increased appreciably as of late in the United States, with MSM comprising the majority of cases. The bacterium causing syphilis, *Treponema pallidum*, is a ciliated microaerophilic spirochete. The primary mode of transmission is direct contact with infected lesions (in the setting of sexual contact) or blood (in the setting of transplacental transmission). The organism proliferates locally in the inoculated area and regional lymph nodes, enters the bloodstream, and disseminates widely to organs and tissues of the reticuloendothelial system. Patients with primary syphilis are at increased risk for HIV transmission and acquisition.

Clinical Manifestations

The natural history of syphilis is divided into primary, secondary, early latent, late latent, and tertiary stages. Primary syphilis begins with a skin chancre at the site of inoculation following an incubation period of 3 to 90 days. The chancre is a firm, nontender, clean-based ulcer that is associated with regional painless lymphadenopathy. If primary syphilis is left untreated, 60% to 90% of patients will go on to the secondary stage. Secondary syphilis occurs 2 to 12 weeks after initial inoculation and is usually associated with fever, rash, mucous membrane lesions, and generalized lymphadenopathy. The rash is often described as copper-colored, may be macular, maculopapular, follicular, or pustular, and frequently involves the palms and soles (Figure 9-9). The mucous membrane lesions ("mucous patches") are typically ulcerative. Dissemination to the central nervous system (CNS) during secondary syphilis is common, although symptomatic meningitis occurs in only 1% to 3% of patients. The facial and auditory nerves may be involved during this stage, resulting in

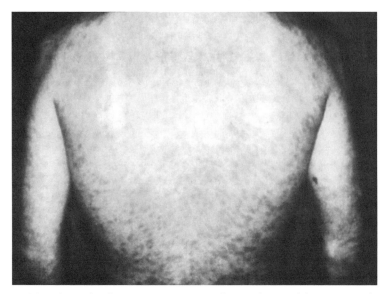

Figure 9-9. Generalized cutaneous eruption of secondary syphilis. (From Hicks CB, et al. Seronegative secondary syphilis in a patient infected with the human immunodeficiency virus (HIV) with Kaposi's sarcoma; a diagnostic dilemma. Ann Intern Med. 1987;107: 492-5; with permission.)

sensorineural hearing loss in some instances. Patients with primary and secondary syphilis are considered highly infectious to their sexual partners.

Latent syphilis is an asymptomatic stage, divided into early latency (within 12 months of the secondary stage), and late latency (beyond 12 months of the secondary stage). There is a 25% chance of relapse to secondary syphilis during early latent syphilis. Perinatal transmission is still possible during the latent stages of syphilis. Natural history studies estimate that tertiary syphilis occurs in 15% to 40% of untreated patients from 10 to 45 years after initial infection. This stage is characterized by an obliterative endarteritis affecting multiple organs, such as the heart and great vessels, brain, skin, bone, and viscera. When cardiovascular disease develops, syphilitic aortitis is the most common finding, with saccular aneurysms of the ascending aorta reported less frequently.

Neurosyphilis is seen in 10% of untreated patients and can occur at any stage. There are five major categories of neurosyphilis: asymptomatic neurosyphilis, syphilitic meningitis, meningovascular disease, parenchymatous neurosyphilis, and gummatous syphilis. Syphilitic meningitis presents within 5 years of infection. Meningovascular syphilis accounts for 10% of cases and can occur in the first 10 years following infection, presenting with multiple small infarcts of the brain and spinal cord. Parenchymatous neurosyphilis is rare in the era of antibiotics; it occurs 5 to 25 years following infection and can present as either tabes dorsalis or general paresis. Gummatous syphilis, also referred to as late benign syphilis, is characterized by the presence of space-occupying lymphocytic and plasma cell infiltrates called "gumma," in the brain, skin, bone, or liver.

Diagnosis

The diagnosis of syphilis is based on clinical findings and serologic evidence of infection. Culture of the organism is not routinely performed for diagnostic purposes. Serologic tests should be interpreted in the same manner as in HIV-seronegative persons. In cases where serology is negative but clinical suspicion is high, a repeat serology or biopsy of skin or mucous membrane lesions should be considered.

Nonspecific treponemal tests (rapid plasma reagin [RPR] and the Venereal Disease Research Laboratory test for syphilis [VDRL]) are used to screen patients. They are quantitative and indicate the degree of disease activity. These tests become positive 4 to 7 days after the chancre appears. Although nonspecific tests can be negative in both primary and tertiary syphilis, they are usually positive in secondary syphilis. False-positive nonspecific treponemal tests can occur in the setting of advancing age, pregnancy, injection drug use, malignancy, autoimmune disease, and other chronic infections. In cases where nontreponemal titers are extremely high (e.g., secondary syphilis), the corresponding assay can be falsely negative and revert to positive when the specimen is diluted ("prozone phenomenon").

Specific treponemal tests (fluorescent treponemal antibody [FTA], treponemal enzyme immunoassay [EIA], *Treponema pallidum* particle agglutination [TPPA] or hemagglutination [TPHA], and microhemagglutination–*Treponema pallidum* [MHA-TP]) are used to confirm the diagnosis of syphilis in the patient with a positive nonspecific test. They are qualitative and remain positive indefinitely, even following antimicrobial treatment. False-positive specific treponemal tests are unusual.

In neurosyphilis, the cerebrospinal (CSF) examination generally shows a modest pleocytosis, increased protein level, and moderately low glucose. The CSF VDRL has a high specificity but low sensitivity (30% to 78%) for the diagnosis of neurosyphilis and can be falsely positive if the specimen is contaminated with blood. A negative test does not exclude neurosyphilis. If the CSF VDRL is negative and CSF indices are suggestive of neurosyphilis, a CSF MHA-TP can be performed. A positive CSF MHA-TP is not diagnostic of neurosyphilis because of passive diffusion from the blood to the CSF. However, if the CSF MHA-TP is negative, neurosyphilis is highly unlikely.

Management

The treatment of syphilis is based upon its disease stage and is the same in HIV-infected patients as the general population (Box 9-3). Penicillin remains the drug of choice. For penicillin-allergic patients, doxycycline (100 mg orally bid for 2 weeks) can be substituted in early-stage syphilis. Penicillin should always be used to treat neurosyphilis, with desensitization performed if there

---

Box 9-3.   Treatment of Syphilis

Primary, Secondary, and Early Latent (<1 Year Duration) Syphilis
• Recommended regimen: 2.4 mIU benzathine penicillin G IM once
• Doxycycline 100 mg twice weekly orally for 2 weeks, if penicillin allergic

Late Latent (>1 Year Duration) and Cardiovascular Syphilis
• Recommended regimen: 2.4 mIU/wk benzathine penicillin G IM for 3 weeks (total 7.2 mIU)
• Doxycycline 100 mg twice weekly orally for 4 weeks, if penicillin allergic

Neurosyphilis*
• Recommended regimen: 18–24 mIU/d aqueous penicillin G IV for 10–14 days
• Alternative: 2.4 mIU/d procaine penicillin IM plus 50 mg probenecid four times daily for 10–14 days
• If patient is penicillin allergic, skin test and desensitize as necessary

---

Adapted from Centers for Disease Control and Prevention. Sexually transmitted disease treatment guidelines 2002. MMWR. 2002;51(RR-6):18–30.
* Following completion of a neurosyphilis regimen, many authorities recommend the administration of 2.4 mIU/wk benzathine penicillin for 3 weeks.

---

is a history of drug allergy. An LP is recommended in patients with syphilis who have neurologic symptoms or signs, a serum VDRL greater than 1:32, treatment failure (see below), late latent infection, or syphilis of unknown duration. Patients treated for syphilis should be followed clinically and serologically on a regular basis. The serum RPR or VDRL usually becomes negative within one year for primary syphilis, two years for secondary syphilis, and five years for tertiary syphilis. If it does not occur, three possibilities should be considered: failure of therapy; reinfection; or a false-positive test result. If failure of therapy is suspected, an LP should be performed. In addition, the patient should be treated for neurosyphilis, if indicated, or re-treated with three weekly doses of benzathine penicillin if the CSF examination is negative. Some patients have persistently detectable RPR or VDRL titers of 1:8 or less ("serofast") despite adequate therapy. While this finding probably does not represent treatment failure in most instances, if the titer rises four-fold or greater above baseline, reinfection is a possible explanation.

Contact tracing should be performed in all patients with early syphilis, and contacts within the prior three months should be treated with penicillin. Contacts of patients with secondary and early latent syphilis should be evaluated and treated as appropriate.

Toxoplasmosis

Epidemiology

In recent years, the incidence of *Toxoplasma gondii* encephalitis has decreased significantly in HIV-infected patients, with the majority of those affected having a CD4 count of less than 50 cells/mm³. Up to 15% of persons in the United States have serologic evidence of prior exposure to toxoplasmosis by a positive serum *Toxoplasma* IgG antibody test; rates of 50% to 75% have been reported in the developing world.

Pathogenesis

Toxoplasma gondii is an obligate intracellular parasite acquired via ingestion of viable oocysts that have been excreted in cat feces and have sporulated in the environment or that were present in infected undercooked meat containing tissue cysts. Person-to-person transmission does not occur. The oocysts transform into replicating trophozoites, which disseminate throughout the body and encyst in tissues. Lack of immunologic containment permits emergence of tachyzoites, which is the proliferative form of the organism. The predilection of the organism for infection in the brain may reflect "sequestering" from immune surveillance. Because toxoplasmosis is generally associated with a positive IgG antibody test, it is thought to represent reactivation of latent infection. Primary infection, however, can occasionally cause CNS or disseminated disease.

Clinical Manifestations

Patients with CNS toxoplasmosis present subacutely, with fever, altered mental status, and other neurologic complaints. Headache occurs in 50% of cases, confusion in up to 52%, fever in up to 47%, seizures in 25%, and focal neurologic abnormalities in 69%. Chorioretinitis, pneumonitis, transverse myelitis, and orchitis have been rarely described.

Diagnosis

Over 95% of patients with CNS toxoplasmosis will have detectable *Toxoplasma* antibodies, with a median IgG titer of 1:256; serum IgM antibody is almost always negative. In patients followed longitudinally, there is no appreciable change in the IgG titer when CNS infection reactivates. A positive IgG titer in a patient with a brain lesion does not establish the diagnosis of toxoplasmosis, but, because the incidence of this infection in patients without detectable antibody is 1% to 3%, a negative result virtually excludes it.

Brain imaging by CT scan with intravenous contrast or MRI with gadolinium is recommended in all patients suspected of having CNS toxoplasmosis. Most patients have two or more contrast-enhancing lesions that are located in the frontal lobes, corticomedullary junction, basal ganglia, thalamus, or pituitary gland (Figure 9-10). Associated edema is common. MRI is more sensitive than CT scan and should be performed in patients with a negative CT if the index of suspicion for toxoplasmosis is high. SPECT and PET scans can sometimes be helpful in distinguishing toxoplasmosis from lymphoma. Differential diagnosis in an HIV-infected patient

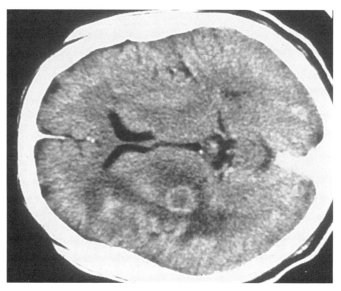

Figure 9-10.   Computed tomography scan of head showing an enhancing lesion in patient with toxoplasmosis.

presenting with CNS complaints who has an abnormal brain imaging study also includes lymphoma, bacterial abscess, cryptococcoma or other fungal infection, mycobacterial infection, and septic emboli.

Examination of the CSF, which should be deferred in the presence of a significant mass lesion, may be helpful in excluding other infectious and malignant processes. The CSF indices associated with toxoplasmosis are variable but generally consist of a mononuclear pleocytosis, a mildly increased protein level, and a normal or low glucose level. CSF *Toxoplasma* IgG antibody and PCR tests have low sensitivities.

Management

Expert consultation is recommended for clinicians with limited experience in the treatment of toxoplasmosis. Empiric therapy is indicated in the presence of multiple contrast-enhancing lesions on brain imaging and a positive *Toxoplasma* IgG serology. Stereotactic CT-guided brain biopsy should be considered if there is no clinical or radiographic improvement within 10 to 14 days of initiation of therapy. If the patient does not have detectable IgG antibody or has an MRI showing a single-mass lesion or nonenhancing lesion(s), brain biopsy should be performed. The causative organisms can be visualized with hematoxylin and eosin or immunoperoxidase stains.

Treatment of toxoplasmosis is successful in up to 85% of cases. Effective drug combinations include sulfadiazine with pyrimethamine or clindamycin with pyrimethamine, with the former regimen demonstrating slightly

---

Box 9-4.   Treatment of Toxoplasmosis

Initial Regimen (6 wk duration)

- Sulfadiazine 1–2 g orally four times daily *and* pyrimethamine 50–75 mg/d orally after loading with 200 mg for 1 day; folinic acid 10–25 mg/d orally should be administered to prevent leukopenia

  or

- Clindamycin 600 mg IV or PO four times daily *and* pyrimethamine 50–100 mg/d orally; folinic acid 10–25 mg/d orally should also be administered

  or

- TMP-SMX (5 mg/kg TMP and 25 mg/kg SMX) IV or PO twice daily

Maintenance Regimen

- Sulfadiazine 0.5–1 g orally four times daily with pyrimethamine 25–50 mg/d orally; folinic acid 10–25 mg/d orally should be administered concurrently
- Clindamycin 300–450 mg orally 3–4 times daily with pyrimethamine 25–50 mg/d orally; folinic acid 10–25 mg/d orally should be administered concurrently
- Atovaquone 750 mg orally twice daily with or without pyrimethamine 25–50 mg/d orally; folinic acid 10–25 mg/d orally should be administered concurrently
- Azithromycin 900–1200 mg orally once daily with pyrimethamine 25–50 mg/d orally; folinic acid 10–25 mg/d orally should be administered concurrently

---

TMP-SMX = trimethoprim-sulfamethoxazole.

---

better success (Box 9-4). Sulfadiazine toxicities may include fever, rash, gastrointestinal complaints, leukopenia, and increased liver function tests; pyrimethamine may cause rash, nausea, or bone marrow suppression (folinic acid should always be coadministered). Alternative regimens include high-dose TMP-SMX, clarithromycin or azithromycin with pyrimethamine, ato-vaquone with pyrimethamine, atovaquone with sulfadiazine, dapsone with pyrimethamine, doxycycline with pyrimethamine, and clindamycin with flucytosine. Patients who require parenteral therapy can be treated with in-travenous TMP-SMX or clindamycin along with oral pyrimethamine.

Adjunctive corticosteroid therapy should be used only if there is signif-icant cerebral edema; it decreases the size of CNS lymphoma lesions and obscures the assessment of therapeutic response. Anticonvulsants should be administered throughout the early treatment period if seizures occur. Consultation with a neurologist is advised for patients who have significant cerebral edema or seizure activity.

Induction doses should be given for 6 weeks and then changed to maintenance therapy, which is essential to prevent relapse. Patients with a suboptimal clinical and radiologic response at 6 weeks and those with ex-tensive disease should continue on induction therapy for a longer period of time. Retrospective data provide support for discontinuing secondary prophylaxis in patients who are asymptomatic, have completed their initial antimicrobial therapy, and have an increase in their CD4 count to more than 200 cells/mm^3 for at least 6 months on ART. Primary prophylaxis of toxoplasmosis is discussed in Chapter 7.

Tuberculosis

Epidemiology

Tuberculosis is one of the most significant infectious diseases in the world, but there has been some progress in controlling it in recent years. According to the World Health Organization (WHO), the overall global TB prevalence has decreased by more than 20% from 1990, and incidence rates have fallen or are stable in 5 of 6 regions of the world. However, in Africa rates have tripled since 1990, increasing 3% to 4% per year, particularly in regions of high HIV seroprevalence. In 2003, there were an estimated 15.4 million TB cases worldwide, including 229,000 in patients who were coinfected with HIV. In developing countries, 50% of HIV-infected patients will contract TB during their lives. TB is responsible for 11% of HIV-related deaths worldwide, making it the leading cause of mortality.

The alarming increase in cases of TB noted in the United States in the mid-1980s was multifactorial, but HIV infection played an important role. At least half of the patients with TB in New York City from 1992 to 1995 were coinfected with HIV and had a median CD4 count of 71 cells/mm³. In the United States, the incidence of TB decreased by 44% between 1993 and 2003 and is now at historically low levels. In 1999, approximately 10% of patients with TB in the US were HIV-infected.

The depletion of CD4 lymphocytes that occurs in HIV infection leads to increased frequency of both primary and reactivation TB and more rapid TB progression. There is a 7% to 10% annual risk of active TB in HIV-infected persons with a positive TB skin test (purified protein derivative [PPD]) compared with a 5% to 10% lifetime risk in seronegative persons with a positive PPD. Co-infected patients also have an accelerated course of HIV infection and decreased survival compared with HIV-infected patients who do not have TB. Activities or occupations that may increase the risk of exposure to and acquisition of TB include urban living, injection-drug use, alcoholism, homelessness, living or working in a correctional institution or medical/chronic care facility, and origin from an endemic country.

Pathogenesis

Primary infection with *Mycobacterium tuberculosis* occurs through inhalation of airborne respiratory droplets that reach the mid- or lower-lung fields. The bacteria are ingested by alveolar macrophages, which spread to regional lymph nodes and then disseminate throughout the body. In the immunocompetent host, primary TB pneumonitis often resolves spontaneously, and reactivation disease involving the lungs or other organs may occur months to years later. In the context of HIV disease, reactivation TB may involve extrapulmonary sites, especially in patients with a low CD4 count.

Clinical Manifestations

The clinical presentation of TB depends in part on the degree of underlying immune dysfunction. In HIV-infected patients with a normal CD4 count, TB is most often the result of reactivation of previous infection, and the presentation usually consists of fever and pulmonary symptoms. Chest x-ray shows pulmonary infiltrates, with or without cavitation, localized to the upper lobes. In patients with a low CD4 count, the presentation of TB is more likely to be atypical and consist of extrapulmonary or disseminated disease. Chest x-ray shows diffuse alveolar and interstitial infiltrates (60%), focal consolidation (30%), or pleural effusion (10%). Twenty-five percent of patients have mediastinal and intrathoracic lymphadenopathy, which may caseate and form abscesses that erode into adjacent structures. Up to 70% of patients with advanced HIV disease have evidence of extrapulmonary infection involving the skin, lymph nodes, CNS, liver, bone marrow, and/or genitourinary tract (Figure 9-11).

Diagnosis

It is more difficult to diagnose TB in HIV-infected patients than in the general population because of atypical clinical presentations, the lower yield of sputum culture, and cutaneous anergy. As HIV infection progresses and cellular immunity declines, the PPD often becomes nonreactive, and chest x-ray findings are more nonspecific. All patients newly diagnosed with HIV

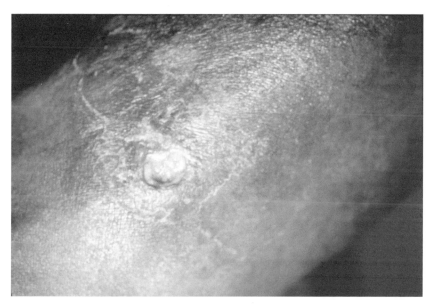

Figure 9-11. Cutaneous tuberculosis in patient with advanced HIV disease. (For color reproduction, see Plate 4 at back of book.)

infection should have an intermediate strength PPD placed; control tests are not necessary. A positive PPD in the context of HIV disease is defined as 5 mm of induration or greater. Such a finding warrants clinical evaluation and a chest x-ray to rule out active TB. Asymptomatic patients with a negative initial PPD should undergo repeat annual testing if there is continued risk of TB exposure. In addition, patients with a negative PPD in the setting of advanced HIV disease (CD4 count < 200 cells/mm^3) should undergo repeat PPD testing if the CD4 count rises in response to ART.

Examination of sputum for acid-fast organisms should be performed if there is evidence of pulmonary disease. However, HIV-infected patients with active TB are more likely to have negative smears than seronegative persons. If the smear demonstrates acid-fast bacilli, PCR techniques are available to distinguish *M. tuberculosis* from atypical mycobacteria. It is important to culture the organism for identification and antibiotic susceptibility testing in order to guide the selection of appropriate therapy. Systems using liquid rather than solid media and radiometric methodology provide rapid and reliable culture results in 1 to 2 weeks, and sensitivity data are generally available one week later.

Tissue biopsy with review of histopathology is sometimes required to confirm the diagnosis of TB. In patients with extrapulmonary disease, needle aspiration can be performed of skin lesions, lymph nodes, or pleural or pericardial fluid to obtain tissue for culture and susceptibility testing. Excisional biopsy should be performed if needle aspiration is nondiagnostic. In the setting of normal immune function, histopathology will demonstrate granulomatous inflammation, but granulomas are poorly formed or absent in the context of immunodeficiency.

Management

Expert consultation is recommended for clinicians with limited experience in the treatment of active TB. A number of issues must be considered in managing patients coinfected with HIV and TB: 1) the optimal duration of treatment of TB is not established; 2) resistance is unusual in the setting of directly observed therapy (DOT) but can occur, particularly with the rifamycins; 3) there are important interactions between TB regimens and ART and significant overlapping toxicities; and 4) immune reconstitution syndrome may occur and can be severe.

Most patients should receive a four-drug therapy with isoniazid (INH), rifampin (RIF), pyrazinamide (PZA), and ethambutol (ETH) for 2 months until culture and sensitivity results are known. If the strain is susceptible, therapy should continue with INH and RIF daily or biweekly (DOT) for 4 additional months if the organism is susceptible. Extrapulmonary and cavitary lung disease is often treated for a total of 9 to 12 months. If multidrug-resistant TB is suspected, initial therapy should consist of 6 or more drugs, depending on the susceptibility data for strains prevalent in the particular region. Infectious disease consultation is strongly recommended. Although there are conflicting reports regarding the likelihood of recurrent TB after appropriate treatment in HIV-infected patients, chronic suppressive therapy is not recommended.

Rifabutin can be substituted for RIF in the treatment of TB in HIV-infected patients. This has particular relevance because rifabutin, unlike RIF, can be used with dosage adjustment in conjunction with protease inhibitors and nonnucleoside reverse-transcriptase inhibitors. RIF should not be used concomitantly with saquinavir, indinavir, nelfinvir, amprenavir, atazanavir, or dual PI combinations using low-dose ritonavir. Rifabutin also is occasionally effective against RIF-resistant strains. Recent data from the CDC suggest that patients treated with rifabutin-based twice-weekly intermittent therapy may be at increased risk for the development of acquired rifamycin resistance. Similar findings were reported with a twice-weekly regimen of INH and RIF. All patients in these studies had a very low CD4 count at the time of TB diagnosis.

Immune reconstitution syndrome is common in patients coinfected with TB and HIV, resulting in a temporary exacerbation of TB symptoms and signs. Patients may present with high fever, lymphadenopathy, worsening pulmonary infiltrates, pleural effusions, and/or progression of lesions. Drug resistance and failure of TB therapy must be ruled out before symptoms are attributed to immune reconstitution. If immune reconstitution is established as the cause, it can be palliated with NSAIDs or corticosteroids.

Baseline laboratory evaluation for patients starting TB therapy should include a complete blood count and liver and renal function tests. Follow-up visits should be scheduled monthly to evaluate clinical progress, reinforce medication adherence, and address any side effects. Patients treated with more than 2 months of ETH should be seen by an ophthalmologist for testing of visual acuity and color discrimination. A monthly sputum sample for smear and culture should be obtained in patients who have pulmonary TB until two consecutive negative cultures have been documented. If sputum cultures remain positive after 3 months of treatment, repeat susceptibility testing should be performed. Antimicrobial prophylaxis for TB is discussed in Chapter 7.

Varicella-Zoster Virus Infection

Epidemiology and Microbiology

Varicella-zoster virus (VZV) is a herpesvirus that presents as chickenpox, usually during childhood, in the absence of vaccine-induced immunity. After primary infection, VZV establishes latency in the dorsal root ganglia of the spinal cord and may reactivate as zoster or "shingles" with age or in the context of immunodeficiency. HIV-infected patients have a frequency of zoster that is three to five times that of the elderly population, and recurrences are also more common.

Clinical Manifestations

Zoster typically presents with a prodrome of pain and paresthesias followed by the development of painful grouped vesicles on an erythematous base in 1 to 2 adjacent dermatomes, usually in the thoracic or trigeminal areas (Figure 9-12). Fever and extradermatomal vesicular lesions are reported occasionally. Zoster may occur shortly after initiation of ART as a manifestation of the immune reconstitution syndrome. One-quarter of HIV-infected patients with zoster, especially those with advanced immunodeficiency, experience complications. These may include meningitis, radiculitis, transverse myelitis, encephalitis, and zoster ophthalmicus.

Acute radiculitis manifesting as severe radicular lower extremity pain has been reported as the prodrome to a zoster outbreak, especially involving a lumbosacral dermatome. Transverse myelitis, a subacute paraplegia with an accompanying sensory level, is an unusual complication of VZV infection. Encephalitis has been reported as a zoster prodromal event, manifesting as headache, fever, and mental status changes. VZV is an important

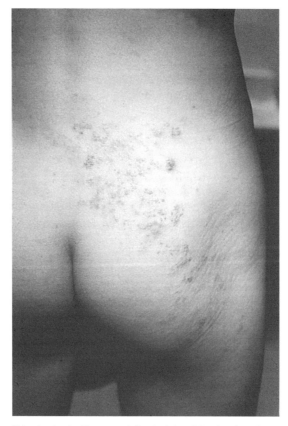

Figure 9-12.   Shingles (varicella-zoster infection) involving lumbar dermatomes.

cause of acute retinal necrosis (ARN) and rapidly progressive herpetic retinal necrosis (RPHRN). ARN is defined by focal necrosis of the retinal periphery anterior to the vascular arcades that progresses circumferentially, resulting in occlusion of the retinal vessels, vitritis, and anterior uveitis. RPHRN occurs more frequently than ARV in advanced HIV disease and is characterized by bilateral multifocal disease with early macular involvement and retinal detachment and tears that may lead to blindness. An episode of zoster usually heralds retinal VZV involvement.

Diagnosis

Zoster can be diagnosed clinically, in most instances, with confirmation by DFA staining of vesicular fluid from a fresh lesion. DFA is more sensitive than viral culture. ARN and RPHRN are diagnosed by their characteristic appearance on ophthalmologic examination. Patients with CNS involvement have a CSF profile suggestive of aseptic meningitis, with a mild-to-moderate pleocytosis and increased protein level. Neurologic disease can be diagnosed by VZV PCR of the CSF, but a negative result does not rule it out. In the case of myelitis and encephalitis, MRI scan shows areas of edema and demyelination in spinal cord and brain, respectively.

Management

Treatment of uncomplicated zoster consists of famciclovir or acyclovir given for 7 to 10 days (see Table 9-6). Valacyclovir has been associated with hemolytic uremic syndrome in patients with advanced HIV disease and should be avoided in this setting. If the patient is extremely ill or neurologic disease is suspected, intravenous acyclovir should be given. Approximately 20% of HIV-infected patients with zoster require hospitalization. Ophthalmic VZV infection requires both systemic and intravitreal therapy, and, although patients with ARN usually respond well, those with RPHRN typically do not. Acyclovir-resistant VZV has been reported in HIV-infected patients, and, if there is no improvement or evidence of progression after 10 days of therapy, an empiric switch to foscarnet is recommended. Postherpetic neuralgia has been reported to occur in almost 20% of HIV-infected patients with zoster; adjunctive corticosteroid therapy has not been demonstrated to prevent it in this setting.

Viral Hepatitis

Overview

Hepatitis A, B, and C infections are common in HIV disease. Because hepatitis A virus (HAV) is transmitted via the fecal-oral route, it is seen mainly in MSM but has also been reported in injection-drug users. Hepatitis B virus

(HBV), which can be spread sexually or through exposure to infected blood, occurs in MSM, heterosexuals, and injection-drug users. Hepatitis C virus (HCV), which is transmitted primarily through exposure to infected blood, is described in injection-drug users, hemophiliacs, and other persons who acquired HIV infection through contaminated blood products. However, recent outbreaks of HCV infection in MSM have demonstrated that the virus can be transmitted via sexual contact as well. Hepatitis A causes acute infection but not chronic liver disease. Hepatitis B causes chronic infection in 20% of HIV-infected patients compared with 4% of affected persons in the general population. Hepatitis C is a chronic infection in the majority of patients and is often associated with progressive liver disease.

Acute viral hepatitis may be asymptomatic or characterized by anorexia, nausea, vomiting, upper abdominal pain, and jaundice; fever is common with HAV infection. Rarely, fulminant hepatitis occurs with rapidly progressive hepatitis dysfunction in patients with acute hepatitis. Physical examination may show a jaundiced patient with tender hepatomegaly. Liver function tests, particularly serum transaminase and bilirubin levels, are increased. Symptoms and signs of acute hepatitis often persist for several weeks before resolution. Patients with HBV or HCV who develop chronic infection may be asymptomatic or have exacerbation of symptoms with variable frequency. Over time, they become at risk for cirrhosis with manifestations of end-stage liver disease and hepatoma.

Acute viral hepatitis is suggested by the clinical presentation in association with abnormal liver function tests. Differential diagnosis includes hepatotoxicity related to alcohol or drugs, infiltrative diseases of the liver, and biliary tract disease. Diagnosis of viral hepatitis is established by serologic tests, which are described below. Chronic hepatitis is defined as lasting 6 months or longer. Liver biopsy may be recommended to establish the extent of disease in patients with chronic hepatitis and to identify those who are candidates for drug treatment. In general, liver function test abnormalities do not correlate with histologic findings.

The management of acute viral hepatitis is supportive. Patients should be asked to maintain adequate oral intake to prevent dehydration and to rest as needed. Expert consultation is recommended for clinicians with limited experience in the treatment of chronic viral hepatitis. Details on the management of HBV and HCV infection are presented below.

Patients with chronic hepatitis should be cautioned about the use of alcohol and other hepatotoxic agents. Because of the potential for transmission of these viruses to other persons, patients with HBV or HCV infection should be advised against sharing razors and other sharp instruments. The importance of practicing safe sex should also be emphasized.

All HIV-infected patients should be tested serologically for HAV, HBV, and HCV infections. Immunization against hepatitis A and B is recommended in those without previous exposure to these pathogens, although the response to these vaccines may be diminished in advanced HIV disease.

If patients do not seroconvert after a standard HBV immunization series, double doses of HBV vaccine and an intensified schedule should be considered. Hepatitis A vaccine is particularly important because of the risk for fulminant hepatitis in HCV-infected patients who subsequently contract HAV.

Hepatitis C Virus

In the United States, 15% to 30% of HIV-infected patients are also infected with HCV, representing approximately 300,000 persons. HIV/HCV coinfection was not recognized as an important problem early in the HIV epidemic because the majority of deaths were caused by other OIs. However, with the introduction of effective ART in the mid-1990's, the mortality from most OIs has decreased significantly, while the number of deaths from end-stage liver disease has increased. HCV-related complications, including decompensated liver disease and hepatoma, are now leading causes of hospitalization and death in HIV/HCV coinfected patients.

All HIV-infected patients should be tested for the presence of antibody to HCV (anti-HCV). Those with advanced HIV disease (CD4 count <100 cells/mm^3) are more likely to have antibody-negative chronic HCV infection, so unexplained increased liver function tests in this setting should also be evaluated with a qualitative HCV RNA assay. All patients with a positive anti-HCV test should have the diagnosis of chronic infection confirmed with a qualitative HCV RNA assay. If the initial HCV RNA test is negative, it should be repeated in 3 to 4 months; if still undetectable, the person does not have chronic HCV infection but should be counseled on avoidance of reexposure. The HCV viral load (quantitative assay) level does not correlate with the degree of liver damage.

HIV/HCV coinfected patients have a three-fold increased risk of progression to decompensated liver disease (bleeding varices, ascites, encephalopathy, high bilirubin) compared with those with HCV alone. Cirrhosis often occurs in 10 to 20 years following exposure compared with 30 to 40 years in those with HCV alone. In a study of nearly 1000 patients with HIV/HCV coinfection, 55% had stage 2 or higher fibrosis (Metavir scale, where a score of 0 is no fibrosis and 4 is cirrhosis) on liver biopsy. Patients with stage 3 or 4 fibrosis were more likely to be over 35 years in age, have a CD4 count of less than 500 cells/mm^3, and drink more than 50 g of alcohol/day. Fifty percent of HIV/HCV coinfected patients die within one year of developing decompensated liver disease compared with five years in those with HCV infection alone. The effect of HCV infection on HIV progression is less clear, but a meta-analysis concluded that coinfected patients had a reduced mean increase in their CD4 count after initiation of ART compared to those with HIV infection alone.

Chronic HCV infection can be effectively managed in many patients with pegylated interferon-alfa in combination with ribavirin (peg-IFN/R). However, determining which patients to treat and when to treat them is not always clear. The APRICOT study reported on 868 patients with HIV/HCV coinfection in 19 countries: 80% were male; 80% were white; median age was 40 years; mean CD4 count was 530 cells/mm^3 (patients with CD4 count < 100 were excluded); 60% had HIV viral load of less than 50 copies/mL; and 60% had HCV genotype 1. The overall sustained virologic response rate (SVR = HCV RNA-negative 6 months after completion of 48 weeks of therapy) for patients with genotype 2 or 3 who received peg-IFN/R was 62%. For patients with HCV genotype 1, the overall SVR was 29%. However, in genotype 1 patients with HCV viral loads of less than 800,000 IU/mL at baseline, the SVR was 60% compared with 18% in those with HCV viral loads of greater than 800,000 IU/mL and in patients who maintained greater than 80% adherence to treatment, the SVR was 39% compared with 11% in those who were less adherent. There was no association between the likelihood of SVR and the CD4 count, having an undetectable HIV viral load, or being on ART in this study. In patients with an early virologic response (EVR = HCV viral load decrease of at least 2 $\log_{10}$ between baseline and week 12 of treatment), 56% were SVR compared with 2% of those who did not achieve an EVR. However, in patients who did not achieve an SVR, over 40% had at least a two score improvement in their histology index on post-treatment liver biopsy.

Adverse events of peg-IFN/R were common and included anemia and neutropenia. It is preferable to support patients with erythropoietin or granulocyte colony stimulating factor rather than reduce the doses of peg-IFN/R if possible. Flu-like symptoms, nausea, diarrhea, and depression have also been frequently reported with anti-HCV treatment. The risk of lactic acidosis is increased when didanosine (ddI) is combined with ribavirin, and there is a "black box" warning against using ddI in this setting. Zidovudine (ZDV) is associated with a substantially increased risk of anemia requiring dose reduction of ribavirin (which can decrease the likelihood of SVR) or need for erythropoietin (which increases treatment costs) and should also be avoided. Abacavir hypersensitivity may be confused with the side effects of peg-IFN/R, so anti-HCV treatment should be delayed at least 4 months after its initiation as part of an ART regimen.

When an HIV-infected patient is diagnosed with chronic HCV infection, the clinician should evaluate for evidence of advanced liver disease by checking synthetic hepatic function (INR, albumin, bilirubin) and obtaining an abdominal ultrasound to look for liver nodularity, splenomegaly, ascites, or portal hypertension. If the patient has stage 2 or greater fibrosis on liver biopsy and does not meet HIV treatment criteria, HCV therapy should be considered. If the patient meets HIV treatment criteria, ART should be initiated first. Patients with HIV/HCV coinfection have a higher risk of hepatotoxicity from ART compared with those with HIV infection alone. In general, antiretroviral drugs to be avoided include ddI and stavudine (d4T), both of which are associated with steatosis, as well as nevirapine, indinavir, and full-dose ritonavir.

Hepatitis B Virus

Serologic evidence of past or current HBV infection is present in up to 80% of HIV-infected patients because of their shared modes of transmission. In the MACS cohort, patients with HIV/HBV coinfection had a 17-fold higher liver mortality rate compared with those with HBV infection alone. All HIV-infected patients should be tested for HBV by measuring antibodies to hepatitis B surface antibody (HBsAb), surface antigen (HBsAg), and core antibody (HBcAb). Isolated HBcAb (with negative HBsAb and HBsAg) is common in HIV-infected patients. Possible explanations for this finding include a false-positive result, being in the "window period" of acute infection, "resolved" infection with loss of HBsAb, the presence of an HBsAg mutant, and HBsAg production below the limit of assay detection. There is a risk of "occult HBV" infection in this setting, so if serum transaminases are increased, the HBV viral load should be measured. If the patient has detectable HBsAg, the clinician should check antibodies to hepatitis B early antibody (HBeAb) and antigen (HBeAg), as well as HBV viral load, to determine the status of HBV replication.

If an HIV/HBV coinfected patient meets criteria for treatment of HIV, an ART regimen should be devised that incorporates drugs also having anti-HBV activity. Lamivudine (3TC), which has been used for the treatment of HBV infection, is associated with a resistance rate of approximately 20% per year when used alone. Emtricitabine (FTC) also has anti-HBV activity, although it has not been as well studied as 3TC. ACTG 5127 compared the anti-HBV drug adefovir with tenofovir (TDF), which has both anti-HIV and anti-HBV activity; results showed TDF to be noninferior. Entecavir, a drug used to treat HBV infection, is not recommended in HIV-infected patients without concomitant antiretroviral therapy because of its potential to induce the M184V mutation, which confers resistance to 3TC and FTC, when given alone. HIV/HBV coinfected patients on ART should be monitored with liver function tests. Decompensation of hepatic disease can be associated with hepatotoxicity from drugs, stopping medications with anti-HBV activity, or seroconversion from HBeAg to HBeAb.

KEY POINTS

- Bacillary angiomatosis, caused by *Bartonella* species, is manifested by skin lesions resembling Kaposi's sarcoma and occasionally visceral involvement.
- Recurrent mucosal candidiasis is common in patients with HIV disease. Treatment usually consists of a topical antifungal drug or oral fluconazole.
- Coccidioidomycosis can occur as a result of reactivation of latent infection in persons who have lived in endemic regions such as the southwestern United States. Common presentations in HIV-infected

patients include disseminated disease and meningitis, the latter of which can lead to severe neurologic sequelae. Treatment consists of intravenous amphotericin B.

- Cryptococcal infection, which involves the meninges and/or lungs, is the most frequent systemic fungal infection in HIV-infected patients. Treatment of meningitis consists of intravenous amphotericin B and flucytosine, followed by oral fluconazole as maintenance therapy.
- Recurrent pneumococcal pneumonia and salmonellosis are two important conventional bacterial infections in HIV-infected patients.
- CMV infection manifests as retinitis, gastrointestinal disease, or a neurologic syndrome in advanced HIV disease. Treatment of retinitis consists of oral valganciclovir or intravenous ganciclovir or foscarnet (sometimes in conjunction with a ganciclovir vitreal implant), followed by oral valganciclovir as maintenance therapy.
- Gastrointestinal parasite infections, including cryptosporidiosis and microsporidiosis, cause chronic diarrhea and weight loss, especially in patients with advanced HIV disease. The effectiveness of anti-microbial treatment varies with the causative pathogen.
- HSV and VZV are responsible for recurrent mucocutaneous disease in HIV-infected patients. Treatment consists of acyclovir or famciclo-vir, with higher doses necessary for VZV infection.
- Disseminated histoplasmosis is reported in HIV-infected patients from endemic regions such as the midwestern United States. It is managed with intravenous amphotericin B followed by oral itracon-azole as maintenance therapy.
- HPV infection manifests as warts that generally respond to topical treatment but recurrence is common. Cervical and anal dysplasia and carcinoma occur with increased frequency in HIV-infected patients.
- LGV infection often presents as proctitis, and early diagnosis is important for its successful treatment.
- Community-acquired MRSA soft tissue infections are becoming in-creasingly common among MSM, and antibiotic sensitivities generally show the organism to be susceptible to TMP-SMX.
- MAC infection presents with constitutional symptoms in the context of advanced HIV disease. Diagnosis is by isolator blood culture or tissue biopsy. Treatment consists of a multidrug antimicrobial regimen.
- Clinical features of PCP include fever, weight loss, nonproductive cough, and dyspnea on exertion. Treatment consists of TMP-SMX or intravenous pentamidine. Corticosteroids are given as well if there is significant pulmonary compromise.
- Syphilis in HIV-infected persons occasionally presents in an atypical fashion but is managed the same as in the general population.
- Toxoplasmosis, which is the most common central nervous system opportunistic infection in HIV-infected patients, presents with focal lesions on brain-imaging studies. Treatment consists of sulfadiazine and pyrimethamine.

- The risk of HIV-infected patients with a positive PPD developing active TB is much higher than that of the general population. Diagnosis may be difficult because of unusual clinical presentations and cutaneous anergy in advanced HIV disease.
- Chronic HCV infection is common in injection-drug users and progresses more rapidly in the context of HIV disease.

SUGGESTED READINGS

General
Treating opportunistic infections among HIV-infected adults and adolescents. Recommendations from CDC, the National Institutes of Health, and the HIV Medicine Association/ Infectious Diseases Society of America. (Available as a living document on AIDSinfo: Department of Health and Human Services website at http://www.aidsinfo.nih.gov.)

Bacillary Angiomatosis
Agan BK, Dolan MJ. Laboratory diagnosis of *Bartonella* infections. Clin Lab Med. 2002;22:937-62.
Koehler JE, Duncan LM. Case records of the Massachusetts General Hospital. Case 30-2005. A 56-year-old man with fever and axillary lymphadenopathy. N Engl J Med. 2005;353: 1387-94.
Koehler JE, Sanchez MA, Tye S, et al. Prevalence of *Bartonella* infection among human immunodeficiency virus–infected patients with fever. Clin Infect Dis. 2003; 37:559–66.
Perkocha LA, Geaghan SM, Yen TSB. Clinical and pathological features of bacillary peliosis hepatitis in association with HIV infection. N Engl J Med. 1990;3232:1581-6.

Candidiasis
Infectious Diseases Society of America. Guidelines for treatment of candidiasis. Clin Infect Dis. 2004;38:161-89.
Klein RS, Harris CA, Small CB, Moll B, Lesser M, Friedland GH. Oral candidiasis in high-risk patients as the initial manifestation of the acquired immunodeficiency syndrome. N Engl J Med. 1984;311:354-8.
Maenza JR, Keruly JC, Moore RD, Chaisson RE, Merz WG, Gallant JE. Risk factors for fluconazole-resistant candidiasis in human immunodeficiency virus-infected patients. J Infect Dis. 1996;173:219-25.

Coccidioidomycosis
Galgiani JN, Ampel NM, Catanzaro A, Johnson RH, Stevens DA, Williams PL. Practice guideline for the treatment of coccidioidomycosis. Infectious Diseases Society of America. Clin Infect Dis. 2000;30:658-61.
Galgiani JN, Catanzaro A, Cloud GA, Higgs J, Friedman BA, Larsen RA, et al. Fluconazole therapy for coccidioidal meningitis. The NIAID-Mycoses Study Group. Ann Intern Med. 1993;119:28-35.

Community-Acquired Pneumonia
Currier JS, Williams P, Feinberg J, et al. Impact of prophylaxis for mycobacterium avium complex on bacterial infections in patients with advanced human immunodeficiency virus. Clin Infect Dis. 2001;32:1615–22.
Flannery B, Heffernan RT, Harrison LH, Ray SM, Reingold AL, Hadler J, et al. Changes in invasive Pneumococcal disease among HIV-infected adults living in the era of childhood pneumococcal immunization. Ann Intern Med. 2006;144:1-9.
Mandell LA, Bartlett JG, Dowell SF, File TM, Musher DM, Whitney CA. IDSA update of practice guidelines for the management of community-acquired pneumonia in immunocompetent adults; 2003. Infectious Diseases Society of America. Clin Infect Dis. 2003;37:1405–33.

Spanish Pneumococcal Infection Study Network (G03/103). Epidemiologic changes in bacteremic pneumococcal disease in patients with human immunodeficiency virus in the era of highly active antiretroviral therapy. Arch Intern Med. 2005;165:1533-40.

Cryptococcosis

Chuck SL, Sande MA. Infections with Cryptococcus neoformans in the acquired immunodeficiency syndrome. N Engl J Med. 1989;321:794-9.

Graybill JR, Sobel J, Saag M, van Der Horst C, Powderly W, Cloud G, et al. Diagnosis and management of increased intracranial pressure in patients with AIDS and cryptococcal meningitis. The NIAID Mycoses Study Group and AIDS Cooperative Treatment Groups. Clin Infect Dis. 2000;30:47-54.

Leenders AC, Reiss P, Portegies P, Clezy K, Hop WC, Hoy J, et al. Liposomal amphotericin B (AmBisome) compared with amphotericin B both followed by oral fluconazole in the treatment of AIDS-associated cryptococcal meningitis. AIDS. 1997;11:1463-71.

Saag MS, Graybill RJ, Larsen RA, Pappas PG, Perfect JR, Powderly WG, et al. Practice guidelines for the management of cryptococcal disease. Infectious Diseases Society of America. Clin Infect Dis. 2000;30:710-8.

van der Horst CM, Saag MS, Cloud GA, Hamill RJ, Graybill JR, Sobel JD, et al. Treatment of cryptococcal meningitis associated with the acquired immunodeficiency syndrome. National Institute of Allergy and Infectious Diseases Mycoses Study Group and AIDS Clinical Trials Group. N Engl J Med. 1997;337:15-21.

Cytomegalovirus Infection

Blanshard C, Benhamou Y, Dohin E, Lernestedt JO, Gazzard BG, Katlama C. Treatment of AIDS-associated gastrointestinal cytomegalovirus infection with foscarnet and ganciclovir: a randomized comparison. J Infect Dis. 1995;172:622-8.

Jacobson MA. Treatment of cytomegalovirus retinitis in patients with the acquired immunodeficiency syndrome. N Engl J Med. 1997;337:105-14.

Jacobson MA, Zegans M, Pavan PR, O'Donnell JJ, Sattler F, Rao N, et al. Cytomegalovirus retinitis after initiation of highly active antiretroviral therapy. Lancet. 1997;349:1443-5.

Spector SA, Wong R, Hsia K, Pilcher M, Stempien MJ. Plasma cytomegalovirus (CMV) DNA load predicts CMV disease and survival in AIDS patients. J Clin Invest. 1998;101:497-502.

Valganciclovir Study Group. A controlled trial of valganciclovir as induction therapy for cytomegalovirus retinitis. N Engl J Med. 2002;346:1119-26.

Gastrointestinal Parasite Infection

Carr A, Marriott D, Field A, Vasak E, Cooper DA. Treatment of HIV-1-associated microsporidiosis and cryptosporidiosis with combination antiretroviral therapy. Lancet. 1998;351:256-61.

Didier ES. Microsporidiosis. Clin Infect Dis. 1998;27:1-7; quiz 8.

Hayes C, Elliot E, Krales E, Downer G. Food and water safety for persons infected with human immunodeficiency virus. Clin Infect Dis. 2003;36:S106-9.

Kotler DP. HIV infection and the gastrointestinal tract. AIDS. 2005;19:107–117.

McGowan I, Hawkins AS, Weller IV. The natural history of cryptosporidial diarrhoea in HIV-infected patients. AIDS. 1993;7:349-54.

Verdier RI, Fitzgerald DW, Johnson WD Jr., Pape JW. Trimethoprim-sulfamethoxazole compared with ciprofloxacin for treatment and prophylaxis of Isospora belli and Cyclospora cayetanensis infection in HIV-infected patients. A randomized, controlled trial. Ann Intern Med. 2000;132:885-8.

Herpes Simplex Virus Infection

Freeman EE, Weiss HA, Glynn JR, Cross PL, Whitworth JA, Hayes RJ. Herpes simplex virus 2 infection increases HIV acquisition in men and women: systematic review and meta-analysis of longitudinal studies. AIDS. 2006;20:73–83.

Levin MJ, Bacon TH, Leary JJ. Resistance of herpes simplex virus infections to nucleoside analogues in HIV-infected patients. Clin Infect Dis. 2004;39(Suppl):S248-S257.

Schacker T, Ryncarz AJ, Goddard J, Diem K, Shaughnessy M, Corey L. Frequent recovery of HIV-1 from genital herpes simplex virus lesions in HIV-1-infected men. JAMA. 1998;280: 61-6.

Histoplasmosis

Karimi K, Wheat LJ, Connolly P, Cloud G, Hajjeh R, Wheat E, et al. Differences in histoplasmosis in patients with acquired immunodeficiency syndrome in the United States and Brazil. J Infect Dis. 2002;186:1655-60.

McKinsey DS, Spiegel RA, Hutwagner L, Stanford J, Driks MR, Brewer J, et al. Prospective study of histoplasmosis in patients infected with human immunodeficiency virus: incidence, risk factors, and pathophysiology. Clin Infect Dis. 1997;24:1195-203.

U.S. National Institute of Allergy and Infectious Diseases Mycoses Study Group. Safety and efficacy of liposomal amphotericin B compared with conventional amphotericin B for induction therapy of histoplasmosis in patients with AIDS. Ann Intern Med. 2002;137: 105-9.

Wheat J, MacWhinney S, Hafner R, MacKinsey D, Chen D, Korzun A, et al. Treatment of histoplasmosis with fluconazole in patients with acquired immunodeficiency syndrome. National Institute of Allergy and Infectious Diseases Acquired Immunodeficiency Syndrome Clinical Trials Group and Mycoses Study Group. Am J Med. 1997;103:223-32.

Wheat J, Sarosi G, McKinsey D, Hamill R, Bradsher R, Johnson P, et al. Practice guidelines for the management of patients with histoplasmosis. Infectious Diseases Society of America. Clin Infect Dis. 2000;30:688-95.

Human Papillomavirus Infection

Daling JR, Weiss NS, Hislop TG, Maden C, Coates RJ, Sherman KJ, et al. Sexual practices, sexually transmitted diseases, and the incidence of anal cancer. N Engl J Med. 1987;317:973-7.

Delmas MC, Larsen C, van Benthem B, Hamers FF, Bergeron C, Poveda JD, et al. Cervical squamous intraepithelial lesions in HIV-infected women: prevalence, incidence and regression. European Study Group on Natural History of HIV Infection in Women. AIDS. 2000;14:1775-84.

Goldie SJ, Kuntz KM, Weinstein MC, Freedberg KA, Welton ML, Palefsky JM. The clinical effectiveness and cost-effectiveness of screening for anal squamous intraepithelial lesions in homosexual and bisexual HIV-positive men. JAMA. 1999;281:1822-9.

Panther LA, Schlecht HP, Dezube BJ. Spectrum of human papillomavirus-related dysplasia and carcinoma of the anus in HIV-infected patients. AIDS Reader. 2005;15:79-91.

Panther LA, Wagner K, Proper J, Fugelso DK, Chatis PA, Weeden W, et al. High resolution anoscopy findings for men who have sex with men: inaccuracy of anal cytology as a predictor of histologic high-grade anal intraepithelial neoplasia and the impact of HIV serostatus. Clin Infect Dis. 2004;38:1490-2.

Lymphogranuloma Venereum

Nieuwenhuis RF, Ossewaarde JM, Götz HM, Dees J, Thio HB, Thomeer MG, et al. Resurgence of lymphogranuloma venereum in Western Europe: an outbreak of Chlamydia trachomatis serovar l2 proctitis in the Netherlands among men who have sex with men. Clin Infect Dis. 2004;39:996-1003.

Van der Bij AK, Spaargaren J, Morré SA, Fennema HS, Mindel A, Coutinho RA, et al. Diagnostic and clinical implications of anorectal lymphogranuloma venereum in men who have sex with men: a retrospective case-control study. Clin Infect Dis. 2006;42:186-94.

Methicillin-Resistant Staphylococcus aureus Infection

Lee NE, Taylor MM, Bancroft E, Ruane PJ, Morgan M, McCoy L, et al. Risk factors for community-associated methicillin-resistant Staphylococcus aureus skin infections among HIV-positive men who have sex with men. Clin Infect Dis. 2005;40:1529-34.

Mathews WC, Caperna JC, Barber RE, Torriani FJ, Miller LG, May S, et al. Incidence of and risk factors for clinically significant methicillin-resistant Staphylococcus aureus infection in a cohort of HIV-infected adults. J Acquir Immune Defic Syndr. 2005;40:155-60.

Mycobacterium avium Complex Infection

Benson CA. Disease due to the Mycobacterium avium complex in patients with AIDS: epidemiology and clinical syndrome. Clin Infect Dis. 1994;18 Suppl 3:S218-22.

Race EM, Adelson-Mitty J, Kriegel GR, Barlam TF, Reimann KA, Letvin NL, et al. Focal mycobacterial lymphadenitis following initiation of protease-inhibitor therapy in patients with advanced HIV-1 disease. Lancet. 1998;351:252-5.

Shafran SD, Singer J, Zarowny DP, Phillips P, Salit I, Walmsley SL, et al. A comparison of two regimens for the treatment of Mycobacterium avium complex bacteremia in AIDS: rifabutin, ethambutol, and clarithromycin versus rifampin, ethambutol, clofazimine, and ciprofloxacin. Canadian HIV Trials Network Protocol 010 Study Group. N Engl J Med. 1996;335: 377-83.

Pneumocystis jiroveci Pneumonia

Beumont MG, Graziani A, Ubel PA, MacGregor RR. Safety of dapsone as Pneumocystis carinii pneumonia prophylaxis in human immunodeficiency virus-infected patients with allergy to trimethoprim/sulfamethoxazole. Am J Med. 1996;100:611-6.

Bozzette SA, Finkelstein DM, Spector SA, Frame P, Powderly WG, He W, et al. A randomized trial of three antipneumocystis agents in patients with advanced human immunodeficiency virus infection. NIAID AIDS Clinical Trials Group. N Engl J Med. 1995;332:693-9.

Bozzette SA, Sattler FR, Chiu J, Wu AW, Gluckstein D, Kemper C, et al. A controlled trial of early adjunctive treatment with corticosteroids for Pneumocystis carinii pneumonia in the acquired immunodeficiency syndrome. California Collaborative Treatment Group. N Engl J Med. 1990;323:1451-7.

Grupo de Estudio del SIDA 04/98. A randomized trial of the discontinuation of primary and secondary prophylaxis against Pneumocystis carinii pneumonia after highly active antiretroviral therapy in patients with HIV infection. Grupo de Estudio del SIDA 04/98. N Engl J Med. 2001;344:159-67.

Kovacs JA, Gill VJ, Meshnick S, Masur H. New insights into transmission, diagnosis, and drug treatment of Pneumocystis carinii pneumonia. JAMA. 2001;286:2450-60.

Masur H. Prevention and treatment of pneumocystis pneumonia. N Engl J Med. 1992;327: 1853-60.

Morris A, Wachter RM, Luce J, Turner J, Huang L. Improved survival with highly active antiretroviral therapy in HIV-infected patients with severe Pneumocystis carinii pneumonia. AIDS. 2003;17:73-80.

Navin TR, Beard CB, Huang L, del Rio C, Lee S, Pieniazek NJ, et al. Effect of mutations in Pneumocystis carinii dihydropteroate synthase gene on outcome of P carinii pneumonia in patients with HIV-1: a prospective study. Lancet. 2001;358:545-9.

Safrin S, Finkelstein DM, Feinberg J, Frame P, Simpson G, Wu A, et al. Comparison of three regimens for treatment of mild to moderate Pneumocystis carinii pneumonia in patients with AIDS. A double-blind, randomized, trial of oral trimethoprim-sulfamethoxazole, dapsonetrimethoprim, and clindamycin-primaquine. ACTG 108 Study Group. Ann Intern Med. 1996;124:792-802.

Salmonellosis

Hoag JB, Sessler CN. A comprehensive review of disseminated Salmonella arizona infection with an illustrative case presentation. South Med J. 2005;98:1123-9.

Hohmann EL. Nontyphoidal salmonellosis. Clin Infect Dis. 2001;32:263-9.

Nelson MR, Shanson DC, Hawkins DA, Gazzard BG. Salmonella, Campylobacter and Shigella in HIV-seropositive patients. AIDS. 1992;6:1495-8.

Syphilis

Goh BT. Syphilis in adults. Sex Transm Infect. 2005;81:448-52.

Gordon SM, Eaton ME, George R, Larsen S, Lukehart SA, Kuypers J, et al. The response of symptomatic neurosyphilis to high-dose intravenous penicillin G in patients with human immunodeficiency virus infection. N Engl J Med. 1994;331:1469-73.

Hook EW 3rd, Marra CM. Acquired syphilis in adults. N Engl J Med. 1992;326:1060-9.

Marra CM, Critchlow CW, Hook EW 3rd, Collier AC, Lukehart SA. Cerebrospinal fluid treponemal antibodies in untreated early syphilis. Arch Neurol. 1995;52:68-72.

Toxoplasmosis

Ammassari A, Scoppettuolo G, Murri R, Pezzotti P, Cingolani A, Del Borgo C, et al. Changing disease patterns in focal brain lesion-causing disorders in AIDS. J Acquir Immune Defic Syndr Hum Retrovirol. 1998;18:365-71.

Dannemann B, McCutchan JA, Israelski D, Antoniskis D, Leport C, Luft B, et al. Treatment of toxoplasmic encephalitis in patients with AIDS. A randomized trial comparing pyrimethamine plus clindamycin to pyrimethamine plus sulfadiazine. The California Collaborative Treatment Group. Ann Intern Med. 1992;116:33-43.

Furrer H, Opravil M, Bernasconi E, Telenti A, Egger M. Stopping primary prophylaxis in HIV-1-infected patients at high risk of toxoplasma encephalitis. Swiss HIV Cohort Study [Letter]. Lancet. 2000;355:2217-8.

Girard PM, Landman R, Gaudebout C, Olivares R, Saimot AG, Jelazko P, et al. Dapsone-pyrimethamine compared with aerosolized pentamidine as primary prophylaxis against Pneumocystis carinii pneumonia and toxoplasmosis in HIV infection. The PRIO Study Group. N Engl J Med. 1993;328:1514-20.

Kovacs JA. Efficacy of atovaquone in treatment of toxoplasmosis in patients with AIDS. The NIAID-Clinical Center Intramural AIDS Program. Lancet. 1992;340:637-8.

Luft BJ, Hafner R, Korzun AH, Leport C, Antoniskis D, Bosler EM, et al. Toxoplasmic encephalitis in patients with the acquired immunodeficiency syndrome. Members of the ACTG 077p/ANRS 009 Study Team. N Engl J Med. 1993;329:995-1000.

Porter SB, Sande MA. Toxoplasmosis of the central nervous system in the acquired immunodeficiency syndrome. N Engl J Med. 1992;327:1643-8.

Skiest DJ. Focal neurological disease in patients with the acquired immunodeficiency syndrome. Clin Inf Dis. 2002;34:103-15.

Zeller V, Truffot C, Agher R, Bossi P, Tubiana R, Caumes E, et al. Discontinuation of secondary prophylaxis against disseminated Mycobacterium avium complex infection and toxoplasmic encephalitis. Clin Infect Dis. 2002;34:662-7.

Tuberculosis

Alpert PL, Munsiff SS, Gourevitch MN, Greenberg B, Klein RS. A prospective study of tuberculosis and human immunodeficiency virus infection: clinical manifestations and factors associated with survival. Clin Infect Dis. 1997;24:661-8.

Havlir DV, Barnes PF. Tuberculosis in patients with human immunodeficiency virus infection. N Engl J Med. 1999;340:367-73.

Shafer RW, Edlin BR. Tuberculosis in patients infected with human immunodeficiency virus: perspective on the past decade. Clin Infect Dis. 1996;22:683-704.

Varicella-Zoster Virus Infection

Balfour HH, Benson C, Braun J, et al. Management of acyclovir-resistant herpes simplex and varicella-zoster virus infections. J Acquir Immune Defic Syndr Hum Retrovirol. 1994;7:254-60.

Gilden DH, Kleinschmidt-DeMasters BK, LaGuardia JJ, Mahalingam R, Cohrs RJ. Neurologic complications of the reactivation of varicella-zoster virus. N Engl J Med. 2000;342:635-45.

Gnann JW. Varicella-zoster virus: atypical presentations and unusual complications. J Infect Dis. 2002;186 (Suppl 1):591-598.

Martínez E, Gatell J, Morán Y, Aznar E, Buira E, Guelar A, et al. High incidence of herpes zoster in patients with AIDS soon after therapy with protease inhibitors. Clin Infect Dis. 1998;27:1510-3.

Ormerod LD, Larkin JA, Margo CA, Pavan PR, Menosky MM, Haight DO, et al. Rapidly progressive herpetic retinal necrosis: a blinding disease characteristic of advanced AIDS. Clin Infect Dis. 1998;26:34-45; discussion 46-7.

Viral Hepatitis

APRICOT Study Group. Peginterferon Alfa-2a plus ribavirin for chronic hepatitis C virus infection in HIV-infected patients. N Engl J Med. 2004;351:438-50.

Graham CS, Baden LR, Yu E, Mrus JM, Carnie J, Heeren T, et al. Influence of human immunodeficiency virus infection on the course of hepatitis C virus infection: a meta-analysis. Clin Infect Dis. 2001;33:562-9.

Miller MF, Haley C, Koziel MJ, Rowley CF. Impact of hepatitis C virus on immune restoration in HIV-infected patients who start highly active antiretroviral therapy: a meta-analysis. Clin Infect Dis. 2005;41:713-20.

Soriano V, Puoti M, Bonacini M, Brook G, Cargnel A, Rockstroh J, et al. Care of patients with chronic hepatitis B and HIV co-infection: recommendations from an HIV-HBV International Panel. AIDS. 2005;19:221-40.

Soriano V, Puoti M, Sulkowski M, Mauss S, Cacoub P, Cargnel A, et al. Care of patients with hepatitis C and HIV co-infection [Editorial]. AIDS. 2004;18:1-12.

Chapter 10

Diagnosis and Management of Opportunistic Cancers

I. Kaposi's Sarcoma
BRUCE J. DEZUBE, MD

II. HIV-Related Lymphomas
JOHN P. DOWEIKO, MD

III. Anogenital Squamous Cell Cancer
JOHN P. DOWEIKO, MD

Conditions that alter cellular immunity, including HIV infection, predispose to the development of neoplasms. Some of the malignancies in HIV-infected persons are AIDS-defining (Box 10-1). These include Kaposi's sarcoma (KS), B-cell lymphomas, and cervical cancer.

Other malignancies are encountered with greater frequency during the course of HIV infection but are not considered AIDS-defining. Among these are Hodgkin's disease and anal cancer, both of which are discussed later in this chapter. The incidence of B-cell acute lymphocytic leukemia and plasma cell dyscrasias is also increased. In addition, T-cell lymphomas and testicular and lung cancers may occur more frequently in HIV-infected persons.

I. KAPOSI'S SARCOMA
BRUCE J. DEZUBE

Epidemiology

Kaposi's sarcoma is the most common neoplasm associated with HIV disease. In the United States, it is 20,000 times more frequent in HIV-infected patients than in the general population and 300 times more frequent than in other immunosuppressed patients.

Box 10-1.   Malignancies in HIV Disease

AIDS-Defining	*HIV-Associated*
• Kaposi's sarcoma	• Hodgkin's disease
• B-cell lymphomas	• Plasma cell dyscrasias
• Cervical cancer	• B-cell acute lymphocytic leukemia
	• T-cell lymphomas
	• Anal cancer
	• Testicular cancer
	• Lung cancer

KS has been described most often in men who have sex with men. Before the advent of effective antiretroviral therapy, KS was an AIDS-defining diagnosis in 20% to 30% of homosexual men but occurred in only 3% of heterosexual injection-drug users, 3% of transfusion recipients, 3% of women and children, and 1% of hemophiliacs. KS is four times more common in an HIV-infected woman with a sexual partner who is a bisexual man than one who is an injection-drug user. The dramatic effect of antiretroviral therapy on the incidence of KS is underscored by a large Swiss study of HIV-infected patients, where the relative risk of developing KS in the years 1997 to 1998 compared with 1992 to 1994 was 0.08 (95% CI, 0.03–0.22).

The early epidemiologic observations noted above suggested that the etiology of KS was infectious. Since then, multiple studies have demonstrated the presence of herpesvirus-like DNA sequences, not only in AIDS-associated KS but also in classic KS and in KS that occurs in HIV-seronegative homosexual men. The discovery of KS herpesvirus (KSHV), also known as human herpesvirus-8 (HHV8), has altered our understanding of this neoplasm. The prevalence of KSHV/HHV8 infection strongly correlates with the number of homosexual partners. Among HIV-infected patients who are seropositive for KSHV/HHV8, the 10-year probability of developing KS is approximately 50%. Among homosexual men, KSHV/ HHV8 is transmitted predominantly by deep kissing in contrast to HIV infection, which is spread by sexual activity, especially receptive anal intercourse.

Pathogenesis

The pathogenesis of AIDS-related KS is multifactorial. It involves KSHV/HHV8, altered expression and response to cytokines, and stimulation of KS growth by the HIV transactivating transduction (TAT) protein, as well as other factors yet to be elucidated. KSHV/HHV8 is necessary, but not sufficient, to cause KS. KSHV/HHV8 encodes proteins that are homologues of interleukin-6 (IL-6), chemokines of the macrophage inflammatory protein family, cell cycle regulators of the cyclin family, and anti-apoptosis genes of the bcl-2 family. The TAT protein promotes the growth of spindle cells of endothelial origin derived from AIDS KS lesions but does so only in the presence of inflammatory cytokines. KSHV/HHV8 has also been demonstrated to induce lymphatic reprogramming of blood vascular endothelium. The synergy between cytokines and the HIV TAT protein, as well as the immunosuppression associated with AIDS, suggests a basis whereby AIDS-related KS is more aggressive than the classic Mediterranean form in which the HIV TAT protein does not play a role. The remarkable findings that KSHV/HHV8 encodes viral IL-6 and IL-6 leads in turn to expression of vascular endothelial growth factor provide a missing link in the chain of events by which the virus produces an inflammatory-angiogenic environment.

Clinical Manifestations

AIDS-related KS has a variable clinical course, ranging from minimal disease presenting as an incidental finding to aggressive disease resulting in significant morbidity and mortality. The management of skin, oral, and gastrointestinal lesions is determined by the presence and degree of symptoms. The psychosocial burden associated with KS may be profound and includes emotional distress and social stigma. In general, KS exhibits a less aggressive presentation in patients on antiretroviral therapy.

The skin lesions appear most often on the lower extremities, face (especially the nose), oral mucosa, and genitalia. Most often, they are papular, ranging in size from several millimeters to several centimeters in diameter, and purple in color (Figure 10-1). They are sometimes elliptical and arranged in a linear fashion along skin "tension lines." Other manifestations of KS are shown in Figure 10-2. Lymphedema, particularly in the face, genitalia, and lower extremities, may be out of proportion to the extent of cutaneous disease related both to vascular obstruction from lymphadenopathy and local cytokine production.

KS in the oral cavity occurs in approximately one-third of patients and is the initial site of disease in about 15%. The location most frequently involved is the palate, followed by the gingiva. Intraoral lesions may become easily traumatized during normal chewing. They may cause pain, bleeding, ulceration, and secondary infection and may interfere with nutrition and speech.

Gastrointestinal involvement is also common in KS and found in 40% of patients at initial diagnosis and up to 80% at autopsy. Involvement can occur in the absence of mucocutaneous disease. Gastrointestinal lesions may cause weight loss, abdominal pain, nausea, vomiting, upper or lower gastrointestinal tract bleeding, or diarrhea in some patients, but others may be asymptomatic. Gastrointestinal tract lesions, recognized by visual inspection on endoscopy, are typically isolated or confluent hemorrhagic

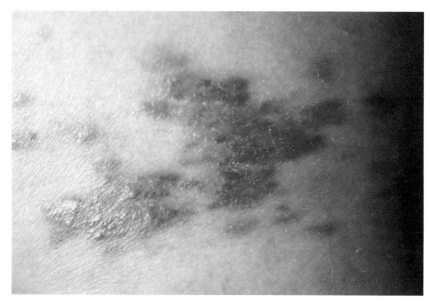

Figure 10-1.   Typical skin lesion of cutaneous Kaposi's sarcoma.

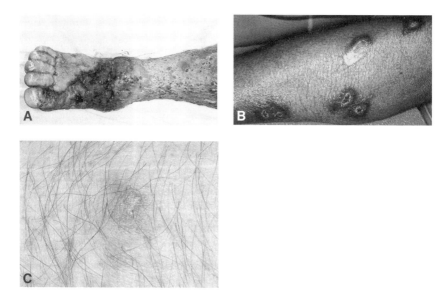

Figure 10-2.   Manifestations of Kaposi's sarcoma: plaque-like lesion with breakdown of overlying skin **(A)**, multiple-colored lesions on leg **(B)**, and lesion with yellow halo **(C)**. (For color reproduction, see Plates 5 to 7 at back of book.) (From van den Brink MR, Dezube BJ. AIDS-Related Kaposi's sarcoma. J Clin Oncol. 1997;15: 1283-4; with permission.)

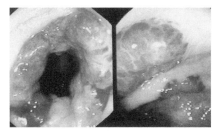

Figure 10-3.   Kaposi's sarcoma can appear as large annular masses with circumferential infiltration and luminal obstruction in the colon and rectum. (For color reproduction, see Plate 8 at back of book.) From van den Brink MR, Dezube BJ. AIDS-Related Kaposi's sarcoma. J Clin Oncol. 1997;15: 1283-4; with permission.)

nodules (Figure 10-3). Because KS lesions tend to be submucosal, they may not be consistently demonstrated on biopsy specimens.

Pulmonary involvement may present as cough, shortness of breath, hemoptysis, chest pain, or as an asymptomatic finding on chest x-ray. Up to 15% of affected patients have no evidence of mucocutaneous KS. Radiographic findings vary greatly and can include nodular, interstitial or alveolar infiltrates, pleural effusion, hilar or mediastinal adenopathy, or an isolated pulmonary nodule. The pleural effusions of KS are associated with visceral pleura lesions that may leak blood. A presumptive diagnosis of pulmonary KS at the time of bronchoscopy can usually be made by visual inspection of lesions. Biopsy should be avoided because of the risk of hemorrhage. Management decisions are guided by the presence of respiratory symptoms and the extent of disease.

Lymph node involvement may be present in patients without evidence of mucocutaneous disease. Autopsy series also have reported KS lesions in the liver, pancreas, heart, testes, and bone marrow.

Two clinical scenarios—KS in the presence of corticosteroid therapy and in the context of an opportunistic infection—are worth highlighting. Corticosteroid therapy has been associated with KS induction and with the exacerbation of pre-existing KS in HIV-infected patients, as well as in HIV-seronegative patients receiving steroids for organ transplantation, autoimmune disorders, or lymphoproliferative diseases. This observation is important because HIV-infected patients may be treated with steroids for a variety of disorders including immune thrombocytopenic purpura and *Pneumocystis jiroveci* (formerly *carinii*) pneumonia. Although not strictly contraindicated in HIV-infected patients with KS, corticosteroids should be used cautiously in this setting. KS lesions may regress upon reduction or withdrawal of steroids. Opportunistic infections have also been associated with KS induction and with the exacerbation of pre-existing KS. High levels of proinflammatory cytokines, which have been demonstrated in this setting, may account for this observation.

Diagnosis

Although an experienced clinician can usually make a presumptive diagnosis of KS, skin biopsy should be performed for confirmation. Early lesions can easily be mistaken for purpura, hematomas, angiomas, dermatofibromas, or nevi. It is especially important to biopsy lesions that are less typical of KS or associated with systemic symptoms to rule out bacillary angiomatosis (BA) (see Chapter 9). Gastrointestinal, pulmonary, lymphatic, and other organ involvement with KS should always be confirmed with biopsy.

Bacillary angiomatosis, which is caused by *Bartonella* species, can be identified by Warthin-Starry silver staining and is managed with antibiotic therapy. Skin lesions of BA appear as multiple red, round papules or nodules, and they may be associated with fever, chills, malaise, anorexia, or headache. Rarely, KS and BA can occur simultaneously in a patient.

Staging and Prognosis

The initial evaluation of a patient with KS consists of a physical examination with special attention to the lower extremities, face, oral mucosa, genitalia, gastrointestinal tract, and lungs. Checking the stool for occult blood should be performed to screen for gastrointestinal lesions. Endoscopy can be reserved for the patient who has gastrointestinal symptoms or occult blood. In a similar fashion, chest x-ray is used to screen for pulmonary lesions. Bronchoscopy can be reserved for the patient who has respiratory symptoms or an abnormal x-ray.

The most commonly utilized staging system for AIDS-related KS was developed by the AIDS Clinical Trial Group (ACTG) of the National Institutes of Health (Table 10-1). Patients are divided into a good- or poor-risk group according to three parameters: extent of tumor (T), immune status (CD4 cell count) (I), and severity of systemic illness (S). In a recent analysis, tumor extent (T) and systemic disease (S) maintained their correlation with survival, whereas CD4 count (I) did not. Importantly, this analysis stratified patients into two main risk categories: those presenting with both poor-risk tumor extension and HIV-related systemic disease (T1S1), who have an increased risk of death, and all other groups (T1S0, T0S1, T0S0).

Treatment

The major management goals for KS are palliation of symptoms; shrinkage of tumor to alleviate edema, organ compromise, or psychological stress; and prevention of disease progression. Treatment options depend greatly on the tumor (extent of disease and rate of growth) and the host (overall medical condition, CD4 count, viral load). In terms of the host, it is important to ascertain any impairment in organ function that will increase the po-

Table 10-1.   Staging System for AIDS-Related Kaposi's Sarcoma

	Good Risk	Poor Risk
Tumor (T)	Confined to skin and/or lymph nodes and/or minimal oral disease (non-nodular KS confined to palate)	Tumor-associated edema or ulceration Extensive oral KS Gastrointestinal KS KS in other non-nodal viscera
Immune status (I)	CD4 cells $\geq$200/mm^3	CD4 cells <200/mm^3
Systemic illness (S)	No history of OI or thrush No "B" symptoms* Karnofsky performance status $\geq$70	History of OI and/or thrush "B" symptoms present Karnofsky performance status <70 Other HIV-related conditions (e.g., neurologic disease, lymphoma)

* "B" symptoms are unexplained fever, night sweats, >10% involuntary weight loss, or diarrhea persisting more than 2 weeks.
Adapted from Dezube BJ. Clinical presentations and natural history of AIDS-related KS. Hematol Oncol Clin North Am. 1996;10:1023-9.

tential for drug-related toxicities and to determine if there are any medications that will increase the likelihood of drug interactions.

Antiretroviral Therapy

KS patients should be prescribed antiretroviral drugs that will maximally suppress the HIV viral load. This recommendation is based on the recognition that effective HIV treatment is associated with regression in the size of existing KS lesions and a decreased frequency of new lesions. Regression of cutaneous and visceral KS has been demonstrated in patients taking protease inhibitor or nonnucleoside reverse-transcriptase inhibitor-based regimens. Antiretroviral therapy also prolongs the time to treatment failure of anti-KS therapies. Immune reconstitution syndrome with KS has been reported in patients with advanced HIV disease upon initiation of antiretroviral therapy.

Local Therapy

Alitretinoin gel 0.1% (9-cis-retinoic acid, Panretin) is the only topical, patient-administered therapy approved for the treatment of KS. Alitretinoin is a naturally occurring retinoid, which, in a placebo-controlled trial, was associated with a shorter time to tumor response, more prolonged duration of response, and more prolonged time to disease progression. Most patients required 4 to 8 weeks of treatment before a response was seen. Baseline CD4 count did not appear to affect treatment response. Dermal irritation, generally mild to moderate, occurred at the site of gel application in some patients. Alitretinoin gel would not be expected to alter the likelihood of development of new lesions in untreated areas.

Other local treatments include intralesional chemotherapy, radiation therapy, laser therapy, and cryotherapy, all of which can be effective at controlling local tumor growth. Vinblastine is probably the most widely used intralesional agent and has a response rate of about 70%. Although treated lesions will not resolve completely, they will usually fade and regress. Radiation therapy can effectively palliate symptomatic disease that is too extensive to be managed with intralesional chemotherapy but not so extensive to warrant systemic therapy. In a series of 36 patients with KS of the feet, a schedule of three fractions a week at 3.5 Gy/fraction to a total dose of 21.0 Gy yielded an overall response rate of 91% and a complete response rate of 80%. Although discomfort from radiation was frequent, it usually resolved within two weeks of completion of the treatment course.

Interferon-alpha

Interferon-alpha is a biological response modifier that is effective in the treatment of cutaneous KS but is rarely used today. Although low doses of interferon (e.g., one million units daily) may be effective when given with nucleoside reverse-transcriptase inhibitors such as zidovudine (ZDV), higher doses are often associated with fever, chills, neutropenia, hepatotoxicity, and cognitive impairment. Poor tumor response and drug-related toxicity are particularly striking in patients with a CD4 count of less than 200 cells/mm^3.

Chemotherapy

Although many older chemotherapeutic agents have been found to be active against KS singly or in combination, current systemic treatment consists of the newer liposomal anthracyclines and paclitaxel. The liposomal formulation of the anthracyclines provides the theoretical advantage of longer plasma half-life, higher tumor drug concentration, and less toxicity in nontarget organs. Overall, it has a higher benefit-to-risk ratio compared with conventional chemotherapy.

The two currently approved liposomal anthracyclines, doxorubicin (Doxil) and daunorubicin (DaunoXome), have become the first-line chemotherapeutic treatment for patients with symptomatic disseminated KS. In randomized multicenter trials, both drugs have been found to be superior to conventional chemotherapy (bleomycin and vincristine with or without nonliposomal doxorubicin) in terms of response rate and toxicity profile. The dose of liposomal doxorubicin is 20 mg/m^2 every 3 weeks; the dose of liposomal daunorubicin is 40 mg/m^2 every 2 weeks.

Both of these liposomal compounds can reliably shrink tumors, lessen edema, and cause the color of lesions to fade in 25% to 59% of patients. Moreover, liposomal doxorubicin is effective in 32% of patients whose tumors have progressed while receiving conventional doxorubicin, suggesting that the liposomal encapsulation increases its efficacy. In general, side effects are quite mild. Alopecia and peripheral neuropathy, in particular, are unusual with these preparations. Furthermore, at higher cumulative doses, they have not typically been associated with the cardiomyopathy that has limited the use of nonliposomal anthracyclines.

Paclitaxel (Taxol), the newest systemic chemotherapeutic agent approved for KS, has shown striking efficacy, even for patients with anthracycline-resistant disease (Table 10-2). The response rates in two phase II trials were 59% and 71%. The median duration of response of 10 months is among the longest observed for any regimen reported for this disease. Paclitaxel is well tolerated, but the higher prevalence of alopecia, myalgia/arthralgia, and bone-marrow suppression, as well as the need for a 3-hour infusion, make it less attractive than liposomal anthracyclines as initial therapy of disseminated disease. Recommended dosing schedules for paclitaxel are 100 mg/m^2 over 3 hours every 2 weeks or 135 mg/m^2 over 3 hours every 3 weeks. The usual premedication regimen for paclitaxel includes diphenhydramine, ranitidine, and a short course of dexamethasone, which can be given orally or intravenously.

The coadministration of some antiretroviral drugs and paclitaxel may be problematic. Metabolism of the protease inhibitors and nonnucleoside reverse-transcriptase inhibitors involves the hepatic cytochrome p450 pathway, which is also important in the oxidation of taxanes to less active metabolites. The profound toxicity noted in at least two patients receiving paclitaxel has been attributed to a toxic interaction between this chemotherapeutic agent and antiretroviral drugs. However, in a pharmacokinetic study, the metabolism of paclitaxel when administered with indinavir, ritonavir, saquinavir, or nevirapine was no different from that of paclitaxel in historical control subjects.

Investigational Agents

Given the highly significant role that angiogenesis plays in the pathogenesis of KS, it is not surprising that many of the angiogenesis inhibitors in development have been or are currently being tested in patients with AIDS-related KS. Angiogenesis inhibitors that have led to durable clinical responses in early clinical trials include fumagillin, thalidomide, the matrix metalloproteinase (MMP) inhibitor COL-3, and the signal transduction inhibitor imatinib (Gleevec). Of note, in early trials of COL-3 in AIDS-related

Table 10-2. Paclitaxel in AIDS-Related Kaposi's Sarcoma

Dose and Schedule	Patients (N)	Response Rate (%)	Median Duration of Response (Months)
100 mg/m^2 every 2 weeks	56	59	10.4
135 mg/m^2 every 3 weeks	28	71	7.4

KS, the tumor response rate was 44%, and treatment was associated with decreased plasma MMP-2 levels. In early trials of imatinib, tumor responses were associated with decreased gene expression of growth factors in serial KS tumor biopsies.

Other potential targets for KS therapies include KSHV/HHV8 and the process of cellular differentiation. A phase II trial of oral 9-cis-retinoic acid in AIDS-related KS resulted in a tumor response rate of 37%. As noted previously, this drug is currently approved as a topical gel for the treatment of cutaneous KS.

KEY POINTS

- Kaposi's sarcoma (KS), the most common tumor arising in HIV-infected patients, is an AIDS-defining condition.
- Recent advances in understanding the pathogenesis of KS have uncovered potential therapeutic targets, including angiogenesis, cellular differentiation, and the KS herpesvirus/human herpesvirus-8.
- AIDS-related KS has a variable clinical course, ranging from minimal disease presenting as an incidental finding to aggressive disease resulting in significant morbidity and mortality. The psychosocial burden associated with KS can be profound.
- Initial evaluation of a KS patient consists of a physical examination, testing of stool for occult blood, chest x-ray, and determination of the CD4 cell count and HIV viral load.
- Antiretroviral therapy is associated with regression in the size of existing KS lesions and a decreased frequency of new lesions.
- Five drugs are currently approved for the treatment of KS: alitretinoin gel for topical administration, and interferon-alpha, liposomal daunorubicin, liposomal doxorubicin, and paclitaxel for systemic administration.
- For patients whose disease merits systemic therapy in addition to antiretroviral therapy, liposomal anthracyclines provide the best benefit-to-risk ratio.

SUGGESTED READINGS

Aboulafia DM. The epidemiologic, pathologic, and clinical features of AIDS-associated pulmonary Kaposi's sarcoma. Chest. 2000;117:1128-45.

AIDS Clinical Trial Group Staging System in the Haart Era—the Italian Cooperative Group on AIDS and Tumors and the Italian Cohort of Patients Naive from Antiretrovirals. AIDS-related Kaposi's sarcoma: evaluation of potential new prognostic factors and assessment of the AIDS Clinical Trial Group Staging System in the Haart Era—the Italian Cooperative Group on AIDS and Tumors and the Italian Cohort of Patients Naive From Antiretrovirals. J Clin Oncol. 2003;21:2876-82.

Bower M, Fox P, Fife K, Gill J, Nelson M, Gazzard B. Highly active anti-retroviral therapy (HAART) prolongs time to treatment failure in Kaposi's sarcoma. AIDS. 1999;13:2105-11.

Cheung L, Rockson SG. The lymphatic biology of Kaposi's sarcoma. Lymphat Res Biol. 2005; 3:25-35.

Cianfrocca M, Cooley TP, Lee JY, Rudek MA, Scadden DT, Ratner L, et al. Matrix metalloproteinase inhibitor COL-3 in the treatment of AIDS-related Kaposi's sarcoma: a phase I AIDS malignancy consortium study. J Clin Oncol. 2002;20:153-9.

Connick E, Kane MA, White IE, Ryder J, Campbell TB. Immune reconstitution inflammatory syndrome associated with Kaposi sarcoma during potent antiretroviral therapy. Clin Infect Dis. 2004;39:1852-5.

Dezube BJ, Pantanowitz L, Aboulafia DM. Management of AIDS-related Kaposi sarcoma: advances in target discovery and treatment. AIDS Read. 2004;14:236-8, 243-4, 251-3.

GICAT. Impact of highly active antiretroviral therapy on the presenting features and outcome of patients with acquired immunodeficiency syndrome-related Kaposi sarcoma. Cancer. 2003;98:2440-6.

Gill PS, Tulpule A, Espina BM, Cabriales S, Bresnahan J, Ilaw M, et al. Paclitaxel is safe and effective in the treatment of advanced AIDS-related Kaposi's sarcoma. J Clin Oncol. 1999; 17:1876-83.

Gill PS, Wernz J, Scadden DT, Cohen P, Mukwaya GM, von Roenn JH, et al. Randomized phase III trial of liposomal daunorubicin versus doxorubicin, bleomycin, and vincristine in AIDS-related Kaposi's sarcoma. J Clin Oncol. 1996;14:2353-64.

Gressen EL, Rosenstock JG, Xie Y, Corn BW. Palliative treatment of epidemic Kaposi sarcoma of the feet. Am J Clin Oncol. 1999;22:286-90.

Koon HB, Bubley GJ, Pantanowitz L, Masiello D, Smith B, Crosby K, et al. Imatinib-induced regression of AIDS-related Kaposi's sarcoma. J Clin Oncol. 2005;23:982-9.

Krown SE, Testa MA, Huang J. AIDS-related Kaposi's sarcoma: prospective validation of the AIDS Clinical Trials Group staging classification. AIDS Clinical Trials Group Oncology Committee. J Clin Oncol. 1997;15:3085-92.

Ledergerber B, Telenti A, Egger M. Risk of HIV related Kaposi's sarcoma and non-Hodgkin's lymphoma with potent antiretroviral therapy: prospective cohort study. Swiss HIV Cohort Study. BMJ. 1999;319:23-4.

Martin JN, Osmond DH. Kaposi's sarcoma-associated herpesvirus and sexual transmission of cancer risk. Curr Opin Oncol. 1999;11:508-15.

Mesri EA. Inflammatory reactivation and angiogenicity of Kaposi's sarcoma-associated herpesvirus/HHV8: a missing link in the pathogenesis of acquired immunodeficiency syndrome-associated Kaposi's sarcoma. Blood. 1999;93:4031-3.

Northfelt DW, Dezube BJ, Thommes JA, Levine R, Von Roenn JH, Dosik GM, et al. Efficacy of pegylated-liposomal doxorubicin in the treatment of AIDS-related Kaposi's sarcoma after failure of standard chemotherapy. J Clin Oncol. 1997;15:653-9.

Northfelt DW, Dezube BJ, Thommes JA, Miller BJ, Fischl MA, Friedman-Kien A, et al. Pegylated-liposomal doxorubicin versus doxorubicin, bleomycin, and vincristine in the treatment of AIDS-related Kaposi's sarcoma: results of a randomized phase III clinical trial. J Clin Oncol. 1998;16:2445-51.

Pauk J, Huang ML, Brodie SJ, Wald A, Koelle DM, Schacker T, et al. Mucosal shedding of human herpesvirus 8 in men. N Engl J Med. 2000;343:1369-77.

Portsmouth S, Stebbing J, Gill J, Mandalia S, Bower M, Nelson M, et al. A comparison of regimens based on non-nucleoside reverse transcriptase inhibitors or protease inhibitors in preventing Kaposi's sarcoma. AIDS. 2003;17:F17-22.

Swift PS. The role of radiation therapy in the management of HIV-related Kaposi's sarcoma. Hematol Oncol Clin North Am. 1996;10:1069-80.

Walmsley S, Northfelt DW, Melosky B, Conant M, Friedman-Kien AE, Wagner B. Treatment of AIDS-related cutaneous Kaposi's sarcoma with topical alitretinoin (9-cis-retinoic acid) gel. Panretin Gel North American Study Group. J Acquir Immune Defic Syndr. 1999;22: 235-46.

Welles L, Saville MW, Lietzau J, Pluda JM, Wyvill KM, Feuerstein I, et al. Phase II trial with dose titration of paclitaxel for the therapy of human immunodeficiency virus-associated Kaposi's sarcoma. J Clin Oncol. 1998;16:1112-21.

II. HIV-Related Lymphomas

JOHN P. DOWEIKO

Hodgkin's Disease

Previous controversy as to whether HIV infection increases the frequency of Hodgkin's disease has been resolved by recent studies that have shown an incidence that is greater than 18-fold that of the general population. Hodgkin's disease occurs most often in patients whose risk behavior is injection-drug use. Its onset is usually later in the course of HIV disease when the median CD4 count has declined to less than 300 cells/mm³.

The presentation of Hodgkin's disease in HIV-infected patients differs from that in the general population. Constitutional symptoms occur in more than 80% of cases, which is much higher than that usually described. Hodgkin's disease is typically more advanced at the time of presentation, with over 75% of patients having stage III or IV disease, and is more aggressive in its course. Extranodal disease occurs in more than 65% of HIV-infected patients compared with about 25% in the general population; more than 50% have bone marrow involvement at the time of presentation.

The histologic spectrum of HIV-related Hodgkin's disease differs from that of the general population. Pathologic types associated with poorer prognosis, such as mixed cellularity and lymphocyte depleted, are encountered in a higher proportion of HIV-infected patients (Table 10-3). In Hodgkin's disease that occurs in the general population, involved tissues are infiltrated with T lymphocytes, whereas the cellular infiltrate in HIV-related Hodgkin's disease is relatively poor in T cells. This finding may account for the more aggressive nature of the disease in this setting. Epstein-Barr virus (EBV) may play a more important role in the pathogenesis of HIV-related Hodgkin's disease because 83% to 100% of these cases have EBV genome within the Reed-Sternberg cells, a much higher proportion than that encountered in the general population.

Despite these differences in the nature of HIV-related Hodgkin's disease, the rate of complete remission may be as high as 80% with standard treatment regimens.

Table 10-3.   Distribution of Pathologic Types of Hodgkin's Disease

Histology	HIV-Infected Population	Seronegative Population
Lymphocyte predominant	1%	5%
Nodular sclerosing	27%	70%
Mixed cellularity	55%	22%
Lymphocyte depleted	12%	1%
Unclassifiable	5%	2%

Non-Hodgkin's Lymphoma

Epidemiology

HIV infection increases the risk of non-Hodgkin's lymphoma (NHL) 60- to 100-fold over that of the general population. Up to 10% of the HIV-infected population will develop NHL, half of which may go unreported. There does not seem to be a correlation between HIV risk behavior and the development of NHL. Since the advent of effective antiretroviral therapy, there has been a significant decrease in the incidence of NHL. However this decline has not been as profound as that seen with KS or opportunistic infections.

HIV-infected patients with the CCR5-32 deletion in the macrophage-tropic receptor not only have a better prognosis with respect to HIV infection but also have less of a tendency to develop NHL. Those with polymorphisms of the CXCR-4 chemokine receptor have an increased risk of developing this neoplasm. The decreased frequency of this receptor in African-Americans may account for the lower incidence of AIDS-related NHL reported in this group.

About 75% of AIDS-related NHL occurs in patients with poorly-controlled HIV infection; however, one-quarter develops even when the viral load is undetectable. In a study of over 82,000 HIV-infected adults, there was an increase in the relative risk of developing a lymphoma of 1.48 for each 100 cells/mm^3 decline in the CD4 count.

Pathogenesis

AIDS-related lymphomas arise from unregulated expansion of cells that are arrested in development and unable to undergo terminal differentiation. AIDS-related NHLs have a different pathogenesis and behavior than lymphomas of similar histology that occur in the HIV-seronegative population. The definition of malignancy in the immunocompetent host, based largely upon clonality, does not strictly apply in the immunosuppressed patient. Not all AIDS-related lymphomas are monoclonal. They result from a combination of factors but not from HIV infection of neoplastic cells (Box 10-2).

During the course of HIV infection, there is chronic stimulation of B cells, resulting in hypergammaglobulinemia and persistent generalized lymphadenopathy. This chronic B-cell stimulation and proliferation increase the chances that a genetic error will occur. The immunosuppression resulting from HIV infection results in a loss of immune surveillance, allowing these aberrant clones of B cells to proliferate instead of being eliminated by the cellular immune system.

The dysregulation of cytokines that occurs during HIV infection is in large part responsible for B-cell proliferation. Two cytokines in particular have special importance. The interleukin-6 level increases early in the course of HIV infection; its duration and amplitude predict the likelihood of lymphoma developing over time. The interleukin-10 (IL-10) level is also

<table>
<tr><td colspan="2">Box 10-2.   Pathogenic Factors for AIDS-Related Lymphoma</td></tr>
</table>

• Chronic B-cell stimulation	• Destruction of lymph nodes
• Immunosuppression and loss of immune surveillance	• Cytokines
• Proto-oncogenes and tumor-suppressor genes	• Other viral infections

markedly increased during HIV infection. This cytokine acts as an autocrine growth factor for lymphoma while simultaneously inhibiting cellular immune response. High levels of IL-10 are associated with a poor prognosis for AIDS-related lymphoma.

Coinciding with chronic stimulation of B cells is the destruction of the dendritic network of the germinal centers of lymph nodes. Dendritic cells exert control over B-cell apoptosis and participate in antigen presentation. This process results in the loss of control of B-cell proliferation and interferes with the ability to mount a specific humoral response.

The DNA rearrangements that occur during B-cell development may activate proto-oncogenes, inactive tumor-suppressor genes, or both. Proto-oncogenes are normal growth-promoting genes, that, when translocated to other areas of the genome, may result in unregulated proliferation of cells. More than 75% of AIDS-related lymphomas have alterations in at least one proto-oncogene. Tumor-suppressor genes are normally expressed and prevent unregulated cellular growth via control of apoptosis. More than 90% of AIDS-related lymphomas have alterations in at least one tumor-suppressor gene.

Another factor in the genesis and progression of AIDS-related lymphoma is the enhanced adhesion of neoplastic lymphocytes to endothelial cells that results from infection of the latter by HIV. It not only brings the malignant cells in close proximity to growth factors produced by the endothelial cells but also accelerates their extravasation into surrounding tissues.

The presence of two other viruses increases the risk of lymphomas in HIV-infected patients. EBV may replicate during HIV infection, inducing polyclonal B-cell proliferation while simultaneously dysregulating tumor-suppressor genes and proto-oncogenes. KSHV/HHV8 possesses genes homologous that are to the human genes that control cell cycling.

Histology

Three histologic types (Burkitt-like, high-grade diffuse large cell, and immunoblastic) comprise almost all AIDS-related lymphomas but account for only about 10% of NHLs in the general population. Small, noncleaved cell lymphomas (Burkitt and non-Burkitt types) constitute about 40% of AIDS-related NHLs. These tumors tend to present at higher CD4 counts than the other types. Large-cell lymphomas account for about 30% of AIDS-related

NHLs. These are the most heterogeneous of lymphomas encountered in HIV disease and contain various proportions of B-cell, T-cell, and macrophage antigens. The remaining 30% of AIDS-related NHLs are immunoblastic-plasmacytoid lymphomas. While diffuse large-cell and immunoblastic lymphomas usually arise in patients with a low CD4 count, small, noncleaved (Burkitt-like) lymphoma occurs at all stages of HIV disease. Rare types of lymphomas encountered in HIV-infected patients include Ki-1 anaplastic lymphoma, angiotrophic large-cell lymphoma, mucosa-associated lymphoid tissue, and Sezary syndrome.

Clinical Manifestations and Diagnosis

The clinical manifestations of AIDS-related NHL are protean with no pathognomonic features. The majority of patients have constitutional symptoms at the time of presentation. These tumors may manifest as a mass lesion, organ failure from tumor infiltration, obstruction, or bleeding. Fever in an HIV-infected patient, particularly if it persists for more than two weeks, may be a sign of lymphoma. At least 80% of patients have stage IV disease at the time of presentation (Table 10-4); the bone marrow is involved in about one third of cases. Bone marrow involvement is more likely with small, non-cleaved (Burkitt-like) lymphoma and is associated with a higher risk of leptomeningeal spread.

The gastrointestinal tract is the most frequent site of extranodal disease. Of patients with gastrointestinal tract NHL, the colon is involved in 46%, the ileum in 39%, and the stomach in 23%. The presenting features of gastrointestinal tract disease include pain and/or weight loss in more than 75% of patients; life-threatening complications, such as bleeding, perforation, and obstruction, occur in about 40% of cases. Studies have shown that patients with gastrointestinal tract NHL tend to survive longer and are more likely to respond to therapy than those with extra-gastrointestinal tract disease. Computed tomography (CT) scanning is the diagnostic test of choice for detection of NHL gastrointestinal tract involvement. At least 80% of CT scan abnormalities consist of solitary lesions of the small intestine that cause annular infiltration, focal wall thickening, and/or cavitation of the gut wall. Hepatic involvement, which occurs in one third of patients, may be

Table 10-4.   Sites of Involvement of AIDS-Related Lymphoma

Site	Involvement*	Site	Involvement*
Lymph nodes	38%	Central nervous system	27%
Lungs	33%	Spleen	23%
Liver	33%	Small bowel	22%
Bone marrow	30%	Large bowel/rectum	21%

* Total is greater than 100% because some patients have multiple sites of involvement.

asymptomatic or present with pain, cholestasis or, less often, increased serum transaminase levels. CT scan generally shows low-attenuation mass lesions.

Standard chest x-rays are abnormal in more than 90% of patients with NHL pulmonary involvement. Findings include pleural effusions in 44%, lobar consolidation in 40%, reticular infiltrates in 24%, mass lesions in 24%, and hilar and/or mediastinal lymphadenopathy in 50%. CT scanning only modestly improves the yield. In patients with pleural effusions, cytology and biopsy are diagnostic in 75% of cases. In those with pulmonary parenchymal involvement, bronchoalveolar lavage or bronchial brushings tend to be of very low diagnostic yield but may be necessary to exclude concurrent opportunistic infection. Although gallium scanning appears sensitive for the detection of intrathoracic NHL, it is nonspecific.

Secondary spread to the central nervous system (CNS), usually as lymphomatous meningitis, is present in up to 20% of NHL patients at the time of presentation. Symptoms and signs may consist of headache, cranial nerve palsies, and, infrequently, meningismus, but almost one quarter of cases are asymptomatic. Leptomeningeal spread is not associated with poorer prognosis. Staging evaluation for AIDS-related NHL should include a lumbar puncture with cerebrospinal fluid (CSF) analysis for cytology, glucose, protein, and EBV DNA by polymerase chain reaction (PCR). The sensitivity and specificity of EBV DNA detection in CSF for CNS involvement are 90% and 100%, respectively. Therapy with intrathecal cytarabine given concurrently with systemic chemotherapy is successful in eradicating disease that has spread to the meninges.

Primary effusion lymphomas, also known as body cavity lymphomas, are a distinct clinical and pathologic subtype of AIDS-related NHL. These high-grade tumors originate in the pleura, pericardium, peritoneum, serosal surfaces, or, rarely, the meninges. They present with a serous (lymphomatous) effusion with no detectable mass lesion. Although primary effusion lymphomas have little propensity to disseminate, they cause local destruction and have a uniformly poor prognosis. Given the unique liquid-phase growth of these tumors, effusions are almost always positive for malignant cells. The neoplastic cells of primary effusion lymphomas may lack surface expression of T-cell or B-cell lymphocyte antigens but contain genomic material from KSHV/HHV8 and frequently from EBV. A previous history of KS increases the risk of developing primary effusion lymphoma.

Primary Central Nervous System Lymphoma

Primary CNS lymphomas represent 20% of all AIDS-related lymphomas but only 2% of lymphomas in the general population. They tend to occur relatively late in HIV disease, with an average CD4 count of 30 cells/mm^3 compared with 190 cells/mm^3 for systemic lymphomas. The majority of these tumors are immunoblastic-plasmacytoid or large-cell histology, and they are always monoclonal. Primary CNS lymphomas rarely spread outside of the CNS, but within the CNS, they may be multifocal.

Unlike systemic AIDS-related NHLs that have secondarily spread to the CNS, wherein the CSF cytology is positive in at least 80% with the first lumbar puncture, leptomeningeal involvement with primary CNS lymphomas is much less common. Here the CSF cytology is positive in only 20% of cases, making this test of very limited diagnostic value.

Primary CNS lymphomas contain genomic material from EBV, which, when detected in the CSF via PCR, may serve as a surrogate marker for this tumor when tissue is unobtainable. Compared with biopsy, its sensitivity is about 84%, with a positive predictive value of almost 100% and a negative predictive value of 93%. Another surrogate marker being investigated for primary CNS lymphoma is CD23 in the CSF. The presence of this soluble B-cell surface antigen is independent of that of EBV DNA and has a sensitivity and specificity of 77% and 94%, respectively.

Primary CNS lymphoma is the second-most common brain space-occupying lesion in patients with AIDS after toxoplasmosis (Box 10-3; see Chapter 9). At the time of presentation, lymphomatous lesions are generally at least 3 cm in size and in a perivascular distribution. On magnetic resonance imaging (MRI) scan, these tumors are hypodense or isodense. The most common locations for primary CNS lymphomas are the cerebral hemispheres, followed by the basal ganglia, cerebellum, and brain stem. Fewer than 10% of these tumors involve the posterior fossa. Lesions in this compartment are more likely infectious in etiology. Unlike primary CNS lymphomas in the general population, these tumors may ring-enhance because their rapid growth results in central necrosis.

Box 10-3.   Characteristics of Central Nervous System Lymphoma and Toxoplasmosis

CNS Lymphoma	Toxoplasmosis
• 5% of AIDS patients	• 15% of AIDS patients
• More chronic illness	• Subacute illness
• 50% of patients have nonfocal symptoms	• Predominantly focal symptoms and signs
• 75% are supratentorial	• Variable location in CNS
• 80% are located deep in the brain	• Basal ganglia commonly involved
• 50% are multifocal on MRI scan	• Usually multiple lesions on MRI scan
• Variable enhancement pattern	• Over 90% enhance
• Lesions may be >3 cm	• Lesions of 1-3 cm common

CNS = central nervous system; MRI = magnetic resonance imaging.

Diagnostic modalities that are being investigated in HIV-infected patients with intracranial mass lesions include thallium-201 and SPECT scanning. In small studies, each modality had a sensitivity that approached 100%, but their specificities were 54% and 69%, respectively. Definitive diagnosis of primary CNS lymphoma in an HIV-infected patient requires a stereotactic brain biopsy. Performed by highly trained staff, this procedure has a yield of up to 88%; morbidity and mortality are 8.4% and 2.9%, respectively.

Treatment

Disseminated disease is encountered in at least 80% of patients with AIDS-related lymphoma at the time of diagnosis. Therefore, staging is of value in only a minority of cases. However, all patients should undergo lumbar puncture to look for occult CNS spread of the tumor.

Optimal treatment for AIDS-related lymphomas has yet to be defined, and there are no established second-line regimens. Although controversial to some extent, the standard therapy is cyclophosphamide, hydroxydauno-mycin (doxorubicin), Oncovin (vincristine), and prednisone (CHOP). When HIV-infected patients are treated with chemotherapy regimens that are used for lymphomas of similar histology in the HIV-seronegative population, complete responses occur less often and are less durable. Comparison between standard-dose and low-dose chemotherapeutic regimens shows a similar complete response rate, time to progression, and median survival, but reduced toxicity with the latter. There seems to be a trade-off between the response rate achieved with the standard-dose regimen and the greater immunosuppression induced by it.

The immunosuppression induced by chemotherapy exceeds the duration of exposure to these drugs. In addition, several drugs used in the treatment of lymphomas may induce or enhance the expression of HIV. Conversely, HIV infection may render lymphocytes resistant to the cytotoxic activity of some antineoplastic agents. During chemotherapy, the CD4 cell count may decline by 50% or more from baseline, necessitating the temporary institution of antimicrobial prophylaxis for opportunistic infections. This effect may persist for several months afterward. Chemotherapy does not seem to affect the likelihood of virologic suppression or the development of HIV resistance mutations.

Zidovudine, originally developed in 1964 as an antineoplastic agent, has anti-proliferative activity when combined with drugs that disrupt thymidylate synthesis such as 5-fluorouracil and methotrexate. In small studies of ZDV, given in higher doses than used today, response rates as high as 80% were achieved. Other nucleoside reverse-transcriptase inhibitors have not shown this effect.

Methyl-glyoxal-*bis* guanlhydrazone (MGBG, mitoguazone) is a noncell cycle-specific cytotoxic agent that was first synthesized in 1898. MGBG inhibits the biosynthesis of polyamines, which are short peptides that are important to

DNA, RNA, and membrane integrity. Monotherapy with this drug is associated with response rates of 29% to 49% in relapsed or refractory AIDS-related lymphomas, with a median survival of 21.5 months for complete responders. MGBG has the advantage of good CNS penetration and relative lack of bone marrow toxicity, but it may cause mucositis, gastrointestinal toxicity, paresthesias, somnolence, and vasodilation. Studies using this drug for initial therapy and in combination with other agents are ongoing.

Daily, low-dose subcutaneous interleukin-2 infusions have been shown to promote expansion of immune effectors such as natural killer cells. Small studies have shown that this treatment may result in down-regulation of lymphoproliferative disorders in HIV-infected patients. Combination antiretroviral therapy must be given concurrently to prevent augmentation of HIV replication.

Another line of investigative therapy of AIDS-related lymphomas involves monoclonal antibodies. The prototype is anti-B4-blocked ricin. The "A" chain of ricin is an enzyme that inactivates ribosomes, and B4 (CD-19) is a B-lineage-restricted surface antigen expressed in more than 95% of AIDS-related B-cell lymphomas. This antibody is given with multiagent chemotherapy. Toxicities include fever, allergic reactions, hepatic dysfunction, and capillary leak syndrome. Rituximab is a monoclonal antibody to the CD20 antigen that is present on at least 95% of AIDS-related lymphomas. Although studies have shown synergy between rituximab and chemotherapy, its role in AIDS-related lymphomas is still undefined. Initial results are mixed, with the potential for greater control of the tumor, offset by an increase in immunosuppression.

The small, noncleaved (Burkitt-like) lymphomas require more intensive chemotherapy such as the CODOX-M/IVAC (Magrath) regimen. Since there are possible interactions between the antineoplastic agents of these regimens and some HIV drugs, temporary discontinuation of antiretroviral therapy should be considered during chemotherapy.

Refractory or relapsed systemic lymphomas have a very poor prognosis, and there are no satisfactory second-line regimens. Consideration should be given to enrolling affected patients in clinical trials. If this is not possible, another option is using a chemotherapy protocol such as platinum-based therapy that is not cross-resistant with the initial regimen.

Primary body cavity lymphomas, despite the fact that they have little propensity to disseminate beyond the site of origin, tend to have a poor prognosis. Local radiation therapy to the affected body cavity may offer palliation. Multi-agent chemotherapy regimens, the most experience being with CHOP, may also be useful. Investigative studies with liposomal doxorubicin and daunorubicin are ongoing. Pegylated liposomal anthracyclines may evade the MDR-1-mediated drug resistance mechanism in primary effusion lymphoma.

Management of primary CNS lymphomas, which consists of radiation therapy with corticosteroids and/or alkylating agents, may increase the length of survival but rarely results in an extended remission. Survival without therapy is 2 to 3 months from the time of presentation compared with 6 to 8 months with therapy. However, palliation of these tumors for up to 18 months has been reported with radiation therapy and control of HIV infection.

An important component of any medical regimen used for the AIDS-related NHLs is the institution of antiretroviral therapy with the goal of attaining an undetectable viral load. Antiretroviral therapy not only enhances the ability of the immune system to deal with aberrant cells but also may increase the radiosensitivity of malignant cells.

Prognosis

In HIV-infected patients treated concurrently with antiretroviral therapy and chemotherapy who achieve a complete remission, the 3-year survival rate is comparable to that of HIV-seronegative patients with lymphomas of similar histology. In addition, the toxicity of chemotherapy (e.g., opportunistic infections) is reduced compared with those treated with chemotherapy alone. The survival benefit is particularly evident in patients who attain at least a 0.5 log decrease in the viral load and at least a 40 cell/mm³ increase in the CD4 count.

Given appropriate therapy, patients with AIDS-related lymphomas with good prognostic features may attain complete remission rates exceeding 50%, with a median survival of at least 18 months. Prognosis is not affected by leptomeningeal disease at the time of diagnosis, the size of the mass lesion, or the presence of constitutional symptoms. However, several adverse prognostic features have been identified, including age greater than 40 years, a CD4 count of less than 100 cells/mm³, and a high serum lactate dehydrogenase (LDH) level at the time of diagnosis (Box 10-4). These characteristics independently increase the hazard ratio by 1.6, 1.7, and 1.8, respectively. Other adverse prognostic factors are a history of injection-drug use; previous therapy with adriamycin, vincristine, or both; and more than one site of disease. The International Prognostic Index (IPI) for aggressive, non-HIV-related lymphomas has also been shown to be valid for AIDS-related lymphomas.

Box 10-4.   Adverse Prognostic Features of AIDS-Related Lymphoma

- Age >40 years
- History of injection-drug use
- Previous therapy with adriamycin or vincristine

- Multiple sites of disease
- CD4 count <100 cells/mm³
- High (>1000 U/dL) serum LDH level

Adverse Prognostic Features	Complete Response Rate	Median Survival
Zero	80%	18 months
One	67%	14 months
Two	57%	11 months
Four	13%	4 months

KEY POINTS

- In HIV-infected patients, Hodgkin's disease is usually more advanced (stage III or IV) at the time of presentation than in the general population.
- Treatment of lymphoma in AIDS patients is less likely to result in a complete response compared with that in HIV-seronegative persons. Chemotherapy induces immunosuppression, and several anticancer agents appear to enhance the expression of HIV.
- HIV infection increases the risk of non-Hodgkin's lymphoma 60- to 100-fold over that of the general population.
- The gastrointestinal tract is the most frequent site of extranodal disease. Patients with gastrointestinal tract lymphoma tend to survive longer and are more likely to respond to therapy than those with extra-gastrointestinal tract disease.
- Although primary CNS lymphomas comprise only 2% of all lymphomas in the general population, they represent 20% of AIDS-related lymphomas.
- Because enhancing immune response is critical to the successful treatment of non-Hodgkin's lymphomas, antiretroviral therapy is an important part of their management.

SUGGESTED READINGS

Cingolani A, Gastaldi R, Fassone L, Pierconti F, Giancola ML, Martini M, et al. Epstein-Barr virus infection is predictive of CNS involvement in systemic AIDS-related non-Hodgkin's lymphomas. J Clin Oncol. 2000;18:3325-30.

Gérard L, Galicier L, Maillard A, Boulanger E, Quint L, Matheron S, et al. Systemic non-Hodgkin lymphoma in HIV-infected patients with effective suppression of HIV replication: persistent occurrence but improved survival. J Acquir Immune Defic Syndr. 2002;30:478-84.

Groupe d'Epidemiologie Clinique du SIDA en Aquitaine. Factors associated with the occurrence of AIDS-related non-Hodgkin lymphoma in the era of highly active antiretroviral therapy: Aquitaine Cohort, France. Clin Infect Dis. 2006;42:411-7.

Groupe d'Etude des Lymphomes de l'Adulte (GELA). Human immunodeficiency virus-related lymphoma: relation between clinical features and histologic subtypes. Am J Med. 2001; 111:704-11.

Kaplan LD. Current status of the treatment of HIV-associated lymphoma. Clin Adv Hematol Oncol. 2005;3:28-29.

Mbulaiteye SM, Biggar RJ, Goedert JJ, Engels EA. Immune deficiency and risk for malignancy among persons with AIDS. J Acquir Immune Defic Syndr. 2003;32:527-33.

Simonelli C, Zanussi S, Cinelli R, Dal Maso L, Di Gennaro G, D'Andrea M, et al. Impact of concomitant antiblastic chemotherapy and highly active antiretroviral therapy on human immunodeficiency virus (HIV) viremia and genotyping in HIV-infected patients with non-Hodgkin lymphoma. Clin Infect Dis. 2003;37:820-7.

Straus DJ. HIV-associated lymphoma: promising new results, but with toxicity. Blood. 2005; 105:1842.

Summaries for Patients. Estimating outcome in patients with HIV-related lymphoma. Ann Intern Med. 2005;143:I28.

Wilson KS, McKenna RW, Kroft SH, Dawson DB, Ansari Q, Schneider NR. Primary effusion lymphomas exhibit complex and recurrent cytogenetic abnormalities. Br J Haematol. 2002; 116:113-21.

III. ANOGENITAL SQUAMOUS CELL CANCER

JOHN P. DOWEIKO

The relative risk of squamous cell carcinomas in HIV-infected patients is 20- to 37-fold that of the general population. Among these malignancies are cancers of the anus and the uterine cervix, the latter being an AIDS-defining diagnosis. Squamous cell cancers of the vulva, penis, oral cavity, and skin also occur with increased frequency in HIV disease.

Pathogenesis

Human papillomavirus (HPV) plays an important role in the pathogenesis of anogenital squamous cell cancers in the HIV-seropositive population (see Chapter 9). Overall, 95% of cervical cancers, 70% of anal cancers, 50% of penile cancers, and 20% of oral cancers are associated with HPV infection. HPV transmission is almost always related to sexual contact. Condom use may help reduce the risk of acquiring and transmitting HPV infection but does not eliminate it. The risk of HPV infection increases with the lifetime number of sexual partners and is higher in uncircumcised males.

Oncogenic strains of HPV, which express oncoproteins and undergo changes in their tumor suppressor genes, are able to integrate into the host genome. Both of these factors promote cell immortality and dedifferentiation. Immunosuppression reactivates latent HPV infection, and the HIV TAT protein increases expression of HPV oncoproteins. Alterations in local immune response and cytokine expression of the anal and genital mucosa caused by HIV infection may result in enhanced susceptibility to HPV and increased expression of HPV oncogenes.

Dysplasia and Carcinoma of the Anus

Squamous cell cancer of the anal canal accounts for only 2% to 3% of malignancies of the lower gastrointestinal tract; 90% of these tumors occur in HIV-infected patients. The relative risk of dysplasia tends to be inversely correlated with the CD4 cell count. Fewer than 50% of patients with dysplasia have a prior history of anogenital warts. The incidence of anal squamous cell cancer may increase with prolonged survival of HIV-infected patients on antiretroviral therapy. Squamous cell cancers of the anal canal in this setting tend to be more aggressive and advance at a faster rate than those in the HIV-seronegative population.

Even high-grade anal dysplasia is usually asymptomatic. As these lesions become malignant, early symptoms may include anal burning, pruritus, or irritation. Bleeding may subsequently develop, and bacterial infections of the anal canal or perirectal area may result from disruption of the mucosa. Mass lesions and ulcers of the anal canal occur late in the course.

Cytology provides a relatively easy way to screen for dysplasia of the anal canal. Despite the absence of formal standards, it seems prudent to perform an anal Pap smear every 6 to 12 months in HIV-infected patients at risk for HPV infection or with a history of anogenital warts (see Chapters 9 and 11). Studies are ongoing to assess the operating characteristics and clinical utility of this test.

Low-grade dysplasia can be followed clinically with anoscopy and colposcopic biopsy every 4 to 6 months. High-grade lesions should be treated with either surgical excision or laser ablation. The management of squamous cell cancer consists of chemotherapy and radiation therapy. The chemotherapy is usually an infusion of 5-fluorouracil with or without mitomycin C during the first few days of radiation therapy. It is important to realize that HIV disease imposes certain limitations on the administration of radiation therapy and chemotherapy, particularly in patients with a CD4 count below 200 cells/mm³. Treatment is associated with an increased risk of damage to normal tissues and delayed healing. In addition, limited bone marrow reserve may preclude the use of standard doses of chemotherapy.

Dysplasia and Carcinoma of the Uterine Cervix

Approximately 95% of uterine cervix neoplasms are squamous cell cancers, which generally arise at the squamocolumnar junction. Only about half of women with cervical cancers have a prior history of anogenital warts.

Cervical dysplasia is usually asymptomatic. Dysplastic squamous cells may evolve into carcinoma in situ over time. Eventually, the malignant cells break through the basement membrane and enter the cervical stroma. Immunosuppression from HIV infection is associated with more aggressive neoplastic disease than that seen in the general population.

Pap smear is used to screen for dysplasia of the cervix. The positive and negative predictive values of an abnormal Pap smear in an HIV-infected woman are 95% and 39%, respectively. Although this test has an overall sensitivity of only 57% to 81% compared with biopsy, its false-negative rate decreases with repeated testing. The Centers for Disease Control and Prevention (CDC) recommends annual Pap smears in most women. However, the more rapid progression of cervical dysplasia in HIV-infected women may merit Pap smears every 6 months, especially in those with prior abnormal results (see Chapters 9 and 11).

Patients with Pap smears showing cellular atypia or dysplasia should be referred to a gynecologist for colposcopy and biopsy if indicated. High-grade lesions are managed with cryotherapy, loop excision, laser therapy, or conization. Women with early stage (up to and including stage IIA) cervical cancer are managed either with radical hysterectomy and pelvic lymphadenectomy or definitive radiation therapy in conjunction with chemotherapy.

KEY POINTS

- Human papillomavirus (HPV) infection plays an important role in the pathogenesis of anogenital squamous cell cancer. HIV infection predisposes not only to an altered susceptibility for HPV infection but also to an increased expression of HPV oncogenes.
- Pap smear screening for dysplasia of the uterine cervix should be performed in HIV-infected women every 6 to 12 months, and regular anal Pap smears should be considered in patients at risk for anal dysplasia.

SUGGESTED READINGS

Klencke B. Invasive anal disease and other non-AIDS defining neoplasms. Presented at Conference on AIDS-Associated Malignancies: Biology and Clinical Management. San Francisco; 1999.

Levine AM, Pieters AS. Non-AIDS defining cancer. In: Summaries of the First National AIDS Malignancy Conference. 28-30 April 1997. Bethesda, MD: National Cancer Institute; pp 18-20.

Northfelt DW, Swift PS, Palefsky JM: Anal neoplasia: pathogenesis, diagnosis, and management. Hematol Oncol Clin North Am. 1996;10:1177-87.

Palefsky JM, Holly EA, Hogeboom CJ, et al. Anal cytology as a screening tool for anal squamous intraepithelial lesions. J Acquir Immune Defic Syndrome Hum Retrovirol. 1997;14: 415-22.

Palefsky JM, Holly EA, Ralston ML, et al. High incidence of anal high-grade squamous intraepithelial lesions among HIV-positive and HIV-negative homosexual and bisexual men. AIDS. 1998;12:495-503.

Palefsky J. Anal squamous intraepithelial lesions in human immunodeficiency virus–positive men and women. Semin Oncol. 2000;27:471-9.

Peddada AV, Smith DE, Rao AR, et al. Chemotherapy and low-dose radiotherapy in the treatment of HIV-infected patients with carcinoma of the anal canal. Int J Radiat Oncol Biol Phys. 1997;37:1101-5.

Unger ER, Vernon SD, Lee DR, et al. Human papillomavirus type in anal epithelial lesions is influenced by human immunodeficiency virus. Arch Pathol Lab Med. 1997;121:820-4.

Chapter 11

HIV Infection in Special Populations

I. Women
RAYMOND O. POWRIE, MD
SUSAN CU-UVIN, MD

II. Men Who Have Sex with Men
BENJAMIN DAVIS, MD

III. African Americans
ERIC P. GOOSBY, MD

IV. Transgender Persons
GREGORY FENTON, MD

V. Injection-Drug Users
JEFFREY H. SAMET, MD, MA, MPH

I. WOMEN
RAYMOND O. POWRIE
SUSAN CU-UVIN

Epidemiology and Transmission of HIV Infection

Women account for nearly half of the 40 million people living with HIV infection worldwide. In the United States, the annual number of AIDS cases increased 15% among women from 1999 to 2003. AIDS is one of the leading causes of death in women of reproductive age. Approximately 60% of HIV-infected women in the United States are African American, and 18% are Hispanic. Initially, injection-drug use was responsible for the majority of HIV cases in women, but heterosexual contact is now the most common mode of transmission.

The care of HIV-infected women is complicated because many come from impoverished communities that traditionally have had poor access to health care. Issues such as childcare, transportation, finances, fear of disclosure, mistrust of doctors, domestic violence, and depression can be significant barriers to medical care. Depression, reported in as many as 60% of HIV-infected women, as well as the other foregoing factors, can adversely affect medication adherence. The importance of effectively addressing this epidemic in women is magnified when one considers that maternal-fetal transmission accounts for nearly all cases of HIV infection in children. While much progress has been made in decreasing overall mortality from HIV disease, this decline has been significantly less pronounced in women than in men.

Clinical Manifestations

Course of HIV Disease

Correcting for differences in access to, and utilization of, health care, it does not appear that gender significantly affects the course of HIV disease. However, evidence does exist that: 1) The initial viral load is not as useful a predictor of clinical progression in women as it is in men; 2) women tend to have lower viral loads for a given CD4 count than men; and 3) women tend to have lower viral loads at the time of seroconversion.

Opportunistic Infections and Sexually Transmitted Diseases

With a few notable exceptions, the spectrum of opportunistic diseases in HIV-infected women and men does not appear to differ. Reports suggest that women with HIV disease are more likely than men to present with herpes simplex virus (HSV) infection, esophageal candidiasis, and wasting syndrome and are less likely to develop Kaposi's sarcoma. For many women, gynecologic conditions may be the initial manifestation of HIV infection. Vaginal candidiasis, bacterial vaginosis, syphilis, HSV infection, and pelvic inflammatory disease (PID) are common and often more difficult to manage than in the HIV-seronegative population. The incidence of cervical dysplasia, and possibly cancer, is also increased.

Candidiasis
Recurrent and/or severe vaginal candidiasis is one of the more common reasons that HIV-infected women seek medical care (see Chapter 9). Treatment with a topical antifungal agent such as clotrimazole (1% cream intravaginally for 7 to 14 days or 2% cream intravaginally for 3 days) or miconazole (vaginal suppository 200 mg daily for 3 days), or oral fluconazole (150 mg single dose tablet) is usually adequate. Preventive therapy with fluconazole 200 mg weekly in HIV-infected women with recurrent vaginal candidiasis has been shown to be effective without resulting in a high rate of fungal resistance.

Bacterial Vaginosis
Bacterial vaginosis is also common in HIV-infected women. The standard regimen, oral metronidazole 500 mg twice daily for 7 days, is generally effective. Studies have shown that untreated bacterial vaginosis may increase HIV shedding in the female genital tract.

Sexually Transmitted Diseases
HIV-infected women should be screened for other STDs at baseline and periodically thereafter if they continue to be at risk. Genital ulcer diseases, such as syphilis and HSV infection, may be more difficult to treat and increase the risk of HIV transmission. Treatment recommendations for syphilis are the same as in the HIV-seronegative population. Treatment of HSV infection with oral acyclovir (400 mg three times daily) or famciclovir (250 mg three times daily) is recommended (see Chapter 9). Both drugs can be used in lower total daily doses as preventive therapy in the setting of frequent recurrences.

Pelvic Inflammatory Disease

The literature is conflicting as to whether PID is more likely to be severe, complicated, or slower to respond to treatment in the context of HIV disease. HIV-infected women with presumed PID should be treated as inpatients with standard drug regimens (e.g., cefoxitin 2 g intravenously every 6 hours plus doxycycline 100 mg intravenously or orally twice daily until improved, then doxycycline 100 mg orally twice daily to complete a 14-day course). Failure to respond to medical management should prompt pelvic ultrasonography to look for evidence of tubo-ovarian abscess and consideration of surgical intervention.

Cervical Dysplasia and Cancer

HIV disease is associated with an increased risk of cervical dysplasia and cancer (see Chapters 9 and 10). Most patients who develop these conditions have a prior history of human papillomavirus (HPV) infection, which is also the cause of anogenital warts. The risk of developing cervical disease is greater in patients with a lower CD4 count and higher viral load.

The Pap smear has been demonstrated to be a useful screening test for cervical dysplasia. Approximately 40% of HIV-infected women will have an abnormal Pap smear at baseline, and 58% will have evidence of HPV infection. A Pap smear should be performed as part of the initial evaluation of all HIV-infected women; it should be repeated 6 months later, and, if normal, repeated at 12-month intervals thereafter. Colposcopy is not recommended as a screening test in this population. More frequent Pap smear evaluations (every 4 to 6 months) are advised if the endocervical component is absent, if there is a history of HPV infection, and after treatment for any cervical lesion. Many experts now recommend screening of HIV-infected women with a cervical HPV DNA assay to help identify those at increased risk for dysplasia.

Women with Pap smear results showing cellular atypia or any degree of cervical dysplasia should be referred to a gynecologist for further diagnostic evaluation. In general, colposcopy and biopsy are performed. Continued close monitoring of HIV-infected women with an abnormal Pap smear is important even after treatment because nearly 50% will have recurrent cervical abnormalities within a year of treatment.

Antiretroviral Therapy

Except in the context of pregnancy, antiretroviral therapy recommendations are the same for women as for men (see Chapter 4). The previously described gender differences in the relationship between CD4 count and viral load have created some concern that women might warrant treatment earlier in the course of HIV disease. However, this observation is not reflected in current antiretroviral therapy guidelines. There is some evidence that long-term toxicities of antiretroviral therapy are different in women than men (see Chapter 5). For example, women may be more likely to experience increased abdominal fat and breast size as part of lipodystrophy syndrome, whereas men are more likely to have fat loss in their limbs and buttocks.

Pregnancy

General Principles

Reproductive decisions in HIV-infected women appear to be no different than those in age-matched seronegative women. Although perinatal transmission of the virus is an important public health concern, the clinician should focus on educating the prospective mother about the potential benefits and risks of pregnancy, answering her questions, and addressing her concerns.

Management of pregnancy in HIV-infected women includes general prenatal care, the appropriate use of antiretroviral and antimicrobial prophylactic therapies in the mother, and monitoring for evidence of disease progression. Optimal care is best accomplished using a multidisciplinary approach involving an obstetrician, HIV specialist and/or internist, nutritionist, and social worker with ready access to a behavioral health specialist. Expert consultation is recommended for clinicians with limited experience in the use of antiretroviral therapy.

Course of HIV Disease

Although pregnancy has been associated with a temporary modest decrease in the CD4 count, this observation does not appear to have a negative impact on the viral load or the prognosis of HIV infection. HIV-infected women may be at increased risk of spontaneous abortion and infertility but, if asymptomatic, are not predisposed to other obstetric complications.

Maternal-Fetal Transmission

In the absence of effective antiretroviral therapy, there is approximately a 25% risk of transmission from the pregnant HIV-infected woman to the newborn. Maternal-fetal transmission of HIV can occur at any stage in gestation, during labor and delivery, and in the postpartum period through breast-feeding. Labor and delivery are responsible for most of the transmission, with direct contact of the infant with maternal blood and cervical secretions as the probable mechanism. This hypothesis is supported by the findings that prolonged rupture of membranes is associated with an increased risk of transmission and that the first born of twins, who spends more time in contact with maternal bodily fluids, is at higher risk of acquiring HIV infection than the second born. Research establishing that elective cesarean section may decrease perinatal transmission provides further evidence. High maternal viral load, low CD4 count, illicit drug use, unprotected sex with multiple sexual partners during pregnancy, maternal anemia, and low infant birth weight are all associated with an increased risk of HIV maternal-fetal transmission.

Antiretroviral Therapy

Antiretroviral therapy in pregnancy has been shown to decrease the rate of perinatal transmission significantly and is generally well tolerated by the mother and fetus (Box 11-1). A landmark study published over a decade ago demonstrated that zidovudine (ZDV) given throughout pregnancy, during labor, and postpartum for 6 weeks to the newborn decreased the rate of transmission by two-thirds. More recent studies have demonstrated that the use of effective combination antiretroviral therapy during pregnancy, which is now the standard of care, can reduce the risk of transmission to less than 2%.

Antiretroviral therapy is recommended in all HIV-infected pregnant women who plan to carry the fetus to term with the goal of achieving virologic suppression. Patients should have the viral load monitored monthly

---

Box 11-1. Antiretroviral Therapy During Pregnancy

- Antiretroviral therapy (ART) is recommended in all pregnant women to decrease the risk of perinatal transmission.
- Goal is suppression of maternal viral load (<1000 copies/mL associated with decreased transmission).
- In women not on ART before pregnancy, consider delaying treatment until the second trimester.
- In women on ART before pregnancy, continue therapy with modification of regimen as warranted on the basis of toxicity or teratogenicity.
- Perform HIV resistance testing before starting ART and in women on ART with detectable viral load.
- Include zidovudine, if possible, in ART regimen.

until it is undetectable and every 2 to 3 months thereafter. Perinatal transmission is rare if the viral load is maintained below 1000 copies/mL. HIV resistance testing is recommended before starting antiretroviral therapy in pregnant women and in women on antiretroviral therapy with a detectable viral load.

For previously untreated HIV-infected pregnant women, three antiretroviral drugs, including ZDV, are initiated after completion of the first trimester. Zidovudine and lamivudine (3TC), in combination with either nelfinavir or lopinavir/ritonavir, is most often prescribed. HIV-infected pregnant women already on an effective antiretroviral regimen should be counseled to maintain therapy because interrupting it, even during the first trimester, may result in a substantial increase in the viral load. Adding ZDV during the second and third trimesters to a non-ZDV-containing regimen should be considered on an individual basis because of its effectiveness in reducing perinatal transmission.

Most antiretroviral drugs are listed as Food and Drug Administration (FDA) pregnancy category B (no evidence of teratogenicity in humans) or C (human teratogenicity has not been demonstrated, but risk cannot be excluded). The one exception is efavirenz (EFV), which is classified as category D (evidence of teratogenicity in humans). Efavirenz use during pregnancy has been associated with significant anomalies in animal studies, case reports, and pregnancy registry data. Women should have a pregnancy test before starting EFV, and women of childbearing potential who are receiving EFV should use two effective methods of birth control. Prospective data on antiretroviral drugs are collected and regularly updated by the antiretroviral pregnancy registry (1-800-258-4263).

Other precautions related to the use of specific antiretroviral drugs in pregnancy are also worth noting. Nevirapine (NVP) can lead to a potentially life-threatening hepatotoxicity in women with a CD4 count of greater than 250 cells/mm^3, and its initiation should be avoided in this setting. Deaths related to lactic acidosis have been reported in pregnant women receiving didanosine (ddI) and stavudine (d4T); therefore, use of this drug combination during pregnancy is contraindicated.

The effectiveness of antiretroviral therapy in decreasing neonatal HIV infection highlights the importance of encouraging all women of childbearing age who are pregnant or considering becoming pregnant to have an HIV antibody test performed. Although no state presently requires testing for HIV infection during pregnancy, some mandate physicians to counsel women at the beginning of their pregnancy and to inform them of the potential benefits of antiretroviral therapy in decreasing the risk of perinatal transmission.

Opportunistic Infection Prophylaxis

Recommendations for initiation and maintenance of prophylaxis of opportunistic infections in pregnant women are standard (see Chapter 7).

Trimethoprim-sulfamethoxazole (TMP-SMX), despite theoretical concerns about its use in pregnancy, has an excellent safety profile when given for *Pneumocystis jiroveci* (formerly *carinii*) pneumonia (PCP) and toxoplasmosis prophylaxis. Isoniazid for TB prophylaxis, azithromycin for *Mycobacterium avium* complex (MAC) prophylaxis, and influenza, pneumococcal, and hepatitis B vaccine preparations can also be given during pregnancy.

Delivery

In general, elective cesarean section is associated with less perinatal HIV transmission than vaginal delivery. The American College of Obstetricians and Gynecologists (ACOG) recommends that the surgical procedure be offered to all HIV-infected pregnant women at 38 weeks gestation but notes that there is no evidence that it will benefit women with a viral load of less than 1000 copies/mL.

Intravenous ZDV should be administered during delivery, and other antiretroviral drugs that the woman has been receiving should be continued throughout parturition. ZDV is also given to the neonate for 6 weeks (Box 11-2). Avoidance of amniocentesis, fetal scalp monitors, artificial rupture of membranes, the use of forceps or vacuum extractor, and fetal blood scalp sampling are all important in decreasing the risk of perinatal transmission during labor and delivery. ACOG also recommends the routine use of prophylactic antibiotics perioperatively to decrease the risk of endometritis.

If a patient presents in labor without knowing her HIV serostatus, every attempt should be made to determine it in a timely fashion. HIV rapid antibody tests are increasingly being used for this purpose. Untreated HIV-infected women in labor and their neonate should receive ZDV as described in Box 11-2. Administration of a single dose of NVP 200 mg to the mother followed by NVP 2 mg/kg to the neonate during the first 72 hours of life may be used as an alternative to or in addition to ZDV. If single-dose NVP is used in the mother, consideration should be given to starting her on a 3 to 7 day course of ZDV with 3TC in an attempt to reduce the likelihood of inducing maternal NVP resistance.

Box 11-2.   Intrapartum and Neonatal Use of Zidovudine (ZDV)

Intrapartum Use

ZDV IV during labor and delivery; 2 mg/kg loading dose over ½ to 1 hour followed by continuous infusion of 1 mg/kg per hour through delivery

Neonatal Use

ZDV syrup 2 mg/kg PO 4 doses/day for 6 weeks; start within 8 to 12 hours of birth. If infant is NPO, ZDV IV (1.5 mg/kg over one-half hour every 6 hours) can be given.

Postpartum Management

Infant bonding should be encouraged in HIV-infected mothers, but contact with maternal body fluids is to be avoided. Patients should be counseled about the options for contraception. Medication adherence may decrease during this transition period, and some women are also at risk for depression.

Breast-Feeding

In the United States, breast-feeding in HIV-infected women is contraindicated because of the increased risk of transmission. However, bottle-feeding is not practical in many resource-limited countries in which acceptable alternatives to breast milk are not available because of poor sanitation, high rates of infectious disease, and economic limitations. In this setting, many experts recommend exclusive breast-feeding of the infant until age 4 to 6 months of age and rapid and complete weaning thereafter.

Neonatal Care

Testing neonates for HIV infection is complicated by the fact that maternal HIV antibodies readily cross the placenta and may be found in the infant for up to 18 months after delivery. HIV infection can be definitively diagnosed through the use of DNA or RNA assays in most infected infants by 1 month of age and in virtually all by 6 months of age. Neonates are considered HIV-infected if two separate blood specimens test positive by polymerase chain reaction (PCR) or viral culture. Ideally, PCR testing should be performed in the neonate within 48 hours of birth, at age 1 to 2 months, and at age 3 to 6 months.

Other Health Issues

Age-appropriate screening and interventions for non-HIV–related conditions, including breast cancer, menopause, osteoporosis, domestic violence, cigarette smoking, and depression, should be performed in HIV-infected women.

Contraceptive counseling in HIV-infected women should include recommendation of a barrier method (male or female condom) to decrease the risk of transmission. Additional methods of contraception should be encouraged to decrease further the risk of an undesired pregnancy. Oral contraceptives may be difficult to give with some nonnucleoside reverse-transcriptase inhibitors and protease inhibitors because of drug interactions. Intrauterine devices have not been recommended in HIV-infected women because of concerns about PID. The use of vaginal spermicidal microbicides such as nonoxynyl-9 is discouraged because they can cause mucosal inflammation, which may increase the risk of HIV transmission.

KEY POINTS

- The number of HIV-infected women in the United States is increasing, and psychosocial and economic barriers to care sometimes complicate their management.
- Correcting for differences in access to and utilization of health care, it does not appear that gender significantly affects the course of HIV disease.
- Cervical dysplasia and cancer are more common in patients with HIV disease and warrant regular Pap smear screening and referral to a gynecologist if any abnormality is found.
- All pregnant women and women considering pregnancy should be encouraged to have HIV antibody testing.
- Antiretroviral therapy is recommended in all HIV-infected pregnant women who plan to carry the fetus to term with the goal of achieving virologic suppression. Perinatal transmission is rare if the viral load is maintained below 1000 copies/mL.
- Elective cesarean delivery may further reduce this risk in HIV-infected women with a viral load > 1000 copies/mL. Breast feeding of neonates is contraindicated except in settings where alternative nutrition is not available.

SUGGESTED WEB SITES

www.aidsinfo.nih.gov. Public Health Service task force recommendations for the use of antiretroviral drugs in pregnant HIV-1 infected women for maternal health and interventions to reduce perinatal HIV-1 transmission in the United States

www.apregistry.com. A national registry for antiretroviral therapy in pregnancy.

SUGGESTED READINGS

Chirenje ZM. HIV and cancer of the cervix. Best Pract Res Clin Obstet Gynaecol. 2005; 19:269-76.

Irwin KL, Moorman AC, O'Sullivan MJ, Sperling R, Koestler ME, Soto I, et al. Influence of human immunodeficiency virus infection on pelvic inflammatory disease. Obstet Gynecol. 2000;95:525-34.

Khoury M, Kovacs A. Pediatric HIV infection. Clin Obstet Gynecol. 2001;44:243-75.

Korn AP. Gynecologic care of women infected with HIV. Clin Obstet Gynecol. 2001;44: 226-42.

Levine AM. Evaluation and management of HIV-infected women. Ann Intern Med. 2002; 136:228-42.

McIntyre J. Preventing mother-to-child transmission of HIV: successes and challenges. BJOG. 2005;112:1196-203.

Moodley J, Wennberg JL. HIV in pregnancy. Curr Opin Obstet Gynecol. 2005;17:117-21.

Prins M, Meyer L, Hessol NA. Sex and the course of HIV infection in the pre- and highly active antiretroviral therapy eras. AIDS. 2005;19:357-70.

Quinn TC, Overbaugh J. HIV/AIDS in women: an expanding epidemic. Science. 2005;308:1582-3.

Sebitloane MH. HIV and gynaecological infections. Best Pract Res Clin Obstet Gynaecol. 2005;19:231-41.

Shetty AK. Perinatally acquired HIV-1 infection: prevention and evaluation of HIV-exposed infants. Semin Pediatr Infect Dis. 2005;16:282-95.

Star J, Powrie R, Cu-Uvin S, Carpenter CC. Should women with human immunodeficiency virus be delivered by cesarean? Obstet Gynecol. 1999;94:799-801.

Sterling TR, Vlahov D, Astemborski J, Hoover DR, Margolick JB, Quinn TC. Initial plasma HIV-1 RNA levels and progression to AIDS in women and men. N Engl J Med. 2001;344:720-5.

Thorne C, Newell ML. The safety of antiretroviral drugs in pregnancy. Expert Opin Drug Saf. 2005;4:323-35.

II. MEN WHO HAVE SEX WITH MEN

BENJAMIN DAVIS

Epidemiology

Men who have sex with men (MSM) continue to account for the largest percentage (63% in 2003) of new HIV infections in the United States. The HIV seroincidence in MSM is estimated to be 1.55 per 100 person-years. However, this burden disproportionately affects communities of color: 50% of newly diagnosed HIV-infected MSM are African-American, 32% are white, and 16% are Hispanic. This disparity is even more pronounced for young MSM. There is geographic variability as well, with HIV incidence rates as high as 8% for MSM in Baltimore and as low as 1.2% for MSM in San Francisco.

Nearly 50% of MSM found to be HIV-infected in a recent nationwide surveillance project were unaware of their serostatus. This percentage was even higher for young MSM. For MSM with unrecognized infection, one half were believed to have contracted it within the last year. Also of note is that 50% of MSM who were unaware of their HIV serostatus reported unprotected anal intercourse, highlighting the urgent need for targeted education, counseling, and testing in this population.

Transmission

Several factors, including recreational drug use, concurrent sexually transmitted diseases (STDs), and lack of knowledge of HIV serostatus, contribute to the high rate of HIV transmission among MSM. Each offers unique opportunities as well as challenges for intervention.

Recreational Drug Use

Recreational drug use, particularly with methamphetamine, has been strongly associated with higher risk sexual behaviors and HIV transmission. Among MSM studied in San Francisco, 53% reported unprotected receptive anal intercourse, and the odds ratio for this behavior was increased two-fold in men who reported using methamphetamine. Among young MSM, the use of alcohol, cocaine, marijuana, and amyl nitrite also increased the risk for unprotected anal intercourse. Unfortunately, methamphetamine use, which is one of the fasting growing addictions in the United States, is notoriously difficult to treat.

Sexually Transmitted Diseases

Sexually transmitted diseases, particularly syphilis and herpes simplex infection, have been shown to increase the risk of HIV transmission and acquisition. Conversely, HIV infection may be associated with more extensive genital ulcer disease and increase the transmission of other STDs.

Alarming increases in STDs have been noted as of late in MSM. The majority of MSM diagnosed with early syphilis are HIV-infected. Of MSM diagnosed with active syphilis, one third present with primary infection with chancres on the penis in 71%, the anus in 22%, and the oropharynx in 8%; two thirds present with secondary syphilis. Of MSM diagnosed with gonorrhea, 59% have urethral infection, 34% rectal infection, and 7% oropharyngeal infection. Of MSM diagnosed with chlamydial infection, 48% have urethral involvement, 48% rectal involvement, and 4% pharyngeal involvement. One inference that may be drawn from these data is that over 60% of STDs in MSM result from oral-anal or oral-genital intercourse, as opposed to anal intercourse. This observation may explain the increasing rates of STDs for MSM who report consistent condom use with anal intercourse.

Another factor hampering the control of STDs is the presence of asymptomatic infections. In a screening study of asymptomatic MSM using nucleic acid amplification techniques for diagnosis, the rates of chlamydial infection by site were 7.9% rectal, 5.2% urethral, and 1.4% pharyngeal, and the rates of gonococcal infection were 6.9% rectal, 6% urethral, and 9.2% pharyngeal. Of note, more than half of chlamydial and gonorrheal infections were nonurethral and would not be detected if only urine specimens were tested. In addition, more than 70% of chlamydial infections would not be detected if men were screened only for gonorrheal infection. Recent outbreaks of a particularly virulent form of chlamydial infection, lymphogranuloma venereum (LGV), have been reported in MSM in Europe and the United States (see Chapter 9). Complications from LGV may include abscess formation, colonic strictures, and lymphedema.

Lack of Knowledge of HIV Serostatus

As noted above, nearly half MSM with HIV infection are unaware of their serostatus, and many are newly infected. Because seroconversion is associated with a high viral load, the risk of transmission during this stage of HIV infection is especially high. Some HIV-infected MSM, in an attempt to protect themselves, may resort to "serosorting," in which they choose to have unprotected sex only with other men who are HIV-infected. However, this activity places them at risk for other STDs and the acquisition of drug-resistant HIV.

Clinical Manifestations

In most respects, the clinical manifestations of HIV infection in MSM are similar to those in other populations. Three prominent exceptions to this rule are the increased prevalence of Kaposi's sarcoma (KS) (see Chapter 10), anal dysplasia/cancer (see Chapters 9 and 10), and skin and soft tissue infections caused by methicillin-resistant *Staphylococcus. aureus* (MRSA) (see Chapter 9). Each of these conditions is caused by pathogens that are prevalent in the gay community.

Kaposi's Sarcoma

Since the beginning of the AIDS epidemic, it has been recognized that KS is much more likely to be diagnosed in MSM compared with other at-risk populations. The development of this neoplasm is strongly linked to Kaposi's sarcoma herpesvirus (KSHV), also known as human herpesvirus-8 (HHV8), which infects up to 35% of HIV-seropositive MSM. Fortunately, the incidence of KS is declining in the United States, and the condition often responds promptly to the initiation of antiretroviral therapy.

Anal Dysplasia and Cancer

Anal dysplasia and cancer, like cervical dysplasia and cancer, are strongly linked to certain strains of human papillomavirus (HPV). Although rates of anal cancer have been increasing in both men and women over the past decade, the rate in MSM with or without HIV infection is dramatically higher (incidence of 35 cases per 100,000 compared with as low as 0.8 per 100,000 in the general population). HIV infection is thought to increase this incidence by at least two-fold. The prevalence of anal cancer does not decline over time as it does for cervical cancer. The most straightforward explanation for this distinction is that women generally acquire high-risk HPV strains as adolescents or young women, whereas MSM continue to acquire them throughout their sexually active lives.

Like cervical cancer, the prognosis of anal cancer is most strongly linked to its stage at diagnosis. Five-year survival rates may be as high as 78% for local disease and as low as 18% for metastatic disease. The most effective management for locally confined anal cancer is a combination of chemotherapy and radiation therapy. Surgery is reserved for relapsing disease.

Anal cancer is believed to go through similar stages of neoplastic transformation as cervical cancer, and an analogous cytologic grading system has been adopted. The sensitivity of anal Pap smears for detecting dysplasia is estimated between 69% and 93%, and the specificity ranges between 32% and 59%. Given the prevalence of dysplasia in MSM, this translates into a positive predictive value of 78% and a negative predictive value of 79%, which are comparable to those for detecting cervical dysplasia in women. Because the anal Pap smear is easy to perform and well tolerated, many practitioners have adopted it for annual screening in sexually active MSM with or without HIV infection, although it is not formally recommended by any organizations.

There is an important difference between anal and cervical neoplasia. Cervical dysplasia can be treated by loop excision of the entire transition zone. This approach has been shown convincingly to decrease the risk of subsequent cervical cancer. Because of anatomic and functional difference between the cervix and the anal canal, there is no directly analogous treatment for anal dysplastic lesions. Several approaches for managing anal dysplasia have been proposed, including electrocautery, infrared coagulation, and the topical application of imiquimod or 5-fluorouracil. Disappointingly, for some of these approaches, the persistence of dysplasia has been reported to be as high as 80%. The hope is that with more research and better treatments for premalignant lesions, anal cancer will begin to decline in incidence.

Methicillin-Resistant Staphylococcus aureus Infection

Community-acquired skin and soft tissue infections caused by MRSA have been increasingly described in recent years. Reports of MRSA infection in MSM began to emerge in 2003, and it has been estimated that their incidence has increased at least six-fold since 2000. Among HIV-infected patients, MRSA infection occurs more frequently in MSM and injection-drug users, and also in patients with a CD4 count below 50 cells/mm³. Risk factors for MRSA infection include having a sex partner with a skin infection, inconsistent condom use, and methamphetamine use. The use of trimethoprim-sulfamethoxazole (TMP-SMX) for opportunistic infection prophylaxis was found to protect against MRSA infection.

The virulence of community-acquired MRSA infection has been well documented. Patients may require hospital admission, treatment with intravenous vancomycin, and incision and drainage of abscesses. Isolates are typically resistant to erythromycin and often to quinolones, but they are frequently susceptible to TMP-SMX, clindamycin, linezolid, and vancomycin. Eradicating skin and nasal carriage of MRSA using topical mupirocin and antibacterial soaps may decrease the frequency of recurrent infections.

KEY POINTS

- Most HIV-infected patients in the United States are MSM, and most new HIV cases occur in MSM.
- African-American MSM are more likely to acquire HIV infection than white or Hispanic MSM but are less likely to be aware of their serostatus.
- Unprotected anal intercourse remains prevalent among HIV-infected MSM, especially in those who are unaware of their serostatus.
- Recreational drug use, particularly with methamphetamine, has been strongly linked to unsafe sexual practices in MSM.
- Other sexually transmitted diseases, such as syphilis and herpes simplex virus infection, are more common in HIV-infected MSM and increase the risk of HIV transmission.
- HIV-infected MSM are at a higher risk of KS, anal dysplasia and cancer, and skin and soft tissue infections caused by MRSA.

SUGGESTED READINGS

Bacon O, Lum P, Hahn J, Evans J, Davidson P, Moss A, et al. Commercial sex work and risk of HIV infection among young drug-injecting men who have sex with men in San Francisco. Sex Transm Dis. 2006;33:228-34.

Brewer DD, Golden MR, Handsfield HH. Unsafe sexual behavior and correlates of risk in a probability sample of men who have sex with men in the era of highly active anti-retroviral therapy. Sex Transm Dis. 2006;33:250-5.

Buchacz K, Greenberg A, Onorato I, Janssen R. Syphilis epidemics and human immunodeficiency virus (HIV) incidence among men who have sex with men in the United States: implications for HIV prevention. Sex Transm Dis. 2005;32:S73-9.

Buchbinder SP, Vittinghoff E, Heagerty PJ, Celum CL, Seage GR 3rd, Judson FN, et al. Sexual risk, nitrite inhalant use, and lack of circumcision associated with HIV seroconversion in men who have sex with men in the United States. J Acquir Immune Defic Syndr. 2005;39:82-9.

Celentano DD, Sifakis F, Hylton J, Torian LV, Guillin V, Koblin BA. Race/ethnic differences in HIV prevalence and risks among adolescent and young adult men who have sex with men. J Urban Health. 2005;82:610-21.

Celentano DD, Valleroy LA, Sifakis F, et al. Associations between substance use and sexual risk among very young men who have sex with men. Sex Transm Dis. 2006;33:265-271.

Centers for Disease Control and Prevention. HIV prevalence, unrecognized infection, and HIV testing among men who have sex with men—five U.S. cities, June 2004-April 2005. MMWR. 2005;54:597-601.

Centers for Disease Control and Prevention. Methamphetamine use and HIV risk behaviors among heterosexual men—preliminary results from five northern California counties, December 2001-November 2003. MMWR. 2006;55:273-7.

Chiao EY, Giordano TP, Palefsky JM, Tyring S, El Serag H. Screening HIV-infected individuals for anal cancer precursor lesions: a systematic review. Clin Infect Dis. 2006;43:223-33.

Chin-Hong PV, Vittinghoff E, Cranston RD, Browne L, Buchbinder S, Colfax G, et al. Age-related prevalence of anal cancer precursors in homosexual men: the EXPLORE study. J Natl Cancer Inst. 2005;97:896-905.

Colfax G, Coates TJ, Husnik MJ, et al. Longitudinal patterns of methamphetamine, popper (amyl nitrite), and cocaine use and high-risk sexual behavior among a cohort of San Francisco men who have sex with men. J Urban Health. 2005;82:62-70.

Kent CK, Chaw JK, Wong W, Liska S, Gibson S, Hubbard G, et al. Prevalence of rectal, urethral, and pharyngeal chlamydia and gonorrhea detected in 2 clinical settings among men who have sex with men: San Francisco, California, 2003. Clin Infect Dis. 2005;41: 67-74.

Lee NE, Taylor MM, Bancroft E, Ruane PJ, Morgan M, McCoy L, et al. Risk factors for community-associated methicillin-resistant *Staphylococcus aureus* skin infections among HIV-positive men who have sex with men. Clin Infect Dis. 2005;40:1529-34.

Mansergh G, Shouse RL, Marks G, Guzman R, Rader M, Buchbinder S, et al. Methamphetamine and sildenafil (Viagra) use are linked to unprotected receptive and insertive anal sex, respectively, in a sample of men who have sex with men. Sex Transm Infect. 2006; 82:131-4.

Mathews WC, Caperna JC, Barber RE, Torriani FJ, Miller LG, May S, et al. Incidence of and risk factors for clinically significant methicillin-resistant Staphylococcus aureus infection in a cohort of HIV-infected adults. J Acquir Immune Defic Syndr. 2005;40:155-60.

MSM-STD-Sentinel Network. Understanding recent increases in the incidence of sexually transmitted infections in men having sex with men: changes in risk behavior from risk avoidance to risk reduction. Sex Transm Dis. 2006;33:11-7.

Young Men's Survey Study Group. Unrecognized HIV infection, risk behaviors, and perceptions of risk among young men who have sex with men: opportunities for advancing HIV prevention in the third decade of HIV/AIDS. J Acquir Immune Defic Syndr. 2005;38:603-14.

III. African Americans

ERIC P. GOOSBY

Epidemiology and Transmission

African Americans in the United States are disproportionately affected by the AIDS epidemic. In 2002, HIV infection was among the top three causes of death in African American men aged 25 to 54 and among the top four causes of death in African American women aged 25 to 54. For African American women aged 25 to 34, it was the leading cause of mortality.

African Americans comprise 13% of the United States population but account for about 50% of new cases of HIV infection and 51% of AIDS-related deaths. Of 145 perinatally HIV-infected infants in the United States in 2004, 105 (73%) were African American, and 63% of children younger than 13 years of age with a new diagnosis of AIDS were African American.

In 2004, the primary mode of HIV transmission in African American men was unprotected sex with other men, followed by heterosexual contact and injection-drug use. In African American women, the primary mode of transmission was heterosexual contact followed by injection-drug use. There is no proven biologic predisposition to HIV infection among African Americans, but there are a number of behavioral and social factors that place them at increased risk for the virus.

Coinfection with sexually transmitted diseases (STDs) has been shown to increase rates of HIV transmission and acquisition. In 2004, STD incidence rates were consistently higher for African Americans than whites: 18.9 times higher for gonorrhea, 15.7 times higher for congenital syphilis, 8.4 times higher for chlamydial infection, and 5.6 times higher for primary and secondary syphilis. Seventy percent of gonorrhea cases and 41% of primary and secondary syphilis cases were among African Americans.

African American women are often not aware of their partner's risks for HIV infection and therefore may not consider themselves at risk. Males who have unprotected sexual contact with multiple partners, are bisexual, or have a history of injection-drug use generally do not discuss this information with their female partners. Thirty-four percent of African American men who have sex with men also reported having sex with women, although only 6% of African American women reported having had sex with a bisexual man. In a study examining sexual practices in African American men who have sex with men, 46% were HIV-infected compared with 21% of whites and 17% of Hispanics. Furthermore, 64% of the African American men, 18% of the Hispanic men, 11% of the white men, and 6% of multiracial/other men were unaware of their HIV serostatus.

The lower socioeconomic status of some African Americans has had a negative effect on their ability to access quality health care. In patients with a diagnosis of AIDS made before 1996, a smaller proportion of African Americans (64%) were alive after ten years compared with American Indians and Alaskan Natives (65%), Hispanics (72%), whites (74%), and Asian and Pacific islanders (81%).

African Americans are twice as likely as whites to have used injection drugs, and HIV infection is more common among African American than white drug users. Twenty-eight percent of African American men will be imprisoned sometime during their life. The "revolving door" experience of entering prison, participating in high-risk behaviors, and returning to the community is an important contributor to the dissemination of HIV infection, other STDs, and viral hepatitis into the African American community.

Management Considerations

There are no proven differences in the natural history of HIV infection among African Americans compared with other populations when corrected for nutritional status, medical comorbidity, and access to and utilization of health care. Anecdotal racial differences in pharmacokinetics, drug toxicity, and drug interactions have not been adequately studied. Standard management recommendations should be followed for all patients, regardless of their race. However, sexually transmitted diseases, viral hepatitis (see Chapter 9), tuberculosis (TB) (see Chapter 9), and lipodystrophy syndrome (see Chapter 6), all of which are more common among African Americans, may pose special problems in this population.

Viral Hepatitis

African Americans are at increased risk for hepatitis B and C virus (HBV and HCV) infections, both of which can be transmitted by injection-drug use. The National Medical Association analyzed 46 published studies on the relationship between ethnicity and viral hepatitis. They concluded that the HBV infection rate is four times higher in African Americans compared with white adolescents. They also reported that there is a higher rate of chronic HBV infection in African Americans compared with whites. African Americans who received blood products before 1992 (when the HCV antibody test first became available) for sickle cell disease are at increased risk for HCV infection. More than 3 million African Americans are in occupations, such as health care, emergency services, and custodial services, which may increase their exposure to HBV and HCV.

Tuberculosis

In 2003, African Americans accounted for 28% of new TB cases in the United States, representing 44% of affected persons born in this country and 13% of affected foreign-born persons. The TB case rate among African Americans (11.5/100000) was more than eight times that of whites (1.4/100000). HIV infection has served to enhance the spread of TB in the African American community.

Lipodystrophy Syndrome

Because of the high frequency of diabetes mellitus, obesity, and hyperlipidemia in African American patients, it is important to monitor the effect of antiretroviral therapy on glucose and lipid metabolism. Overall, African Americans are 1.8 times more likely than whites to have diabetes mellitus. Thirteen percent of African Americans 20 years of age and older have diabetes mellitus, and one-third of them are undiagnosed. The National Health and Nutrition Examination Survey III reported that 45% of African American men and 46% of African American women have total cholesterol levels greater than 200 mg/dl. In addition, 15% of African American men and 18% of African American women have total cholesterol levels greater than 240 mg/dl. These multiple cardiac risk factors are likely responsible for the increased morbidity and mortality from coronary artery disease reported in the African American population.

Family, Community, and Church

The African American community depends on family and religious institutions as important sources of support. However, creating an environment in which the individual feels comfortable discussing behaviors (e.g., homosexuality, injection-drug use) not accepted by the community has been a challenge. The stigma associated with these behaviors may prevent persons at risk for or infected with HIV from accessing health care. However, in recent years, some African American churches, often in partnership with local and national government agencies, have taken an active role in addressing the devastating impact that HIV infection has had on their communities. Church-based organizations have established HIV counseling and testing programs, social support services, and home-based care services. Medication adherence support has also been made available through grassroots organizations and churches in the African American community.

KEY POINTS

- African Americans in the United States are disproportionately affected by the AIDS epidemic. It is the leading cause of mortality for African American women aged 25 to 34 years.
- There are no proven differences in the natural history of HIV infection among African Americans compared with other populations when corrected for nutritional status, medical comorbidity, and access to, and utilization of, health care.
- Sexually transmitted diseases, viral hepatitis, tuberculosis, and lipodystrophy syndrome, all of which are more common among African Americans, may pose special problems in this population.
- In recent years, African American churches, often in partnership with local and national government agencies, have taken an active role in addressing the devastating impact that HIV infection has had on their communities.

SUGGESTED READINGS

Asher CR, Topol EJ, Moliterno DJ. Insights into the pathophysiology of atherosclerosis and prognosis of black Americans with acute coronary syndromes. Am Heart J. 1999;138: 1073-81.

Backus LI, Boothroyd D, Deyton LR. HIV, hepatitis C, and HIV/HCV co-infection in vulnerable populations. AIDS. 2005;19 Suppl 3:S13-19.

Bangsberg DR, Hecht FM, Charlebois ED, Zolopa AR, Holodniy M, Sheiner L, et al. Adherence to protease inhibitors, HIV-1 viral load, and development of drug resistance in an indigent population. AIDS. 2000;14:357-66.

Cowie CC, Port FK, Wolfe RA, Savage PJ, Moll PP, Hawthorne VM. Disparities in incidence of diabetic end-stage renal disease according to race and type of diabetes. N Engl J Med. 1989;321:1074-9.

Ferdinand KC. Coronary heart disease and lipid-modifying treatment in African American patients. Am Heart J. 2004;147:774-82.

Fleming DT, Wasserheit JN. From epidemiological synergy to public health policy and practice: the contribution of other STDs to sexual transmission of HIV infection. Sex Transm Infect. 1999;75:3-17.

Funnyé AS, Ganesan K, Yoshikawa TT. Tuberculosis in African Americans: clinical characteristics and outcome. J Natl Med Assoc. 1998;90:73-6.

Harris MI, Klein R, Cowie CC, Rowland M, Byrd-Holt DD. Is the risk of diabetic retinopathy greater in non-Hispanic blacks and Mexican Americans than in non-Hispanic whites with type 2 diabetes? A U.S. population study. Diabetes Care. 1998;21:1230-5.

Leigh BC, Stall R. Substance use and risky sexual behavior for exposure to HIV. Issues in methodology, interpretation, and prevention. Am Psychol. 1993;48:1035-45.

Millett G, Malebranche D, Mason B, Spikes P. Focusing "down-low:" bisexual black men, HIV risk and heterosexual transmission. J Natl Med Assoc. 2005:97:52S-59S.

Montgomery J, Mokotoff ED, Gentry AC, Blair JM. The extent of bisexual behavior in HIV-infected men and implications for transmission to their female sex partners. AIDS Care. 2003;15:82-837.

Roberts KJ. Physician-patient relationship, patient satisfaction and ARV medication adherence among HIV-infected adults attending a public health clinic. AIDS Patient Care STDS. 2002:16:43-50.

Sanders EC 2nd. New insights and interventions: churches uniting to reach the African American community with health information. J Health Care Poor Underserved. 1997;8: 373-5; discussion 375-6.

Stone VE. Strategies for optimizing adherence to highly active antiretroviral therapy: lessons from research and clinical practice. Clin Infect Dis. 2001;33:865-72.

IV. TRANSGENDER PERSONS

GREGORY FENTON

Transgender persons often receive suboptimal medical and mental health care. The reasons for this observation are many and include insensitivity by clinicians, lack of trust, cost of health care, fear of exposure, and stigma. Unfortunately, data on HIV-infected transgender patients are limited. Primary care providers are uniquely situated to make a positive difference in the life of a transgender person in providing direct care or serving as an important link to specialty services. This section provides an overview of health care for transgender persons and presents management strategies for those who are HIV-infected.

Violence is common in transgender populations, and depression and suicide rates are also high. Transgender youth are especially at risk, given the frequency of homelessness, lack of marketable job skills, sexual behaviors, and substance use. They may be more inclined to use hormones and silicone from the street, placing them at increased risk for infections and other medical conditions. HIV infection is yet another risk that these youth face.

Terminology

In order to provide care for a transgender person, it is important to understand the relevant terms. Sexual orientation and gender identity are different. Sexual orientation refers to one's feelings about self related to physical attraction towards others. It can exist along a continuum. Terms that are used to describe sexual orientation include gay, lesbian, bisexual, and straight. Gender identity refers to one's sexual self-perception. Transgender is another variant of gender identity. For transgender persons, their genetic sex may not coincide with their gender identity. It can be thought of as being an umbrella term that encompasses transsexuals, cross-dressers, and others. Additional lay terms include MTF (male to female), FTM (female to male), transman, transwoman, transperson, two-spirit, boi, bi-gendered, gender bender, and person of transexperience. These descriptions may change over time for a given individual.

Epidemiology

Transgender persons, particularly MTFs of color, are thought to be at high risk for HIV infection. Studies indicate a seroprevalence rate in the MTF population of between 14% and 47%, and it may be as high as 68% for those involved in sex work. Sexual practices and needle-sharing (e.g., hormone therapy, silicon injection, substance use) are believed to be major risk behaviors in this population; social stigma and marginalization may be contributing factors as well. For FTMs, the seroprevalence rate is between 2% and 3%. In one study, it was found that FTMs were less likely to use condoms the last time they had sex but were more likely than MTFs to have engaged in recent high-risk sexual activity.

Management Considerations

Primary care providers have an important responsibility in preventing morbidity and mortality in this population. The initial task is to gain the trust of a transperson and engage the individual in care. Trust can be enhanced by making sure that patients feel welcomed. Specific measures may include providing intake forms with appropriate gender choices, conveying a clear message that confidentiality is respected, and being careful of assumptions about people regarding their gender and sexuality. Reflections of inclusiveness can be as simple as providing transperson-sensitive pamphlets or displaying posters. Unisex bathrooms can go a long way in making everyone feel more comfortable. All patients should be asked by what salutation and name they would like to be addressed. It is critical that all staff members be trained in culturally competent care.

Once a transperson is engaged, the clinician can refer to protocols that have been established for medical care. The Harry Benjamin International Gender Dysphoria Association, Dr. Sheila Kirk, Tom Waddel Clinic, and others have contributed to this literature. At the core of these protocols is an assessment of the psychosocial issues, including mental health and social supports, with which a transgender person presents. The next step involves a physical assessment. The breasts, prostate, and ovaries warrant careful attention because of an increased risk of cancer associated with hormonal therapies. For patients in whom estrogens may be prescribed, the pretreatment laboratory evaluation should consist of a complete blood count, fasting glucose, liver function tests, free testosterone level, and prolactin level. For patients in whom androgens may be prescribed, the pretreatment laboratory evaluation should consist of a complete blood count, liver function tests, and fasting lipid profile.

Once the psychosocial, physical, and laboratory data are compiled, the next step is consideration of medical and/or surgical interventions to achieve physical change. For many patients, hormone therapies or hormone blockers are an important component of the medical intervention.

Estrogen therapy is the preferred approach for MTFs and can be administered orally or by skin patch or injection; anti-androgens such as spironolactone are also often used. Physical changes, which may take months to a few years to occur, include increased breast size, softer skin, and testicular atrophy. A provider may encounter patients who want quicker and more pronounced physical changes, but these requests should be discouraged because of the increased risk of toxicity, including thromboembolic disease and cancer, from higher dose estrogens. Some physical changes, such as infertility, may be irreversible. Liver function tests and prolactin levels should be monitored in patients on estrogen therapy. Surgical procedures for MTFs include orchiectomy, vaginoplasty, breast augmentation, tracheal shave, and face reconstruction.

For FTMs, testosterone therapy, which can be administered by injection or skin gel or patch, is generally preferred. Physical changes may include a deepening voice, increased strength and lean muscle mass, facial hair, and loss of menses. Temporal balding may also occur in some patients. Changes in voice and hair distribution may be permanent, and some patients may experience polycystic ovaries, vaginal atrophy, and acne vulgaris. If vaginal spotting or bleeding occurs after menses has stopped, further evaluation, including pelvic ultrasound and endometrial biopsy, may be warranted. A complete blood count, fasting lipid profile, and liver function tests should be monitored in patients on testosterone therapy. Surgical procedures for FTMs include hysterectomy, oophorectomy, and breast reduction.

As transgender persons age, they may be at increased risk from chronic medical conditions. For instance, hypertension and a hypercoagulable state from estrogen therapy may predispose to coronary artery and thromboembolic diseases, respectively. Hyperlipidemia associated with testosterone therapy may also increase the likelihood of coronary artery disease. Despite these concerns, a retrospective analysis of MTFs and FTMs who were on treatment for many years showed that the interventions were generally safe. MTFs did have some increased risk of thromboembolic disease, but FTMs experienced no significant morbidity. The mortality in both groups was the same as in the general population.

Clinicians should be cognizant of potential drug interactions in HIV-infected transgender patients on hormone therapy. Many drugs, including antiretroviral agents and estrogens, are metabolized via the cytochrome p450 enzyme system in the liver. Protease inhibitors (PIs) generally inhibit this system, but some can induce it. For example, ritonavir has the greatest inhibitory effort, while tipranavir is an inducer. Some nonnucleoside reverse-transcriptase inhibitors (NNRTIs) can inhibit these enzymes, and others induce them. Specifically, indinavir (PI), atazanavir (PI), and efavirenz (NNRTI) can potentially increase estrogen levels, whereas nelfinavir (PI), lopinavir/ritonavir (PI), and nevirapine (NNRTI) may decrease them. It should also be noted that hormone therapy may sometimes affect antiretroviral drug levels.

KEY POINTS

- Transgender patients experience significant health disparities that are even more problematic if they are HIV-infected.
- Transgender persons, particularly MTFs of color, are thought to be at high risk for HIV infection.
- An awareness of transgender-specific medical, mental health, and psychosocial issues is important for their optimal care.
- Primary care providers can refer to protocols from The Harry Benjamin International Gender Dysphoria Association and other organizations on the medical care of transgender persons.
- Clinicians should be aware of potential interactions between antiretroviral drugs and hormonal therapies in the management of HIV-infected transgender patients.

SUGGESTED READINGS

Bockting W, Kirk S, eds. Transgender and HIV: Risks, Prevention, and Care. Binghamton, NY: Haworth Press; 2001.

Clements-Nolle K, Marx R, Guzman R, et al. HIV prevalence, risk behaviors, health care use, and mental health status of transgender persons in San Francisco: implications for public health intervention. Am J Public Health. 2001;91:915-21.

Elifson KW, Boles J, Posey E, et al. Male transvestite prostitutes and HIV risk. Am J Public Health. 1993;83:260-2.

Feldman J, Bockting W. Transgender health. Minn Med. 2003;86:25-32.

Harry Benjamin International Gender Dysphoria Association (Standards of care, 6th version). 2001. http://www.hbigda.org/soc.htm.

Kenagy GP, Hsieh CM. The risk less known: female-to-male transgender persons' vulnerability to HIV infection. AIDS Care. 2005;17:195-207.

Moore E, Wisniewski A, Dobs A. Endocrine treatment of transsexual people: a review of treatment regimens, outcomes, and adverse effects. J Clin Endocrinol Metab. 2003;88:3467-73.

National Coalition of Anti-Violence Programs. Anti-Lesbian, Gay, Bisexual, and Transgender Violence in 2004.

Nemoto T, Sausa LA, Operario D, Keatley J. Need for HIV/AIDS education and intervention for MTF transgenders: responding to the challenge. J Homosex. 2006;51:183-202.

Protocols for Hormonal Reassignment of Gender from the Tom Waddell Health Center, 2001.

Simon PA, Reback CJ, Bemis CC. HIV prevalence and incidence among male-to-female transsexuals receiving HIV prevention services in Los Angeles County [Letter]. AIDS. 2000;14:2953-5.

van Kesteren PJ, Asscheman H, Megens JA, Gooren LJ. Mortality and morbidity in transsexual subjects treated with cross-sex hormones. Clin Endocrinol. 1997;47:337-42.

Xavier J. Final Report of the Washington Transgender Needs Assessment Survey, Washington, DC; 2000.

V. Injection-Drug Users

JEFFREY H. SAMET

HIV-infected injection-drug users (IDUs) present many challenges to the clinician. In addition to managing HIV infection and its consequences, the primary care provider often needs to address coinfection with hepatitis C virus (HCV), chronic pain management, high-risk drug use and sexual behaviors, mental health disorders, and social problems. Cocaine, methamphetamine, alcohol, and benzodiazepine abuse, which are common in IDUs, may also require attention.

Epidemiology

Injection-drug use has been identified as a risk behavior in 34% of AIDS patients in the United States through 2003. In men, it accounts for 32% of cases, and in women, it accounts for 41% of cases. Additional women are at risk through sexual contact with IDUs. Worldwide, injection-drug use as mode of transmission for HIV infection has been reported in over 100 countries. Eighty percent to 90% of HIV cases in Russia and 44% in China are in IDUs in contrast to only 5% of cases in Australia. The difference in HIV seroprevalence rates among IDUs is attributable to the local nature of drug use, the level of awareness of HIV risk in the population, and the availability of prevention programs. In the United States, HIV seroprevalence among IDUs entering drug treatment centers varies by region, with New York City reporting a 20% to 30% rate and Los Angeles reporting about a 1% rate. Injection-drug use accounts for two to three times the proportion of AIDS cases among African Americans and Hispanics than among whites.

Behavioral Aspects

Use of injection drugs may involve heroin (which is an opioid agonist), cocaine combined with heroin ("speed-balling"), cocaine alone, or more recently, methamphetamine. Heroin is typically used 4 to 6 times a day in a dependent individual to prevent withdrawal symptoms. Cocaine use is more variable but may be as frequent as 10 to 20 times a day in a binge pattern. The onset of action of intravenous cocaine is almost instantaneous, peaking in minutes and leaving the individual with intense craving for more drug within an hour of its use. Methamphetamine has a more prolonged half-life, resulting in its use two to three times a day until there is physical exhaustion or lack of availability of the drug. Withdrawal symptoms of opioids, cocaine, and methamphetamine are listed in Box 11-3. Noninjection use of heroin commonly progresses to injection use within one year. In addition, noninjection heroin, cocaine, and methamphetamine use may be associated with medical complications, risky sexual behaviors, and social impairment. Alcohol and benzodiazepines are other substances that are commonly abused by IDUs.

Addressing both drug- and sex-related high-risk behaviors for the transmission of HIV infection is important in IDUs. It is estimated that one third to one half of IDUs share needles and that over one half have unsafe sex. However, behavior change is possible among IDUs, and efforts should be made to address the need for consistent condom and sterile needle use (see Boxes 2-2 and 2-3 in Chapter 2). Drug treatment and abstinence represent the optimal outcomes with regard to substance abuse, but these goals are often achieved incrementally. In many communities, one important element has been the implementation of needle-exchange programs (NEPs), which has been documented to decrease HIV transmission among IDUs. Patients should be made aware of the locations, hours, and rules of local NEPs

---

Box 11-3.   Withdrawal Syndromes for Opioids, Cocaine, and Methamphetamine

Opioid Withdrawal

Vital signs	Tachycardia, hypertension, fever
Central nervous system	Craving, restlessness, insomnia, muscle cramps, yawning, miosis
Eyes, nose	Lacrimation, rhinorrhea
Skin	Perspiration, piloerection
Gastrointestinal	Nausea, vomiting, diarrhea

Cocaine/Methamphetamine Withdrawal

Crash	Depression, fatigue
Withdrawal	Anxiety, high craving
Extinction	Normalization of mood, episodic craving

From O'Connor PG, Samet JH, Stein MD. Management of hospitalized intravenous drug users: role of the internist. Am J Med. 1994;96:551-8; with permission.

and of the means for obtaining clean needles in states where it is legal. Addressing alcohol use as a means of decreasing high-risk behaviors in IDUs is also important.

HIV Antibody Testing

Screening IDUs for HIV infection is essential given its high prevalence in this population. HIV-infected persons often present for medical care years after contracting the infection. The optimal frequency of HIV antibody testing in IDUs is not well defined, but, among individuals engaging in high-risk behaviors, every 6 to 12 months appears reasonable. Learning of a positive HIV antibody test may be a trigger for relapse to drug use, but it has also been associated with recovery among active users. HIV antibody testing in a hospitalized IDU may represent a unique opportunity to engage the patient who does not receive regular medical care. Utilizing rapid testing techniques or establishing a protocol in which HIV antibody test results can be easily obtained after hospitalization is important.

Addressing Drug Abuse in Clinical Practice

Caring for a patient who uses injection drugs requires the clinician to address the issue of substance abuse on a regular basis. The primary care provider should explore the adverse consequences of drug and alcohol use on personal health, family, work, and social relationships. This history, together with an assessment of whether loss of control occurs when using the drug and whether symptoms of withdrawal occur when it is not used, enables the categorization of drug abuse or dependence (Table 11-1). Once the diagnosis is clear, determining the patient's perception of his or her drug or alcohol use and the need and perceived ability to change behavior should be assessed (Example: "Do you think that your drug use is a problem?").

This assessment allows the clinician to tailor the approach to the patient as opposed to either ignoring the substance abuse issue or just saying, "Stop using drugs." For example, an IDU who has no interest in ceasing heroin use may be receptive to the message not to share "works" (injection paraphernalia) and receiving information about NEPs. The IDU can also be counseled that, if sharing of needles occurs, they should be disinfected in bleach (flushed first with clean water, then soaked for at least one minute in full-strength bleach, followed by another thorough rinse with water), although this practice is not as safe as using sterile paraphernalia.

The individual who has decided to seek substance abuse treatment may want to learn what options are available. A patient struggling in recovery may benefit from practical advice about avoiding situations that have led to relapse in the past. A person in stable recovery can receive supportive

Table 11-1.   Diagnostic Criteria for Drug Abuse and Dependence

Abuse (≥1 Needed for 12 Months)	*Dependence (≥3 Needed)*
1. Recurrent substance use resulting in failure to fulfill major role obligations at work, school, or home	1. Tolerance
	2. Withdrawal
2. Recurrent substance use in situations in which it is physically hazardous	3. Substance often taken in larger amounts over a longer period than intended
3. Recurrent legal problems related to substance use	4. Any unsuccessful effort or a persistent desire to cut down or control substance use
4. Continued substance use despite having persistent or recurrent social or interpersonal problems caused or exacerbated by the effects of the substance	5. Much time spent in activities necessary to obtain the substance or recover from its effects
	6. Important social, occupational, or recreational activities given up or reduced because of substance use
and	7. Continued substance use despite knowledge of having had persistent or recurrent physical or psychological problems that are likely to be caused or exacerbated by the substance
Never having met criteria for dependence	

recognition of the substantial effort required to maintain it. Such an approach will help engage and maintain the patient in medical care.

When considering treatment options for a heroin-dependent patient, both nonpharmacologic and pharmacologic approaches are possible. If a nonpharmacologic approach is chosen, substance abuse care after detoxification typically involves individual, family, and/or group counseling. In addition, participation in a self-help group such as Narcotics or Alcoholics Anonymous (NA or AA) can be an important support. While effective pharmacologic approaches exist for opioid dependence, none has been demonstrated for cocaine or metamphetamine dependence.

Opioid substitution therapy is the standard of care for heroin dependence. It is based on the principle of substituting a long-acting, orally effective opioid for shorter-acting opioids. Methadone, the major drug used in this therapeutic approach, has been shown to relieve symptoms of heroin withdrawal. With proper dosing, typically in the 60 to 100 mg/day range, craving for heroin abates, and the effects of heroin use are blocked. Since its introduction in the 1960s, methadone maintenance has almost exclusively been restricted to narcotic treatment programs approved by federal agencies that provide methadone, counseling, medical evaluation, and urine toxicology screening.

Buprenorphine, a partial opioid agonist/antagonist, is a relatively new drug with proven efficacy in the treatment of opioid dependence. Its increasing use for maintenance therapy allows patients to receive both HIV and addiction care in the same medical setting from clinicians who have received appropriate training. Patients without significant psychiatric disease, alcoholism, and other drug dependence are the optimal candidates for this approach. Counseling and urine toxicology screening are important components of care.

Management Considerations

Antiretroviral Therapy

The indications for antiretroviral therapy in HIV-infected IDUs are the same as those in other patients. The rate of clinical and immunologic progression of HIV disease in IDUs appears comparable to that of nondrug users. The IDU in recovery, with or without pharmacologic support (e.g., methadone or buprenorphine), should be considered for antiretroviral therapy in the same manner as a patient without this history. The decision whether to start antiretroviral therapy in the active drug user should be individualized based upon the following considerations:

1. Optimal adherence with initial regimens offers the best chance of avoiding the development of resistant virus.
2. Maximal likelihood of viral suppression is achieved by 95% medication adherence.
3. Active drug users have worse adherence than those in recovery from drug use or those without a drug use history.
4. Most deaths from HIV infection do not occur until the CD4 count falls below 50 copies/mm^3.

For example, these facts may lead the clinician to delay recommending antiretroviral therapy to an active IDU with a CD4 count of 250 cells/mm^3 and viral load of 30,000 copies/mL. This same person, however, with a CD4 count of 50 cells/mm^3 may not be able to wait until optimal adherence can be achieved.

The interaction of methadone with antiretroviral drugs can have important clinical implications. The most notable drug interactions involve those medications that induce hepatic metabolism via the cytochrome p450 pathway. In particular, the use of efavirenz and nevirapine may require increased methadone dosing. No specific formula exists for these modifications, but one should be cognizant of the need to monitor for symptoms and signs of opioid withdrawal as dose adjustments are made. Interactions of antiretroviral drugs with buprenorphine are less clearly delineated.

Hepatitis C Infection

A large majority of HIV-infected IDUs are also infected with HCV (see Chapter 9). It is clear that coinfected patients have a more rapid progression to cirrhosis, and morbidity from hepatic disease attributable to HCV has become more common since the advent of effective antiretroviral therapy. The decision whether to treat HCV infection in the HIV-infected IDU is complicated. Factors to consider include the effectiveness and tolerability of pegylated interferon in combination with ribavirin, the patient's commitment to such a regimen, and the potential for reinfection after treatment with relapsing drug use. Expert consultation is recommended for clinicians with limited experience in the management of chronic viral hepatitis.

Pain Control

The issue of pain control often arises in the care of HIV-infected IDUs. Pain in these patients can be of an acute or chronic nature. Acute severe pain with a clear underlying etiology, such as shingles or a documented injury, pre-sents little therapeutic dilemma. Narcotic medications may be required and should be given if the patient does not decline treatment for fear of relapse to drug use. In this case, the dose of the opioid will often be higher and the medication administered more frequently if the patient is physiologically tolerant to it as a result of his or her drug use or treatment with methadone or buprenorphine.

Management of chronic pain or acute pain without a clear etiology requires a careful history and physical examination, the use of nonnarcotic analgesics if possible, circumspection about prescribing narcotic analgesics, and setting reasonable expectations regarding their use and the likelihood of treatment success. The dual agenda of treating a patient's pain while not facilitating addictive use of prescription medications is challenging. Nonetheless, when a decision is made to use narcotic drugs for chronic pain management, establishing an unambiguous written agreement ("contracting") may help minimize its potential pitfalls.

KEY POINTS

- Thirty-four percent of AIDS cases in the United States have been associated with injection-drug use.
- Among IDUs engaging in high-risk behaviors, HIV antibody testing at 6 to 12 month intervals is recommended.
- The clinical approach to drug abuse should be tailored. It may consist of offering nonpharmacologic (e.g., Narcotics Anonymous) and/or pharmacologic (e.g., methadone) treatment options. For the patient who is not ready to abstain from drugs, clinicians should use the encounter to discuss the importance of sterile needles and to provide information on needle exchange programs.
- The rate of clinical and immunologic progression of HIV disease in IDUs appears comparable to that of non-drug users.

- The IDU in recovery should be considered for antiretroviral therapy in the same manner as any other patient. The decision whether to start antiretroviral therapy in the active drug user should be individualized.
- Hepatitis C infection affects a majority of HIV-infected IDUs and is associated with a more rapid progression to cirrhosis.

SUGGESTED READINGS

Abdala N, Gleghorn AA, Carney JM, Heimer R. Can HIV-1 contaminated syringes be disinfected? J Acquir Immune Defic Syndr. 2001;28:487-94.

Alford D, Compton P, Samet JH. Acute pain management for patients receiving maintenance methadone or buprenorphine therapy. Ann Intern Med. 2006;144:127-34.

Fisher JD, Fisher WA, Cornman DH, Amico RK, Bryan A, Friedland GH. Clinician-delivered intervention during routine clinical care reduces unprotected sexual behavior among HIV-infected patients. J Acquir Immune Defic Syndr. 2006;41:44-52.

Kapadia F, Vlahov D, Donahoe RM, Friedland G. The role of substance abuse in HIV disease progression: reconciling differences from laboratory and epidemiologic investigations. Clin Infect Dis. 2005;41:1027-34.

Khalsa JH, Kresina T, Sherman K, Vocci F. Medical management of HIV-hepatitis C virus coinfection in injection drug users. Clin Infect Dis. 2005;41:S1-S6.

Krupitsky EM, Horton NJ, Williams EC, Lioznov D, Kuznetsova M, Zvartau E, et al. Alcohol use and HIV risk behaviors among HIV-infected hospitalized patients in St. Petersburg, Russia. Drug Alcohol Depend. 2005;79:251-6.

Needle RH, Burrows D, Friedman SR, Dorabjee J, Graziele T, Badrieva L, et al. Effectiveness of community-based outreach in preventing HIV/AIDS among injection drug users. Int J Drug Policy. 2005;16:45-57.

Palepu A, Tyndall M, Yip B, O'Shaughnessy MV, Hogg RS, Montaner JSG. Impaired virologic response to highly active antiretroviral therapy associated with ongoing injection drug use. J Acquir Immune Defic Syndr. 2003;32:522-6.

Rees V, Saitz R, Horton NJ, Samet JH. Association of alcohol consumption with HIV sex- and drug-risk behaviors among drug users. J Substance Abuse Treat. 2001;21:128-34.

Samet JH, Freedberg KA, Savetsky JB, et al. Understanding delay to medical care for HIV infection: the long-term non-presenter. AIDS. 2001;15:77-85.

Stein MD, Hanna L, Natarajan R, et al. Alcohol use patterns predict high-risk HIV behaviors among active injection drug-users. J Substance Abuse Treat. 2000;18: 359-63.

Urbina A, Jones K. Crystal methamphetamine, its analogues, and HIV infection: medical and psychiatric aspects of a new epidemic. Clin Infect Dis. 2004;38:890-4.

Vlahov D, Safaien M, Shenghan L, et al. Sexual and drug risk-related behaviours after initiating highly active antiretroviral therapy among injection drug users. AIDS. 2001;15:2311-6.

Chapter 12

Antiretroviral Post-Exposure Prophylaxis

MICHAEL T. WONG, MD
SONIA NAGY CHIMIENTI, MD

This chapter addresses post-exposure prophylaxis (PEP) in two settings: 1) occupational exposures for health care workers (HCWs), including first responders, hospital workers, dental staff, and research personnel; and 2) nonoccupational exposures in persons having unprotected sex, survivors of sexual assault, and in persons sharing needles or other drug paraphernalia. Prevention of mother-to-child transmission is discussed in Chapter 11.

Occupational Post-Exposure Prophylaxis

In addition to understanding PEP measures, it is incumbent upon all health-care institutions and HCWs to recognize the need for, and adherence to, preventive measures to limit exposure to blood and body fluids in all staff who are potentially at risk.

Epidemiology

An estimated 600,000 to 800,000 occupationally acquired percutaneous injuries occur annually in the United States. The majority of these injuries are in nursing and ancillary care staff. The mechanisms of injury differ by profession. The predominant nursing injuries are associated with hollow-bore needles, including recapping (25%), giving injections (14%), phlebotomy (14%), IV manipulations (14%), needle disposal (9%), and finding an errant needle (19%). Physician injuries are largely procedure-related (suturing [21%] or while operating on a patient [23%]).

As of 2005, 106 cases of HIV seroconversion had been reported in the occupational setting worldwide. These include 57 in the United States, 35 in Europe, and 14 elsewhere. An additional 238 cases were suspected but lacked the necessary supportive epidemiologic or exposure data. The types of exposures of persons who seroconverted in the United States are as follows: Forty-eight had a percutaneous (puncture/cut injury) exposure, 5 had a mucocutaneous (mucous membrane and/or skin) exposure, 2 had both percutaneous and mucocutaneous exposures, and 2 had an unknown route of exposure. Forty-nine health care workers were exposed to HIV-infected blood, 3 to concentrated virus in a laboratory, 1 to visibly bloody fluid, and 4 to an unspecified fluid. By occupation, the majority were nurses or laboratory workers; there have been no reported cases in physicians who do procedures. Placed in context, these seroconversions occurred in the setting of 28,010 reported exposures to blood and body fluids in the United States over the same time period.

Transmission Risk Factors

The risk of seroconversion after an exposure from an HIV-infected source patient ranges substantially, from no risk after a small splash event to intact skin to 0.3%-0.5% after a percutaneous injury (Table 12-1). In prospective studies and one metaanalysis of prospective studies involving occupational exposure to blood or body fluids from source patients known or later found to be HIV-infected, the average risk of transmission following a percutaneous injury was estimated to be 0.3% (95% confidence interval [CI]: 0.006% to 0.5%). Although episodes of HIV transmission after nonintact skin or mucous membrane exposure have been documented, transmission by this route is rare, and the risk has been estimated as less than 0.1% (95% CI, 0.05-0.1%).

To place these figures in perspective, the estimated average risk for HIV seroconversion following an unprotected sexual encounter with an HIV-infected partner is as high as 1 in 200 exposures, and the risk following receipt of a blood product in the United States is less than 1 in 1,000,000 exposures. The risk for transmission after exposure to fluids other than blood from HIV-infected persons also has not been quantified but is probably considerably lower than that for blood exposures.

A variety of factors affect the risk of HIV transmission after an occupational exposure. Nearly all reported HIV seroconversion events from percutaneous injuries have been the result of deep hollow-bore needle exposures. In a retrospective case control study of HCWs who had percutaneous injuries, the risk for HIV infection was found to be increased with exposure to a larger quantity of blood from the source patient (as indicated

Table 12-1.   Relative Risk of HIV Seroconversion after Blood or Body Fluid Exposure to an HIV-Infected Source Patient

Route	Relative Risk (95% Confidence Intervals)
Percutaneous	0.3% (0.5-0.006%)
Cutaneous (intact skin)	0.1%
Mucous membrane or nonintact skin	0.1% (0.1-0.005%)

by a device visibly contaminated with the patient's blood), a procedure that involved a needle being placed directly in a vein or artery, or a deep injury (greater than 1 cm in depth). The risk also was increased for exposure to blood from the source patient with advanced HIV disease, possibly reflecting a higher HIV plasma viral load and/or other factors (e.g., the presence of syncytia-inducing HIV strains).

The use of a source patient viral load for assessing HIV transmission risk has not been established. While plasma HIV viral load reflects the level of cell-free virus in the peripheral blood, latently infected CD4-bearing cells (circulating T-cells, stem cells, or macrophages) might transmit infection in the absence of viremia. A viral load below the lower limit of detection probably indicates a lower risk of transmission but does not exclude it.

Some evidence exists regarding the possibility that host defenses influence the risk for HIV infection. A study of HIV-exposed but uninfected HCWs demonstrated an HIV-specific cytotoxic T-lymphocyte (CTL) response when peripheral blood mononuclear cells were stimulated in vitro with HIV-specific antigens. Similar CTL responses have been observed in other groups who experienced repeated HIV exposure without resulting infection. Among potential explanations for this observation is that the host immune response may prevent establishment of HIV infection after a percutaneous exposure or that the CTL response might simply be a marker for exposure.

Prevention of Exposure

Unquestionably, the most effective way of avoiding exposure to blood or body fluids is by the appropriate use of barrier protection. Universal precautions were first recommended in 1987. These precautions differ from earlier guidelines in that they assume blood or body fluids from any person entering into a healthcare environment may be infected with a pathogen. Fluid-resistant or fluid-impermeable gowns, approved gloves, and eye/face wear should be used to prevent splash events. Facial protection should include either closed eye goggles or face shields incorporated into surgical masks. Corrective glasses do not serve as appropriate protective eye wear. In spite of these recommendations, splash-protective equipment is used less than 50% of the time.

The protective nature of gloves has been demonstrated in an in vitro model. A variety of injuries were simulated using hollow-bore devices (18 to 25 gauge needles) and solid-bore suture needles (2-0 to 5-0) at various depths of injury (0.5 cm up to 2.5 cm) in the absence or presence of single and double latex gloves and single nonlatex gloves. Not only was the volume of blood transferred across a percutaneous injury directly related to the size of the offending needle and depth of injury, but also it was substantially greater with hollow-bore than solid-bore needles. When evaluated for protection, gloves decreased the volume of blood transferred in such an injury by at least 50%, with latex and nonlatex types proving to be roughly equivalent.

Rationale for Post-Exposure Prophylaxis

The Centers for Disease Control and Prevention (CDC) identifies four issues, our understanding of which provides the rationale for PEP: 1) HIV pathogenesis, particularly the time course of early infection; 2) the biological plausibility that infection can be prevented or ameliorated by using antiretroviral drugs immediately following exposure; 3) direct or indirect evidence of the efficacy of specific agents; and 4) the risk and benefit of PEP for the exposed HCW.

The virology and immunology of early infection have led to a greater understanding of the effects of PEP following an exposure to an HIV-infected source patient. Animal data have been useful in elucidating the immune responses to exposure and early infection. However, extrapolation of data acquired from nonhuman primate studies to humans is difficult at best. As a family, retroviruses are highly species-specific. Early studies were performed using the simian immunodeficiency virus (SIV). While this virus has substantial sequence homology with HIV, it rarely infects humans and does not always respond to the drugs used in the treatment of HIV infection.

The first study supporting antiretroviral therapy in the context of HIV exposure was the landmark ACTG 076, in which perinatal HIV infection was reduced by 67% with the use of zidovudine (ZDV) during pregnancy and labor. While maternal viral load reduction occurred, it was not maximally suppressed in many subjects, indicating that other factors may be responsible for the effectiveness of ZDV in this setting. To date, the only published data regarding occupational exposures is a retrospective case control study demonstrating an 81% (95% CI: 43% to 94%) reduction in HIV seroconversion among HCWs who sustained significant blood or body fluid exposures to HIV-infected source patients and took ZDV monotherapy compared with a matched population that received no therapy.

Treatment Failure

In a large international surveillance report covering the period from 1990 to 2005, 24 occupationally acquired HIV infections occurred in HCWs receiving PEP. Monotherapy with ZDV was prescribed in 17/24 (71%) cases, dual therapy with ZDV plus didanosine (ddI) was prescribed in 2/24 (8%), and three or more drugs were used in the remainder (21%). In most cases, the injury-associated device was a large-gauge hollow-bore needle, and medications were started within 2 hours of the exposure (75%). Regimen changes were required early in three instances (12.5%). Seroconversion occurred at a median of 55 days (range 20 to 131 days), although the majority (71%) occurred between weeks 6 and 12. Factors that influenced the outcome included: 1) the size of inoculum, 2) source patient viral load at the time of injury, 3) delay in evaluation of the HCW, 4) delay in initiation of therapy, 5) short duration of PEP, and 6) inability to tolerate the medications.

Evaluation of the Exposed Patient

The decision whether to recommend PEP in an occupational setting is based upon risk assessment of the exposure. On one extreme, if the HCW was wearing appropriate protective equipment and the exposure was not significant, PEP is unnecessary even if the source patient has advanced HIV disease. Conversely, if the injury was deep and the source patient was HIV-infected and had a recent genotype test showing drug resistance, PEP with drugs that are effective against the resistant virus would be recommended.

Exposure risk assessment consists of identification of the nature of the injury and the type of body fluid (Table 12-2). Important information includes:

Table 12-2.   Assessment of HIV Occupational Exposure

Exposure Type/Source	Comments
Injury	
Percutaneous injury	The majority of reported exposures are through percutaneous injuries. No HIV seroconversions have been reported in health care settings from a percutaneous solid-bore needle injury. Assessment should include
	1. Type of instrument
	a) Hollow-bore >18 gauge
	b) Hollow-bore <18 gauge
	c) Solid-bore, large gauge
	d) Other sharp
	2. Depth of injury
	a) >0.5 cm
	b) <0.5 cm
	3. Presence of source-patient blood or body fluid defined above
	a) Yes
	b) No (minimal or no risk)
Splash exposure to mucous membrane or open wound	Seroconversion has been documented after splash exposure to the eyes.
Splash injury to skin surface	No HIV seroconversions have been reported after a splash to intact skin. However, PEP should be considered when prolonged contact to a large volume of blood occurs in a health care worker or first responder if the individual is unable to wash off the area within several minutes of exposure.
Body Fluid	
HIV-positive tissue culture	Most highly infectious source. All laboratories that perform HIV virology or immunology research should inform their affiliated employee health programs of this activity so that PEP can be instituted rapidly should an occupational exposure occur.

(cont'd)

Table 12-2.   Assessment of HIV Occupational Exposure (cont'd)

Exposure Type/Source	Comments
Body Fluid (cont'd)	
Blood or blood-tinged fluid	Most infectious of source patient fluids
Vaginal or seminal fluid	Infectivity related to duration of exposure
Fluids from body cavities	Examples include fluids aspirated during arthrocentesis, thoracentesis, or paracentesis. HIV has been isolated from CSF, and, although no seroconversions have been reported after a splash exposure from HIV-positive patients, CSF should be considered potentially infectious.
Urine, saliva, tears, sweat	Unless these are blood-tinged, risk of HIV exposure is minimal.
Source	
Known HIV-positive person	Factors associated with transmission include viral load and type of virus (e.g., syncytia-forming vs. non-syncytia-forming). These data are usually not available at the time of evaluation. Medication history and HIV resistance test results, if available, should be obtained.
Person with unknown HIV serostatus	Persons with unknown HIV serostatus represent the majority of exposures. PEP should be started and maintained while the source is tested for HIV after in-formed consent. If there are no concerns about acute retroviral syndrome* and the source is found to be HIV-negative, PEP can be discontinued.
Unknown	Examples include a percutaneous injury from an unseen needle extending from a disposal container and a per-cutaneous injury from a stray needle with blood or body fluid in waste.
Known HIV-negative or low-risk person	This type of exposure poses no HIV risk. However, confirming low-risk status is a priority and should not be assumed under any circumstances.

CSF = cerebrospinal fluid.

* Acute retroviral syndrome manifestations may include fever, generalized adenopathy, pharyngitis, headache, rash, myalgia, and arthralgia.

Percutaneous Injury

1. Hollow-bore vs. solid-bore device
2. Gauge of the device
3. Depth of the injury
4. Use of personal protective equipment

Mucocutaneous or Cutaneous Exposure or Splash

1. Volume of exposure
2. Exposure to mucocutaneous tissue or open wound
3. Duration of exposure
4. Use of personal protective equipment

Type of Body Fluid

1. Blood from an HIV-infected source
2. Blood-tinged fluid from an HIV-infected source
3. Other potentially infectious body fluids, such as seminal or vaginal secretions, breast milk, and, in rare circumstances, cerebrospinal fluid, from an HIV-infected source

Source Assessment

In addition to the nature of the injury and the type of body fluid, assessment of exposure requires information on the source, which is categorized as follows:

1. Known HIV-infected patient
2. Potentially HIV-infected patient (e.g., exhibits symptoms consistent with HIV seroconversion)
3. Unknown HIV serostatus
4. Unknown source (e.g. injury from needle with blood in the hub sticking out of sharps container)
5. Known HIV-negative or low-risk patient

The assessment outlined above is synthesized into a decision to 1) not treat, 2) treat with two drugs, or 3) treat with more than two drugs. The CDC has provided detailed tables to guide this process (Tables 12-3 and 12-4).

Choice of Antiretroviral Drugs

Dual-drug regimens consist of two nucleoside reverse-transcriptase inhibitors (NRTIs), usually ZDV and lamivudine (3TC), *or* the nucleotide reverse-transcriptase inhibitor tenofovir (TDF) and 3TC or emtracitabine (FTC). In general, these are prescribed as a combination pill (ZDV/3TC [Combivir] or TDF/FTC [Truvada]). Dual-drug regimens are used in less severe percutaneous exposures to class 1 source patients and in most mucous membrane and intact skin exposures.

Triple-drug regimens previously consisted of the protease inhibitor (PI) indinavir (IDV) or nelfinavir (NFV) given in combination with two NRTIs. More recent guidelines substitute lopinavir/ritonavir (LPV/RTV) for IDV or NFV. The decision to add a PI to the basic regimen should be made only in high-risk settings.

Other "nonconventional" antiretroviral drug combinations may be indicated in very specific circumstances. These are usually recommended in the setting of a high-risk exposure to blood or body fluid from a source patient who is highly drug-experienced or has a genotype test indicating the presence of multi-drug resistance. Such decisions should be made with the consultation of an HIV expert.

Table 12-3. **Recommended HIV Post-Exposure Prophylaxis (PEP) for Percutaneous Injuries**

| | Infection Status of Source | | | |
Exposure Type	HIV-positive, Class 1*	HIV-positive, Class 2*	Source of Unknown HIV Status†	Unknown Source§	HIV-Negative
Less severe¶	Recommend basic 2-drug PEP	Recommend expanded ≥3-drug PEP	Generally, no PEP warranted; however, consider basic 2-drug PEP** for source with HIV risk factors††	Generally, no PEP warranted; however, consider basic 2-drug PEP** in settings in which exposure to HIV-infected persons is likely	No PEP warranted
More severe§§	Recommend expanded 3-drug PEP	Recommend expanded ≥3-drug PEP	Generally, no PEP warranted; however, consider basic 2-drug PEP** for source with HIV risk factors††	Generally, no PEP warranted; however, consider basic 2-drug PEP** in settings in which exposure to HIV-infected persons is likely	No PEP warranted

* HIV-positive, class 1—asymptomatic HIV infection or known low viral load (e.g., <1500 copies/mL). HIV-positive, class 2—symptomatic HIV infection, acquired immunodeficiency syndrome, acute seroconversion, or known high viral load. If drug resistance is a concern, obtain expert consultation. However, initiation of PEP should not be delayed.

† For example, deceased source person with no samples available for HIV testing.

§ For example, a needle from a sharps disposal container.

¶ For example, solid needle or superficial injury.

** The recommendation "consider PEP" indicates that PEP is optional; a decision to initiate PEP should be based on a discussion between the exposed person and the treating clinician regarding its potential risks and benefits.

†† If PEP is offered and administered and the source is later determined to be HIV-negative, PEP should be discontinued.

§§ For example, large-bore hollow needle, deep puncture, visible blood on device, or needle used in patient's artery or vein.

From Occupational PEP Guidelines. Updated US Public Health Service guidelines for the management of occupational exposures to HIV and recommendations for postexposure prophylaxis. MMWR. September 30, 2005/Vol. 54/No. RR-9.

Table 12-4.   Recommended HIV Post-Exposure Prophylaxis (PEP) for Mucous Membrane and Nonintact Skin Exposures*

Exposure Type	Infection Status of Source				
	HIV-positive, Class 1†	HIV-positive, Class 2†	Source of Unknown HIV Status§	Unknown Source¶	HIV-Negative
Small volume**	Consider basic 2-drug PEP††	Recommend basic 2-drug PEP	Generally, no PEP warranted§§	Generally, no PEP warranted	No PEP warranted
Large volume¶¶	Recommend basic 2-drug PEP	Recommend expanded ≥3-drug PEP	Generally, no PEP warranted; however, consider basic 2-drug PEP†† for source with HIV risk factors§§	Generally, no PEP warranted; however, consider basic 2-drug PEP†† in settings in which exposure to HIV-infected persons is likely	No PEP warranted

* For skin exposures, follow-up is indicated only if evidence exists of compromised skin integrity (e.g., dermatitis, abrasion, or open wound).

† HIV-positive, class 1—asymptomatic HIV infection or known low-viral load (e.g., <1500 copies/mL). HIV-positive, class 2—symptomatic HIV infection, AIDS, acute seroconversion, or known high viral load. If drug resistance is a concern, obtain expert consultation. However, initiation of PEP should not be delayed.

§ For example, deceased source person with no samples available for HIV testing.

¶ For example, splash from inappropriately disposed blood.

** For example, a few drops.

†† The recommendation "consider PEP" indicates that PEP is optional; a decision to initiate PEP should be based on a discussion between the exposed person and the treating clinician regarding its potential risks and benefits.

§§ If PEP is offered and administered and the source is later determined to be HIV-negative, PEP should be discontinued.

¶¶ For example, a major blood splash.

From Occupational PEP Guidelines. Updated US Public Health Service guidelines for the management of occupational exposures to HIV and recommendations for postexposure prophylaxis. MMWR. September 30, 2005/Vol. 54/No.RR-9.

Drug Toxicity

The toxicities of antiretroviral drugs are described in Chapter 4. It is important to note that some side effects are experienced more frequently when the medications are provided in PEP compared with treatment settings. For example, the reported occurrence of nausea, vomiting, anorexia, and diarrhea was over 50% in ZDV-containing PEP regimens and resulted in the discontinuation of the drug in over one-third of those treated. The reasons for this disparity are not clear but may be related to the differences in free and bound drug levels in HIV-infected and uninfected persons. A number of pharmacokinetic studies have demonstrated greater serum concentrations of PIs when given to HIV-seronegative volunteers. Serious toxicities reported on PEP have included nephrolithiasis, hepatitis, and pancytopenia. The use of nevirapine (NVP), which has been associated with Stevens-Johnson syndrome, rhabdomyolysis, and fulminant hepatitis should be avoided in PEP regimens. Long-term toxicities from PEP have not been described.

Timing and Duration of Therapy

Ideally, PEP should be initiated within 1 to 2 hours of the injury. Earlier animal studies suggested that PEP is substantially less effective when started more than 24 to 36 hours post-exposure, while more recent studies with TDF indicate some protection from infection when used as long as 72 hours later. The interval after which no benefit is gained from PEP is undefined. Therefore, PEP should be considered for high-risk exposures even when the interval exceeds 72 hours. The optimal duration of PEP is unknown, but four weeks is generally recommended.

Counseling and Follow-Up

Counseling of HCWs should include discussion about the low risk of HIV transmission at home from nonintimate activities to help decrease anxiety. Other important discussion topics include: 1) safer sex practices during the observation period or until it is determined that the source patient is HIV-seronegative and not seroconverting; 2) temporary removal of an organ donor card from the wallet; and 3) the potential side effects of prescribed drugs.

An HIV antibody test should be performed at baseline. If the source patient is unknown or identified as HIV-infected, the HCW should return for follow-up testing at 6 weeks, 3 months, and 6 months following the injury. Seroconversions after 6 months are extremely rare, having been reported only in the setting of hepatitis C virus (HCV) infection from the same blood exposure. Assessment of hematologic, renal, and hepatic function should be performed at baseline and 2 weeks into treatment. Screening for other pathogens, such as syphilis, hepatitis B virus (HBV), and HCV, is also warranted. An HIV viral load is generally not useful in this setting.

Nonoccupational Post-Exposure Prophylaxis

The remainder of this chapter summarizes the data upon which nonoccupational post-exposure prophylaxis (NPEP) is based and provides an overview of published guidelines. The primary care provider may be the first point of contact for an exposed patient. It is incumbent upon each clinician to know either when and how to administer NPEP or where to refer patients for care if another setting is more appropriate.

In July 1997, the CDC convened a meeting to determine whether or not guidelines should be issued on the use of NPEP. The following year, the Department of Health and Human Services (DHHS) released a statement saying that there was insufficient evidence to provide recommendations regarding NPEP. However, since that time, the use of NPEP in the setting of sexual, injection-drug use, and other nonoccupational exposures to HIV has increased. In response to this trend, the DHHS published guidelines for NPEP in January 2005.

Epidemiology

There have been many reports over the past decade documenting the management of exposures to blood and body fluids outside of the occupational setting. A retrospective review of emergency department visits for 1436 exposures over a 6-year period indicated that 78% were nonoccupational. In adults, 73% of the exposures were from human bites, while in adolescents and children, 81% of the exposures involved sexual contact. Antiretroviral drug prophylaxis was prescribed on 143 occasions, 51 of which were for nonoccupational exposures.

Sexual assault is not uncommon, and survivors are understandably concerned about the potential for HIV transmission, as well as other sexually transmitted diseases (STDs). A study in the early 1990's reported that 13% of women had been raped sometime during their lives and that 60% of these sexual assaults occurred in those under the age of 18 years. Some men are also at risk for rape. Approximately 5% of rape victims evaluated in the emergency department in a Memphis sexual assault program were men, 80% of whom were incarcerated. A 1999 crime survey from the United States Department of Justice reported that 11.6% of rapes in persons older than 12 years involved men.

The risk of HIV transmission following different types of nonoccupational exposures varies. Needle-sharing injection-drug use confers the highest risk of transmission, estimated at 67 per 10,000 exposures. The greatest risk from an unprotected sexual act occurs with receptive anal intercourse, estimated at 1 per 200 exposures. The risks of transmission with other forms of unprotected sexual intercourse are much lower: 10 per 10,000 exposures for receptive vaginal intercourse, 6.5 per 10,000 exposures for insertive anal intercourse, and 5 per 10,000 exposures for insertive vaginal intercourse. A study of prison inmates estimated that the HIV seroprevalence rate in persons convicted of sexual assault was 1% compared with 3% for all inmates and 0.3% in the general male population. These data support the assumption that the risk of HIV transmission may be relatively low in survivors of sexual assault.

Effectiveness

Randomized trials evaluating the effectiveness of NPEP have not been conducted and are not likely to be for ethical reasons. However, available data from animal and perinatal transmission studies suggest that NPEP may be effective. There are also numerous published observational studies suggesting that the rate of HIV seroconversion following the use of NPEP is low. Available data suggest that NPEP may be at least somewhat effective in higher risk populations.

A study in Brazil of a high-risk cohort of MSM and bisexual men reported that the HIV seroincidence was 0.7/100 person-years in subjects who received NPEP compared with 4.1/100 person-years in those who did not. Another group from Brazil reported that there were no HIV seroconversions in 180 female survivors of sexual assault who were treated with NPEP within 72 hours compared with 4 seroconversions (2.7%) in 145 women who did not receive it. A feasibility trial conducted in San Francisco evaluating the efficacy of NPEP for 401 sexual and needle-sharing exposures reported no seroconversions in any group, regardless of whether NPEP had been prescribed or completed. The NPEP guidelines published in 2005 compiled data from registries from Australia, France, Switzerland, and the United States and reported that there were no seroconversions in 2000 NPEP cases despite the fact that 350 source patients were confirmed to be HIV-seropositive. In 2005, a study of NPEP in a high-risk cohort in San Francisco reported that post-exposure prophylaxis may not be completely effective in preventing HIV transmission. In it, HIV-seronegative persons with high-risk sexual or injection-drug use exposures were provided 28 days of NPEP in a nonrandomized fashion. Of 702 evaluable subjects, there were 7 (1%) HIV seroconversions. Three of these were confirmed as possible NPEP failures based on a negative HIV antibody test and an undetectable viral load at baseline and the lack of subsequent high-risk exposures.

Concerns Regarding the Use of NPEP

Increased Risky Behavior

The increasing availability of NPEP has resulted in a variety of concerns. Patients may increase risky behavior, believing that HIV transmission can be easily prevented following an exposure. The recent increased incidence of STDs in some populations gives credence to this concern, but there is little evidence to indicate that the availability of NPEP is responsible.

Researchers in San Francisco collected data on sexual and drug use behaviors in patients who received a course of NPEP for a high-risk exposure. Patients were queried regarding risk behavior 3 months prior to and 6 and 12 months following NPEP. Seventy-two percent of subjects reported a decrease in high-risk behavior at 12 months following the course of NPEP, and 14% reported an increase in high-risk behavior. At 12 months, 17% of subjects had received a second course of NPEP for a subsequent high-risk exposure. A similar rate of repeated treatment for high-risk exposures was seen in a Boston cohort.

Drug Toxicity

Data from occupational PEP case reports and registries indicate that drug toxicity is common. Side effects include nausea, headache, diarrhea, and fatigue. Serious complications such as nephrolithiasis and hepatitis have also been reported. Given these risks, clinicians should be cautious about prescribing NPEP when the risk of HIV transmission is low. Adverse events occur in approximately 22% of NPEP cases and lead to treatment cessation at rates similar to occupational PEP.

Selection of Resistant Virus

Resistant HIV strains have been documented in some patients who have received NPEP, although it is unclear whether resistant virus was transmitted or if resistance was related to NPEP.

Cost of Implementation

Studies have been published demonstrating that NPEP is cost-effective in at least some clinical settings. In a French report, NPEP prevented 3.4 infections and saved 27.7 quality adjusted life years (QALYs) at a net cost of $1.8 million. For receptive anal sex with HIV-infected partners, NPEP saved $9400 per QALY (cost-effective defined as <$20,000 per QALY). For receptive anal sex with gay male partners of unknown serostatus, NPEP was also cost-effective. For other sexual exposures with partners of unknown serostatus, the cost-effectiveness ratios were more than $1 million per QALY. In this cohort, these lower risk exposures represented 49% of those for which NPEP was prescribed.

Management of the Exposed Patient

The exposed patient should be HIV antibody tested at baseline and should be considered seronegative until the results of testing are obtained. The specific nature of the exposure should be determined in order to assess the risk for HIV transmission, and the HIV serostatus of the source patient should be obtained whenever possible. Factors that should be elicited in sexual assault survivors include the type of sexual exposure (anal, vaginal, oral; receptive, insertive), the presence of trauma, the number of assailants, and the timing of the sexual assault relative to presentation for care.

The exposed patient should be evaluated for pre-existing HIV infection with an antibody test; other STDs, including gonorrhea, chlamydial infection, trichomoniasis, and syphilis; and HBV and HCV infections. Sexual assault survivors who receive preventive treatment for STDs should be evaluated 1 to 2 weeks afterward, and testing for them should be repeated in symptomatic patients. In most cases, HBV vaccination in patients who are not immune is sufficient for protection against transmission. Use of emergency contraception should be offered to all women who have been sexually assaulted.

The DHHS recommends that a 28-day course of treatment be provided for any exposure to blood or body fluids from persons who are known to be HIV-seropositive if the exposure represents a "substantial risk for HIV transmission" and if that exposure occurred less than 72 hours prior to presentation for care. An algorithmic approach to NPEP is presented in Figure 12-1. The guidelines define a substantial risk as having occurred when all three of the following conditions have been met:

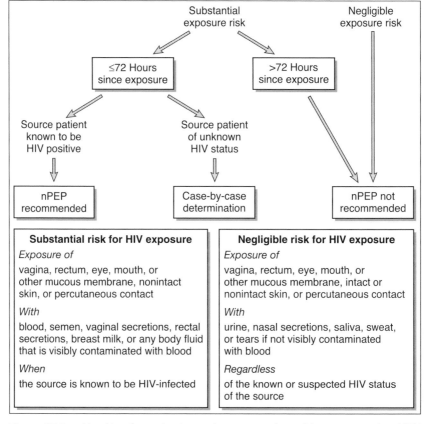

Figure 12-1.   Algorithm for evaluation and treatment of possible nonoccupational HIV exposures.

1. Exposure of a mucous membrane, nonintact skin, or percutaneous contact
2. Exposure to blood, semen, vaginal secretions, rectal secretions, breast milk, or any body fluid visibly contaminated with blood
3. Exposure to a person known to be HIV-infected

If the HIV serostatus of the source patient is unknown, there is no recommendation for or against the use of NPEP, and treatment decisions should be individualized. Patients who present for care more than 72 hours after the exposure and those who have sustained an exposure that is of negligible risk should not be treated with NPEP.

Choice of Antiretroviral Drugs

Treatment with a triple-drug regimen containing an NNRTI or PI is generally recommended (Table 12-5). For the NNRTI regimen, ZDV/3TC or TDF/FTC is given in conjunction with efavirenz (EFV). For the PI regimen, LPV/RTV is substituted for EFV. If the source patient is known to be HIV-infected and the antiretroviral drug history and viral resistance profile are known, selection of an NPEP regimen should be guided by this information. Case reports suggest that regimens containing TDF may be better tolerated than those containing ZDV, with less nausea and fewer headaches. Assessment of hematologic, renal, and hepatic function should be performed at baseline and two weeks into treatment.

Counseling and Follow-Up

Patients who exhibit high-risk behavior should be counseled regarding the options of sexual abstinence, reduction in the number of partners, consistent condom use for all sexual activity, abstinence from injection-drug use, and use of sterile needles if abstinence from drugs is not possible (see Chapter 2). Patients should also be counseled regarding the use of barrier protection with sexual partners during the course of NPEP until negative follow-up HIV antibody testing (at 6 weeks, 3 months, and 6 months) has been documented. In addition, patients should be educated regarding the symptoms and signs of the acute retroviral syndrome (see Chapter 1) and instructed to return for evaluation should these develop.

KEY POINTS

- The most effective way of avoiding exposure to blood or body fluids is by the appropriate use of barrier protection.
- As of 2005, 106 cases of HIV seroconversion had been reported in the occupational setting worldwide. The majority were nurses or

Table 12-5.   Antiretroviral Regimens for Nonoccupational Post-Exposure Prophylaxis of HIV Infection

Preferred Regimens	
NNRTI-based	Efavirenz[†] plus (lamivudine or emtricitabine plus (zidovudine or tenofovir)
PI-based	Lopinavir/ritonavir plus (lamivudine or emtricitabine) plus zidovudine

Alternative Regimens	
NNRTI-based	Efavirenz plus (lamivudine or emtricitabine) plus abacavir or didanosine or stavudine[§]
PI-based	Atazanavir plus (lamivudine or emtricitabine) plus (zidovudine or stavudine or abacavir or didanosine) or (tenofovir plus ritonavir [100 mg/day])
	Fosamprenavir plus (lamivudine or emtricitabine) plus (zidovudine or stavudine) or (abacavir or tenofovir or didanosine)
	Fosamprenavir/ritonavir[¶] plus (lamivudine or emtricitabine) plus (zidovudine or stavudine or abacavir or tenofovir or didanosine)
	Indinavir/ritonavir[**] plus (lamivudine or emtricitabine) plus (zidovudine or stavudine or abacavir or tenofovir or didanosine)
	Lopinavir/ritonavir plus (lamivudine or emtricitabine) plus (stavudine or abacavir or tenofovir or didanosine)
	Nelfinavir plus (lamivudine or emtricitabine) plus (zidovudine or stavudine or abacavir or tenofovir or didanosine)
	Saquinavir/ritonavir plus (lamivudine or emtricitabine) plus (zidovudine or stavudine or abacavir or tenofovir or didanosine)
Triple NRTI	Abacavir plus lamivudine plus zidovudine (only when an NNRTI- or PI-based regimen cannot or should not be used)

NNRTI = non-nucleoside reverse-transcriptase inhibitor; NRTI = nucleoside reverse-transcriptase inhibitor; PI = protease inhibitor.

[†] Efavirenz should be avoided in pregnant women and women of child-bearing potential.

[§] Higher incidence of lipoatrophy, hyperlipidemia, and mitochondrial toxicity associated with stavudine than with other NRTIs.

[¶] Low-dose (100-400 mg) ritonavir.

[**] Use of ritonavir with indinavir may increase risk for renal adverse events.

Source: Department of Health and Human Services. Guidelines for the Use of Antiretroviral Agents in HIV-Infected Adults and Adolescents, October 29, 2004 revision. Available at http://www.aidsinfo.nih.gov/guidelines/default_db2.asp?id=50. This document is updated periodically; refer to Web site for updated versions.

laboratory workers; there have been no reported cases in physicians who do procedures.

- The risk of seroconversion following an exposure from an HIV-infected patient ranges substantially, from no risk following a small splash event to intact skin to 0.3-0.5% following a percutaneous injury.

- Factors that increase the likelihood of seroconversion from a percutaneous injury include the type of needle (large-gauge, hollow-bore), the depth of the injury, and the presence of advanced HIV disease in the source patient.
- Post-exposure use of antiretroviral drugs is effective at reducing the risk of HIV seroconversion based upon animal data and a case-control human study. It should be initiated as soon as possible after exposure. Common drug combinations for low- to moderate-risk exposures are ZDV/3TC *or* TDF/3TC or TDF/FTC. EFV or LPV/RTV is added for high-risk exposures. Treatment is continued for 4 weeks.
- Counseling and appropriate laboratory testing should be performed at baseline and follow-up visits.
- The risk of HIV transmission following different types of nonoccupational exposures varies but is in a similar range as occupational exposures.
- Animal data and epidemiologic studies in humans support the effectiveness of nonoccupational PEP, but a randomized clinical trial has not been performed.
- Concerns regarding nonoccupational PEP include increased risky behavior, drug toxicity, selection of resistant virus, and the cost of implementation.
- For nonoccupational PEP, a three-drug regimen containing an NNRTI or PI is generally recommended. The management considerations described for occupational PEP are also applicable to nonoccupational PEP.

SUGGESTED READINGS

Occupational Post-Exposure Prophylaxis
Beltrami EM, Luo C-C, Dela Torre N, Cardo DM. HIV transmission after an occupational exposure despite post-exposure prophylaxis with a combination drug regimen [Abstract P-S2-62]. In: Program and abstracts of the 4th Decennial International Conference on Nosocomial and Healthcare-Associated Infections in conjunction with the 10th Annual Meeting of SHEA. Atlanta: CDC, 2000:125-6.
Cardo DM, Culver DH, Ciesielski CA Srivastava PU, Marcus R,Abiteboul D, et al. A case-control study of HIV seroconversion in health care workers after percutaneous exposure. Centers for Disease Control and Prevention Needlestick Surveillance Group. N Engl J Med. 1997;337:1485-90.
CDC. Serious adverse events attributed to nevirapine regimens for post-exposure prophylaxis after HIV exposures—worldwide. 1997-2000. MMWR. 2001;49:1153-6.
CDC. MMWR, Updated USPHS Guidelines for the Management of Occupational Exposure to HBV, HCV and HIV and Recommendations for Post-exposure Prophylaxis, 2001;50 (RR11):1-42.
CDC. MMWR, Updated U.S. Public Health Service guidelines for the management of occupational exposure to HIV and recommendations for post-exposure prophylaxis, 2005; 54 (RR9): 1-24. http://www.cdc.gov/mmwr/preview/mmwrhtml/rr5409a1.htm

CDC. HCHSTP-Division of HIV/AIDS Prevention Fact Sheet; Preventing Occupational HIV Transmission to Health Care Workers, February 2006: http://www.cdc.gov/hiv/pubs/facts/hcwprev.htm

Gerberding JL. Management of occupational exposures to blood-borne viruses. N Eng J Med. 1995;16:444-51.

Henderson DK, Fahey BJ, Willy M, Schmitt JM, Carey K, Koziol DE, et al. Risk for occupational transmission of human immunodeficiency virus type 1 (HIV-1) associated with clinical exposures. A prospective evaluation. Ann Intern Med. 1990;113:740-6.

Jochimsen EM. Failures of zidovudine postexposure prophylaxis. Am J Med. 1997;102:52-5; discussion 56-7.

Mast ST, Woolwine JD, Gerberding JL. Efficacy of gloves in reducing blood volumes transferred during simulated needlestick injury. J Infect Dis. 1993;168:1589-92.

Ridzon R, Gallagher K, Ciesielski C, Ginsberg MB, Robertson BJ, Luo CC, et al. Simultaneous transmission of human immunodeficiency virus and hepatitis C virus from a needle-stick injury. N Engl J Med. 1997;336:919-22.

Sperling RS, Shapiro DE, Coombs RW, Todd JA, Herman SA, McSherry GD, et al. Maternal viral load, zidovudine treatment, and the risk of transmission of human immunodeficiency virus type 1 from mother to infant. Pediatric AIDS Clinical Trials Group Protocol 076 Study Group. N Engl J Med. 1996;335:1621-9.

Wang SA, Panlilio AL, Doi PA, White AD, Stek M Jr., Saah A. Experience of healthcare workers taking postexposure prophylaxis after occupational HIV exposures: findings of the HIV Postexposure Prophylaxis Registry. Infect Control Hosp Epidemiol. 2000;21:780-5.

Nonoccupational Post-Exposure Prophylaxis

CDC. Sexually Transmitted Diseases Treatment Guidelines 2002. MMWR 2002:51 (No. RR-06):1-82.

CDC. Antiretroviral Post-exposure Prophylaxis After Sexual, Injection-Drug Use, or Other Nonoccupational Exposure to HIV in the United States. MMWR 2005:54 (No. RR-02); 1-20.

De Santis M, Carducci B, De Santis L, Cavaliere AF, Straface G. Periconceptional exposure to efavirenz and neural tube defects. Arch Intern Med. 2002;162:355.

Dumond J, Yeh R, Patterson K, Corbett A, Jung BH, Rezk N, et al. First Dose and Steady-state Genital Tract Pharmacokinetics of Ten Antiretroviral Drugs in HIV-infected Women: Implications for Pre- and Post-Exposure Prophylaxis. [Abstract 129]. Presented at the 13th Conference on Retroviruses and Opportunistic Infections, Denver, Colorado, February 5-8, 2006. http://www.retroconference.org/2006/Abstracts/26114.HTM

Hamers FF, Lot F, Larsen C, and Laporte A. Cost-effectiveness of prophylaxis following non-occupational exposure to HIV infection in France. [Abstract 230]. Presented at the 8th Conference on Retroviruses and Opportunistic Infections, Chicago, Illinois, February 4-8, 2001. http://www.retroconference.org/2001/abstracts/default.htm

Harrison LH, do Lago RF, Moreira RI, Mendelsohn AB and Schechter M. Post-sexual-exposure chemoprophylaxis (PEP) for HIV: a prospective cohort study of behavioral impact. [Abstract 225]. Presented at the 8th Conference on Retroviruses and Opportunistic Infections, Chicago, Illinois, February 4-8, 2001. http://www.retroconference.org/2001/abstracts/default.htm

Martin JN, Roland ME, Bamberger JD, Chesney MA, Kahn JO, Coates TJ et al. Post-exposure prophylaxis (PEP) for sexual exposure to HIV does not lead to increases in high risk behavior: The San Francisco PEP Project. [Abstract 224]. Presented at the 8th Conference on Retroviruses and Opportunistic Infections, Chicago, Illinois, February 4-8, 2001. http://www.retroconference.org/2001/abstracts/default.htm

Pinkerton SD, Holtgrave DR. Prophylaxis after sexual exposure to HIV [Letter]. Ann Intern Med. 1998;129:671; author reply 672.

Pinkerton SD, Holtgrave DR, Bloom FR. Postexposure treatment of HIV [Letter]. N Engl J Med. 1997;337:500-1.

Rabaud C, Burty C, Valle C, Christian B, Penalba C, Prazuck T, et al. Post-exposure prophylaxis of HIV infection: comparison of tolerability of 4 PEP regimens. [Abstract 905]. Presented at the 13th Conference on Retroviruses and Opportunistic Infections, Denver, Colorado, February 5-8, 2006. http://www.retroconference.org/2006/Abstracts/26277. HTM

Rakai Project Team. Probability of HIV-1 transmission per coital act in monogamous, heterosexual, HIV-1-discordant couples in Rakai, Uganda. Lancet. 2001;357:1149-53.

Roland ME, Neilands TB, Krone MR, Katz MH, Franses K, Grant RM, et al. Seroconversion following nonoccupational postexposure prophylaxis against HIV. Clin Infect Dis. 2005; 41:1507-13.

Spaulding A, Salas C, Cleaver D, Grundy M, Macalino G, Marcussen P, and Rich J. HIV seroprevalence in male sexual offenders in Rhode Island: implications for post-exposure prophylaxis. [Abstract 229]. Presented at the 8th Conference on Retroviruses and Opportunistic Infections, Chicago, Illinois, February 4-8, 2001. http://www.retroconference.org/2001/abstracts/default.htm

Winston A, McAllister J, Amin J, Cooper DA, Carr A. The use of a triple nucleoside-nucleotide regimen for nonoccupational HIV post-exposure prophylaxis. HIV Med. 2005;6:191-7.

Management Resources

National Clinician's Postexposure Prophylaxis Hotline. Managed by the University of California, San Francisco (phone 888-448-4911, or Internet at www.ucsf.edu/hivcntr).

Occupational PEP Registry, 1996-1999; Final Report.
http://www.cdc.gov/ncidod/dhqp/pdf/bbp/pep/PEPRegistry.pdf

Chapter 13

HIV Global Epidemiology

MEGAN O'BRIEN, PhD
ELIZABETH A. McCARTHY, MPH

Overview of the Epidemic

By the end of 2005, the Joint United Nations Programme on HIV/AIDS (UNAIDS) estimated that 38.6 million people worldwide were living with HIV, more than 90% of them in developing countries. In 2005, 4.1 million people acquired new HIV infections, and AIDS caused the deaths of 2.8 million people. Women comprised 48% of adult HIV cases, and 6% of persons living with HIV were children under the age of 15 (Table 13-1).

The prevalence of HIV cases varies across regions, and case distribution is disproportionate to population distribution (Figure 13-1). For instance, Sub-Saharan Africa comprised less than 10% of the global population aged 15 to 49 in 2005 but accounted for approximately 60% of HIV cases in this group. In 2005, Sub-Saharan Africa was the home of 63% of people living with HIV, 66% of people newly infected with HIV, 76% of women with HIV, and 71% of people who died of AIDS in the world. In contrast, East Asia represented about 25% of the global population aged 15 to 49 in 2005 but accounted for just 2.6% of persons living with HIV in this group. Although the adult HIV prevalence was just 0.6% in South and Southeast Asia, there were approximately 7.6 million people living with HIV in this region, representing about 20% of cases in the world. North America, Latin America, Eastern Europe and Central Asia, and East Asia each had between 0.7 and 1.6 million people living with HIV. Although the 330,000 people living with HIV in the Caribbean constitute less than 1% of global cases, the adult prevalence rate of 1.6% in this region is among the highest in the world, exceeded only by Sub-Saharan Africa.

The majority of people worldwide are in settings with low HIV prevalence. In 2005, about 86% of the world's population aged 15 to 49 was living in a country with an adult prevalence rate of 1% or lower, 13% in a country with a rate of between 1.1% and 10%, and less than 2% in one of the 10 countries (all in Sub-Saharan Africa) where the rate exceeded 10%. Table 13-2 lists the 10 countries with the greatest adult HIV prevalence rates in 2005, and Table 13-3 lists the 10 countries with the greatest number of HIV cases in 2005. Globally, the incidence of HIV infection appears to have stabilized after peaking in the late 1990s. Consequently, the prevalence has

Table 13-1. Global Summary of the HIV Epidemic in 2005

Region	Adults and Children Living with HIV	Adult Women Living with HIV	Adult Prevalence (%)	Percent of Adults Living with HIV Who Are Women (%)	Adult and Child Deaths from AIDS
Global	38.6 million [33.4–46.0 million]	17.3 million [14.8–20.6 million]	1.0 [0.9–1.2]	48	2.8 million [2.4–3.3 million]
Sub-Saharan Africa	24.5 million [21.6–27.4 million]	13.2 million [11.4–15.1 million]	6.1 [5.4–6.8]	59	2.0 million [1.7–2.3 million]
South and Southeast Asia	7.6 million [5.1–11.7 million]	2.2 million [1.3–3.5 million]	0.6 [0.4–1.0]	30	560,000 [370,000–810,000]
Latin America	1.6 million [1.2–2.4 million]	480,000 [340,000–760,000]	0.5 [0.4–1.2]	30	59,000 [47,000–76,000]
Eastern Europe and Central Asia	1.5 million [1.0–2.3 million]	420,000 [270,000–680,000]	0.8 [0.6–1.4]	28	53,000 [36,000–75,000]
North America	1.3 million [770,000–2.1 million]	310,000 [170,000–550,000]	0.8 [0.5–1.1]	26	18,000 [11,000–26,000]
East Asia	680,000 [420,000–1.1 million]	190,000 [110,000–330,000]	0.1 [<0.2]	28	33,000 [20,000–49,000]
Western and Central Europe	720,000 [550,000–950,000]	200,000 [150,000–290,000]	0.3 [0.2–0.4]	28	12,000 [<15,000]
North Africa and the Middle East	440,000 [250,000–720,000]	190,000 [95,000–350,000]	0.2 [0.1–0.4]	48	37,000 [20,000–62,000]
Caribbean	330,000 [240,000–420,000]	160,000 [100,000–220,000]	1.6 [1.1–2.2]	53	27,000 [19,000–36,000]
Oceania	78,000 [48,000–170,000]	35,000 [17,000–86,000]	0.3 [0.2–0.8]	47	3,400 [1,900–5,500]

Source: UNAIDS, 2006 Report on the Global AIDS Epidemic

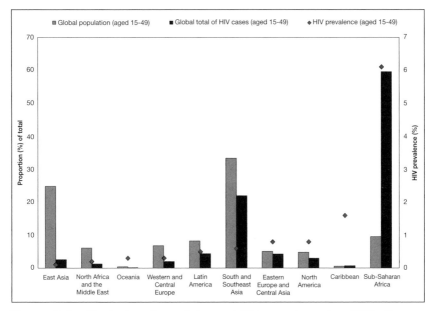

Figure 13-1. Distribution of population and HIV cases by region, 2005. (Sources: Population estimates are from US Census Bureau International Data Base; HIV prevalence estimates are from UNAIDS 2006 Report on the Global AIDS Epidemic.)

Table 13-2.   Countries with the Highest Adult HIV Prevalence in 2005

Country	Estimated Adult HIV Prevalence (%)
Swaziland	33.4
Botswana	24.1
Lesotho	23.2
Zimbabwe	20.1
Namibia	19.6
South Africa	18.8
Zambia	17.0
Mozambique	16.1
Malawi	14.1
Central African Republic	10.7

Source: UNAIDS, 2006 Report on the Global AIDS Epidemic

remained at about 1% since 2001. However, even with a stable prevalence, population growth and improved survival have resulted in an increasing number of people living with HIV each year (Figure 13-2).

The proportion of women with HIV infection has been increasing slowly over the last 20 years, accounting for 35% of adult cases in 1985 and

Table 13-3.   Countries with the Greatest Number of HIV Cases in 2005

Country	Approximate Number of People Living with HIV
India	5,700,000
South Africa	5,500,000
Nigeria	2,900,000
Mozambique	1,800,000
Zimbabwe	1,700,000
Tanzania	1,400,000
Kenya	1,300,000
United States	1,200,000
Zambia	1,100,000
Uganda	1,000,000
Democratic Republic of the Congo	1,000,000

Source: UNAIDS, 2006 Report on the Global AIDS Epidemic

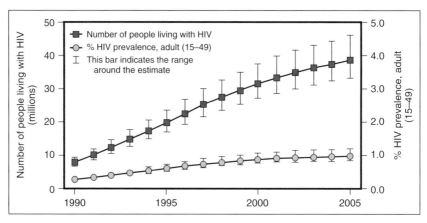

Figure 13-2.   Global trend in HIV prevalence. (Source: UNAIDS 2006 Report on the Global AIDS Epidemic.)

48% in 2005. Women accounted for more than 45% of adults with HIV in Sub-Saharan Africa (59%), the Caribbean (53%), North Africa and the Middle East (48%), and Oceania (47%) in 2005. The increasing proportion of HIV-infected women indicates a shift in the nature of epidemic, reflecting, in part, sociocultural differences between males and females. Because of gender inequities, women are often less able to protect themselves by abstaining from sex or using a condom during sex.

The proportion of youth aged 15 to 24 with HIV infection is also increasing in many regions of the world, and young women are particularly at risk because of the culture of silence surrounding sexuality, exploitive intergenerational sex, and violence against women in relationships.

Most children in the world with HIV infection acquired it through mother-to-child transmission. As a result, the epidemiology of pediatric HIV is similar to that of women of child-bearing age, with adjustments made for fertility and the availability of services to prevent vertical transmission. By the end of 2005, it was estimated that 87% of children under the age of 15 living with HIV were in Sub-Saharan Africa. Up to 35% of children born to HIV-seropositive mothers globally had been reported in the past to have acquired the infection, but this rate has been reduced to 1% to 2% in regions of the world where obstetric care and antiretroviral drugs are available.

In 2005, the majority of people with HIV infection lacked access to antiretroviral therapy. Advocacy and funding for treatment in resource-limited settings has increased substantially since about 2001, and prices of drugs and laboratory equipment and reagents have been reduced as a result. It was estimated that about 1.3 million people in low- and middle-income countries were receiving treatment at the end of 2005, representing about 20% of the estimated 6.8 million people requiring it. The impact of increasing access to treatment on the global epidemic remains to be determined, but programs in South Africa, Uganda, Cote d'Ivoire, and Haiti have demonstrated that antiretroviral therapy leads to higher rates of HIV testing and condom use. In addition, effective treatment, by lowering the amount of virus in the body, may lead to reduced HIV transmission. Extended survival of people with HIV may contribute to higher HIV prevalence, but this effect may be offset by reductions in prevalence if new infections are prevented.

Characterization of the Epidemic

HIV epidemics are characterized in as low-level, concentrated, or generalized. Appreciating these differences not only affects our understanding of the epidemic but also how prevention, care, and treatment programs are designed. In a low-level epidemic, HIV cases are reported in subpopulations, but the prevalence rate in any group does not consistently exceed 5%. Many terms are used to refer to subpopulations, including core groups, marginalized groups, vulnerable groups, and high-risk groups. Subpopulations may be identified by location, age, profession, structural factors such as poverty, or behavior. Low-level epidemics are usually observed where infections are confined to persons in high-risk networks, such as commercial sex workers, injection-drug users, men having sex with men, or in settings in which HIV was recently introduced. In a concentrated epidemic, the HIV prevalence rate among pregnant women in urban areas does not exceed 1%, but it consistently exceeds 5% in at least one subpopulation.

Concentrated epidemics are heterogeneous, with high transmission within certain subpopulations but minimal transmission within the general population. This concentrated epidemic state is considered a critical "tipping point," as the higher prevalence among subpopulations compared to a low-level setting increases the likelihood that transmission will cross over into the general population. A generalized epidemic is one in which the HIV prevalence rate among pregnant women consistently exceeds 1% (adult prevalence above 1% may be also used). In this instance, HIV is firmly established among sexually active adults through heterosexual transmission, although subpopulations may continue to experience higher prevalence rates than the general population.

The transition from a concentrated epidemic to a generalized epidemic is commonly thought to be facilitated by "bridge" populations that link subpopulations to the general population. Examples of bridge populations include male clients of commercial sex workers who also have regular partners, injection-drug users who share contaminated needles and also have unprotected sex with partners outside the risk group, and men who have sex with both men and women. Once an epidemic has moved into the general population, interventions focused on preventing HIV transmission among subpopulations may no longer be adequate to control it.

Methodology of Global Estimates

Global data on the HIV epidemic are published by UNAIDS in cooperation with national governments. UNAIDS uses surveys of pregnant women accessing antenatal services, population-based surveys, sentinel surveillance among high-risk groups, case reporting, vital registration systems, and other surveillance data to estimate HIV prevalence.

Surveillance of pregnant women accessing antenatal services is the key source of data for estimating HIV prevalence in generalized epidemics because they represent a cross-section of healthy, sexually active women in the general population. Validation studies suggest that estimates derived from antenatal clinics provide a good approximation of HIV prevalence among men and women aged 15 to 49. Potential drawbacks to this methodology are that pregnant women represent women having unprotected sex and may differ from those who consistently use condoms or abstain from sex; HIV-infected women experience declining fertility as their disease progresses and thus may be underrepresented in the sample; and surveillance may exclude women who access care from private facilities or who do not access antenatal services. To estimate the adult prevalence of HIV infection, antenatal clinic surveillance data are adjusted to reflect changes in fertility in HIV-infected women and different rates of HIV infection for men and women, and they may be stratified by geographic or epidemiologic characteristics of the population. Estimates of the probability of survival with HIV infection are used in conjunction with prevalence estimates to derive estimates of HIV incidence and AIDS-related deaths. Estimation of HIV prevalence, incidence, and AIDS-related deaths in children are based on the HIV prevalence among pregnant women, the probability of mother-to-child transmission, and the probability of survival in HIV-infected children.

Where epidemics are low-level or concentrated, estimation of HIV prevalence relies on data from sentinel surveillance among high-risk groups, such as men who have sex with men, commercial sex workers, and injection-drug users, as well as voluntary testing and counseling sites, antenatal screening, and case reports. Derivation of the adult HIV prevalence requires estimation of the prevalence for each high-risk group and estimation of the size of each group. When warranted, these estimations are done separately for different geographic areas. Since 2000, population-based HIV prevalence surveys have become increasingly available, especially in Sub-Saharan Africa. They have provided important new data resulting in substantial revisions in the prevalence estimates.

An understanding of the methods of estimation and presentation is required for meaningful interpretation of the data. The accuracy of each estimate is a function of the quality and coverage of the surveillance data, as well as the estimations used to adjust them. UNAIDS provides plausibility ranges for each estimate that reflect the degree of uncertainty around the point estimate. They are calculated separately for each country based on the nature of the epidemic, the quality of surveillance data, and the number of steps or assumptions required to derive an estimate. Changes in HIV/AIDS estimates over the years may reflect, to varying degrees, an increase in the amount and improvement in the quality of data from expanded surveillance systems, the evolution of estimation methods, and real differences in the nature of the epidemic. Variations in regional estimates reflect these contributing factors and may also be related to changing country classifications over time or across sources or inclusion or exclusion of countries based on data availability.

The latest data available from UNAIDS are estimates for the year 2005. Although UNAIDS presents plausibility ranges, for simplicity, point estimates were used in this chapter for discussions in the text and country-level calculations. To describe variations among countries, we used the UNAIDS 2005 estimates of national HIV prevalence among people aged 15 to 49 and population estimates for the mid-year 2005 population aged 15 to 49 from the United States Census Bureau International Database. Adult HIV prevalence was available for 148 countries. For 19 countries, the point prevalence was known only to be less than 0.1%. In these instances, we set the prevalence rate as 0.1% for calculations, so the estimates of HIV cases may be higher than the actual numbers.

Regional Epidemiology

Sub-Saharan Africa

UNAIDS estimated that there were 24.5 million adults and children living with HIV in Sub-Saharan Africa in 2005, representing about 63% of the global total. Approximately 6.1% of adults were HIV-infected, and about 59% of HIV-seropositive adults were female. There were 2.0 million deaths related to AIDS (see Table 13-1).

The latest release of country-level HIV prevalence data by UNAIDS for 2005, which included data for 42 countries in Sub-Saharan Africa, indicated that the epidemic was generalized in most countries; only six (Comoros, Madagascar, Mauritius, Mauritania, Senegal, and Somalia) had an estimated adult prevalence below 1% (Figure 13-3). There was wide variation across the region, with adult prevalence rates ranging from 0.1% in Comoros to 33.4% in Swaziland. Approximately 54% of people with HIV were residing in five countries: South Africa (22%); Nigeria (12%); Zimbabwe (7%); Mozambique (7%); and Tanzania (6%).

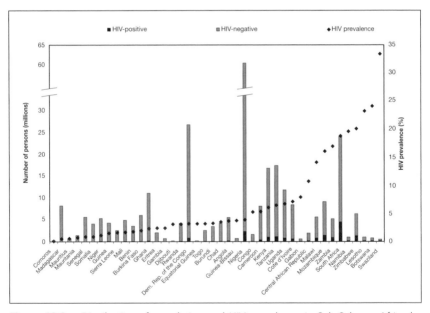

Figure 13-3.   Distribution of population and HIV prevalence in Sub-Saharan Africa by country, 2005. Note: UNAIDS estimated the adult HIV prevalence to be <0.1% in Comoros. HIV prevalence estimates were not available in 2005 for Liberia or Ethiopia, but prevalence was estimated to be in the range of 2.0% to 5.0% for Liberia and 0.9% to 3.5% for Ethiopia. Sources: Population estimates are from the US Census Bureau International Data Base. HIV prevalence estimates are from the UNAIDS 2006 Report on the Global AIDS Epidemic.

The most affected sub-region has been Southern Africa, which contains nine countries (Botswana, Lesotho, Malawi, Mozambique, Namibia, South Africa, Swaziland, Zambia, and Zimbabwe) with an estimated HIV prevalence among adults above 11%. Recent trends suggest a declining prevalence in only one country, Zimbabwe, and marked increases in prevalence in Mozambique, Namibia, South Africa, and Swaziland. South Africa, in particular, has been experiencing a rapidly expanding epidemic. With a population of about 24 million people between the ages of 15 to 49 and an HIV prevalence in this group of 18.8%, it was home to over 5.5 million HIV-infected people, which is nearly a quarter of the cases in Sub-Saharan Africa and second in number only to India worldwide.

In East Africa, adult HIV prevalence ranged from 0.9% in Somalia to 6.7% in Uganda. Recent trends suggest a declining prevalence of HIV in Kenya and stabilization of prevalence elsewhere in the sub-region. In West and Central Africa, adult prevalence ranged from 0.7% in Mauritania to 10.7% in the Central African Republic, the only country outside of Southern Africa with an estimated adult HIV prevalence exceeding 8%. Recent trends of prevalence among pregnant women suggest a stabilization of new infection rates. This sub-region contains Nigeria, which represents approximately 21% of the adult population of Sub-Saharan Africa and is home to 61 million people aged 15 to 49. The adult prevalence of 3.9% translated into about 2.9 million HIV-infected people, a number exceeded only by South Africa and India.

South and Southeast Asia

UNAIDS estimated that there were 7.6 million adults and children living with HIV in South and Southeast Asia in 2005, representing about 20% of the global total. Approximately 0.6% of adults were HIV-infected, and about 30% of HIV-seropositive adults were female. There were 560,000 deaths related to AIDS (see Table 13-1).

Compared to the generalized epidemic in sub-Saharan Africa, HIV infection in South and Southeast Asia is primarily concentrated in subpopulations characterized by injection-drug users and commercial sex workers. Evidence of a shift toward generalization of the epidemic in this region is cause for concern since it contains about one-third of the global adult population. Adult prevalence in 2005 was above 1% in three countries: Cambodia, Myanmar, and Thailand (Figure 13-4). The combined number of HIV cases among people aged 15 to 49 in these countries represented about 14% of the total cases in this group in the region. Thailand's prevention program has focused on the commercial sex industry, with a resulting decrease from 140,000 new infections in 1991 to 21,000 in 2003. However, their adult overall prevalence rate of 1.4% masks an increasing rate among injection-drug users, reported to be as

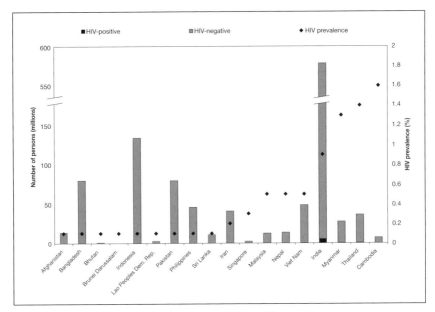

Figure 13-4. Distribution of population and HIV prevalence in South and Southeast Asia by country, 2005. Note: UNAIDS estimated the adult HIV prevalence to be <0.1% in Brunei Darussalam, Bhutan Sri Lanka, and the Philippines. Sources: Population estimates are from the US Census Bureau International Data Base. HIV prevalence estimates are from the UNAIDS 2006 Report on the Global AIDS Epidemic.

high as 45% in one study and representing a shift toward generalization of the epidemic.

India, with an adult HIV prevalence rate of less than 1% but a population aged 15 to 49 of over 1 billion people, was home to about 5.7 million HIV-infected people in 2005. This was the highest disease burden in the world. Within India, there is considerable variation in HIV prevalence and the pattern of the epidemic. Sexual transmission is the most common route. Although the epidemic is low-level in the majority of states, there is evidence that HIV is moving from high-risk groups into the general population, resulting in an increased incidence in rural settings and among women. As of 2003, three states, Goa, Gujarat, and Pondicherry, were experiencing a concentrated epidemic, and 6 states (Manipur and Nagaland in the north, and Andhra Pradesh, Karnataka, Maharashtra, and Tamil Nadu in the south) were experiencing a generalized epidemic. The epidemic in the southern states has been mostly via heterosexual transmission. In the northern states, the prevalence rate is highest among injection-drug users.

Latin America

UNAIDS estimated that there were 1.6 million adults and children living with HIV in Latin America in 2005, representing about 4% of the global total. Approximately 0.5% of adults were HIV-infected, and about 30% of HIV-seropositive adults were female. There were 59,000 deaths related to AIDS (see Table 13-1).

The HIV epidemic in Latin America is primarily concentrated among men who have sex with men, injection-drug users, and commercial sex workers, and in urban areas and along transport routes. Increasing prevalence among women and a decreasing male-to-female ratio among those with AIDS suggests that the epidemic is expanding into the general population in several countries. The adult prevalence of HIV was above 1% in four countries (Belize, Guyana, Honduras, and Suriname) in 2005, but the combined number of people aged 15 to 49 with HIV infection represented just 5% of the total cases in this group in Latin America. Meanwhile, close to 70% of HIV cases among people aged 15 to 49 in the region were in four countries: Brazil (38%), Mexico (12%), Colombia (10%), and Argentina (9%).

Eastern Europe and Central Asia

UNAIDS estimated that there were 1.5 million adults and children living with HIV in Eastern Europe and Central Asia in 2005, representing about 4% of the global total. Approximately 0.8% of adults were HIV-infected, and about 28% of HIV-seropositive adults were female. There were 53,000 deaths related to AIDS (see Table 13-1).

Many countries in the Eastern Europe and Central Asia region are in a low-level phase of the epidemic, with cases primarily among injection-drug users, commercial sex workers, incarcerated persons, and youth. About 90% of HIV cases among people aged 15 to 49 in the region in 2005 were in the Russian Federation (64%) and the Ukraine (25%). Ukraine has the highest prevalence (1.4%), followed by Estonia (1.3%), the Republic of Moldova (1.1%), and the Russian Federation (1.1%). Notably, prison populations in the Russian Federation have an HIV prevalence that is four times the national rate. The epidemic in the Russian Federation, while still concentrated, shows signs of becoming increasingly generalized and, like other countries in the region, appears to be driven by heterosexual transmission.

North America

UNAIDS estimated that there were 1.3 million adults and children living with HIV in North America in 2005, representing about 3% of the global total. Approximately 0.8% of adults were HIV-infected, and about 26% of HIV-seropositive adults were female. There were 18,000 deaths related to AIDS (see Table 13-1).

The epidemic in North America is primarily concentrated in men who have sex with men, injection-drug users, and, to a growing extent, people of color. The epidemic in this region is driven predominantly by the United States, which contained about 90% of the people aged 15 to 49 in 2005 and about 95% of those aged 15 to 49 with HIV infection. African Americans comprised 12.5% of the population in the United States but 48% of new HIV cases in 2003; AIDS is among the top three causes of death among African American men aged 25 to 54 and is the leading cause of death among African American women aged 25 to 34.

East Asia

UNAIDS estimated that there were 680,000 adults and children living with HIV in East Asia in 2005, representing about 2% of the global total. Approximately 0.1% of adults were HIV-infected, and about 28% of HIV-seropositive adults were female. There were 33,000 deaths related to AIDS (see Table 13-1).

Similar to South and Southeast Asia, East Asia's epidemic is primarily concentrated among injection-drug users and commercial sex workers. Estimated adult HIV prevalence rates were 0.1% or less for all countries in the region in 2005. China was home to about 90% of people aged 15 to 49 and 90% of HIV cases in the same age group. Transmission via injection-drug use was responsible for about 44% of HIV cases in China in 2003. HIV prevalence among women has increased in recent years, reflecting the bridging of transmission from commercial sex workers and injection-drug users into the general population.

Western and Central Europe

UNAIDS estimated that there were 720,000 adults and children living with HIV in Western and Central Europe in 2005, about 2% of the global total. Approximately 0.3% of adults were HIV-infected, and about 28% of HIV-seropositive adults were female. There were 12,000 deaths related to AIDS (see Table 13-1).

Among the countries in Western and Central Europe with data from 2005, France, Italy, and Spain together accounted for about 60% of HIV cases among people aged 15 to 49. These three countries, together with Switzerland and Portugal, had the highest adult prevalence in the region. In the Western Europe sub-region, the epidemic is shifting, with heterosexual contact now the leading cause of new infections, particularly among women. Men having sex with men remained the leading risk behavior in Denmark, Germany, Greece, and the Netherlands in 2004. A substantial number of reported HIV cases were among people or sexual partners of people from regions (predominantly Sub-Saharan Africa) with generalized epidemics. This trend was responsible for about 62% of the 8879 reported HIV cases from heterosexual transmission in the sub-region in 2004.

Central Europe has remained minimally affected by the HIV epidemic. Among cases reported in the sub-region in 2004 with a known transmission cause, heterosexual contact was the most frequent (50%), followed by injection-drug use (22%) and men having sex with men (21%). In contrast to Western Europe, only 9% of the 302 reported HIV cases in the sub-region in 2004 from heterosexual transmission were among people or sexual partners of people from countries with generalized epidemics.

North Africa and the Middle East

UNAIDS estimated that there were 440,000 adults and children living with HIV in North Africa and the Middle East in 2005, representing about 1% of the global total. Approximately 0.2% of adults were HIV-infected, and about 48% of HIV-seropositive adults were female. There were 37,000 deaths related to AIDS (see Table 13-1).

Transmission is predominantly through unprotected sex. Most of the region is experiencing a low-level epidemic, with higher prevalence rates among diffuse subpopulations characterized by injection-drug use, commercial sex workers, and men having sex with men. According to 2005 estimates, 78% of HIV cases among people aged 15 to 49 in the region were in Sudan, where just 18% of people in this age group lived, which also had the highest (1.6%) prevalence in the region. Prevalence in all other countries in the region did not exceed 0.1%.

The Caribbean

UNAIDS estimated that there were 330,000 adults and children living with HIV in the Caribbean in 2005, representing less than 1% of the global total. Approximately 1.6% of adults were HIV-infected, and about 53% of HIV-seropositive adults were female. There were 27,000 deaths related to AIDS (see Table 13-1).

Among the countries with available data in 2005, Haiti had the highest adult HIV prevalence (3.8%) and the greatest number of cases (about 190,000) among people aged 15 to 49. Haiti contained just 22% of the population aged 15 to 49 among countries in the region with data but about 59% of HIV cases in the same age group. Approximately 21% of people aged 15 to 49 with HIV were living in the Dominican Republic (1.1% adult prevalence rate), and fewer than 10% were in each of the remaining countries, where adult prevalence ranged from 1.5 to 3.3%, with the exception of Cuba (0.1%).

Oceania

UNAIDS estimated that there were 78,000 adults and children living with HIV in Oceania in 2005, representing less than 1% of the global total. Approximately 0.3% of adults were HIV-infected, and about 47% of HIV-seropositive adults were female. There were 3400 deaths related to AIDS (see Table 13-1).

Country-level data for 2005 are available for Australia, Fiji, Papua New Guinea, and New Zealand. In these countries, adult prevalence was highest in Papua New Guinea (1.8%) and estimated to be about 0.1% in the others. Papua New Guinea contained about 18% of the population aged 15 to 49 among countries in the region but 80% of HIV cases in the same age group. Australia was home to about 65% of people aged 15 to 49 and 16% of HIV cases in the same age group. Transmission in Papua New Guinea appears related to heterosexual commercial and casual sex networks. In contrast, the epidemic in Australia has been characterized by transmission among men having sex with men; however, heterosexual transmission has increased in recent years, leading to more new HIV cases in women.

KEY POINTS

- 38.6 million people worldwide were living with HIV at the end of 2005.
- 4.1 million people acquired new HIV infections during 2005, and 2.8 million people died of an AIDS-related cause.
- Sub-Saharan Africans represent about 10% of the global population, but they constitute 63% of the people with HIV, 66% of new HIV infections, 76% of women with HIV, 87% of children with HIV, and 71% of those who died from AIDS.
- The global incidence of HIV infection stabilized after peaking in the late 1990s, and the prevalence has been constant at about 1% since 2001. However, the total number of people living with HIV is still increasing.
- The proportion of women among adults with HIV infection continues to grow as transmission crosses over from concentrated epidemics into the general population.

SUGGESTED READINGS

EuroHIV (2005) HIV/AIDS Surveillance in Europe: End-year report 2004, No. 71. European Centre for the Epidemiological Monitoring of AIDS.

Grassly NC, Morgan M, Walker N, Garnett G, Stanecki KA, et al. (2004) Uncertainty in estimates of HIV/AIDS: the estimation and application of plausibility bounds. Sex Transm Infect. 80 Suppl 1: i31-38.

National AIDS Control Organization (2005) An Overview of the Spread and Prevalence of HIV/AIDS in India. Government of India, Ministry of Health and Family Welfare.

National AIDS Control Organization (2004) Annual Report, 2002-2003, 2003-2004. Government of India, Ministry of Health and Family Welfare.

Punpanich W, Ungchusak K, Detels R. (2004) Thailand's response to the HIV epidemic: yesterday, today, and tomorrow. AIDS Educ Prev 16: 119-136.

UNAIDS (2006) 2006 Report on the global AIDS epidemic. Geneva: Joint United Nations Programme on HIV/AIDS (UNAIDS).

UNAIDS (2005) Understanding the latest estimates of the global AIDS epidemic: background on methodology. Geneva: Joint United Nations Programme on HIV/AIDS (UNAIDS).

UNAIDS/UNFPA/UNIFEM (2004) Women and HIV/AIDS: Confronting the Crisis. Geneva and New York: Joint United Nations Programme on HIV/AIDS (UNAIDS), United Nations Population Fund (UNFPA), and United Nations Development Fund for Women (UNIFEM).

UNICEF (2005) Children: the missing face of AIDS. New York: The United Nations Children's Fund (UNICEF).

Walker N, Grassly NC, Garnett GP, Stanecki KA, Ghys PD. Estimating the global burden of HIV/AIDS: What do we really know about the HIV pandemic? Lancet. 2004;363:2180-2185.

WHO (2006) Progress on global access to antiretroviral therapy, an update on "3 by 5." Geneva: World Health Organization (WHO).

Chapter 14

Clinical Considerations in Developing Countries

LISA A. COSIMI, MD

More than 20 years into the AIDS epidemic, there are over 40 million people living with HIV infection worldwide. Despite the availability of antiretroviral therapy in developed countries and increasing access to it in developing counties, the epidemic continues to grow. As evidence, 4.9 million new infections and 3.1 million deaths were reported in 2005 (see Chapter 13). Two-thirds of HIV-infected people live in Central and Sub-Saharan Africa, and there are a growing number of cases in Eastern Europe and in Central and East Asia. With the increasing mobility of the global community, it is important for physicians to be cognizant of issues related to the worldwide epidemic. This chapter addresses the clinical manifestations of HIV infection around the world, particularly focusing on conditions that are seen less commonly in developed countries. Clinical manifestations of HIV infection in the developed world are discussed in Chapter 8, opportunistic infections in Chapter 9, and opportunistic cancers in Chapter 10.

Course of HIV Disease

The manifestations of early HIV infection appear to be similar in developing and developed countries, but disease progression is often more rapid in the former. There is a consensus that poverty is to some degree responsible for this disparity, although its effect may be difficult to quantify. Given the relative lack of medical infrastructure and services in many developing countries, HIV-infected patients may delay seeking health care and present with more advanced disease. There is often higher mortality from treatable conditions, such as community-acquired pneumonia, compared to that reported in developed countries.

Although there has been considerable debate, it is believed that the time from HIV seroconversion to the onset of AIDS is similar in developing and developed countries. However, multiple studies have demonstrated that survival is shorter in the former, with an average of 9 months in patients with advanced disease reported in developing countries compared to

20 months in developed countries. It is unknown whether this disparity is related only to inadequate health resources or whether specific factors such as malnutrition and untreated opportunistic infections play a role.

Clinical Manifestations

Respiratory

Respiratory complications of HIV infection are described worldwide. The most common etiologies reported are tuberculosis (TB) and pneumonias caused by *Streptococcus pneumoniae* and *Pneumocystis jiroveci* (formerly *carinii* [PCP]). Other respiratory pathogens reported in developed countries occur less frequently in developing countries.

Gastrointestinal

Diarrhea is the most common cause of morbidity in HIV-infected persons worldwide. It may be caused by bacterial, viral, or parasitic infections or be a manifestation of drug toxicity. *Cryptosporidium parvum* and microsporidia are frequently reported in HIV-infected patients in developing countries. In addition, non-typhoid *Salmonella* is common in areas where sanitation is poor and can be a cause of chronic diarrhea. In advanced HIV disease, diarrhea may be a manifestation of TB or *Mycobacterium avium* complex (MAC) infection.

Genitourinary

Herpes simplex virus infection, which may be severe and recurrent in patients with advanced HIV disease, is common worldwide. In the past, likely related to the lack of surveillance and a short survival time, the incidence of cervical dysplasia was not reported to be high in developing countries. However, with a growing epidemic and the increasing availability of antiretroviral therapy, it is expected that HIV-infected women will be living longer and that more cervical disease will be identified.

Neurologic

Meningitis associated with TB and cryptococcal infection is common throughout the world. In Thailand, cryptococcal disease is the most common reason for hospitalization of HIV-infected patients. Space-occupying lesions are also seen worldwide, and although definitive diagnosis is not made in many cases, they are generally attributed to toxoplasmosis, TB, and lymphoma.

Fever

One of the most common clinical manifestations of HIV infection is fever without localizing symptoms or signs. The differential diagnosis is broad and depends on the patient's degree of immunodeficiency and geographic location, but TB should always be considered. Other common etiologies include non-typhoid *Salmonella* infection and pneumococcal bacteremia. In African series, bacteremia has been reported in up to 42% of HIV-infected patients presenting with fever. Fungal causes include cryptococcal infection, histoplasmosis, and *Penicillium marneffei* (PM) infection (see below). PCP may present with fever, and, although less common in developing countries, should be considered in the differential diagnosis. In patients living in or traveling from the Mediterranean region and other endemic areas, visceral leishmaniasis (VL) (see below) should be included in patients with advanced immunodeficiency. MAC and cytomegalovirus (CMV) infections are also in the differential diagnosis.

Neoplastic Diseases

Kaposi's sarcoma, caused by Kaposi's sarcoma herpesvirus/human herpesvirus-8 (KSHV/HHV8), and non-Hodgkin's lymphoma are the most common neoplastic complications of HIV infection worldwide. There is marked regional variation with regards to the prevalence of KSHV/HHV8 infection. It is described in East and Central Africa but rarely reported in Southeast Asia. Limited data from Africa suggest that non-Hodgkin's lymphoma occurs at a lower prevalence than that reported in developed countries prior to the advent of effective combination antiretroviral therapy. However, this observation may be the result of patients dying earlier from other causes or the lack of diagnostic capabilities.

Selected Infections

Tuberculosis

Tuberculosis is the most important cause of morbidity and mortality in HIV-infected patients worldwide and the leading cause of death in this population in Sub-Saharan Africa. In 2005, the World Health Organization (WHO) declared the TB epidemic in Africa to be a regional emergency. TB control methods appear to be failing, and incidence rates have been increasing every year. In addition to Africa, expanding TB epidemics have been reported in India, Eastern Europe, and Southeast Asia. TB should be considered in the differential diagnosis of a wide range of clinical manifestations in HIV-infected patients who have emigrated from developing countries.

Clinical Manifestations

As described elsewhere, the interaction between TB and HIV disease is complex. TB is associated with higher HIV viral load levels, more rapid HIV disease progression, and increased mortality. In addition, HIV-infected patients with *Mycobacterium tuberculosis* infection are much more likely to develop active TB and, in advanced HIV disease, to have atypical pulmonary manifestations and extrapulmonary involvement. This broad disease spectrum often makes the diagnosis and treatment of TB in developing countries, where patients often present for care late, problematic.

Management

Treatment recommendations for TB are described elsewhere, and expert consultation is advised for clinicians with limited experience in its management. The increasing availability of antiretroviral therapy in developing countries may play an important role in addressing the TB epidemic. Antiretroviral therapy reduces the risk of active TB through restoration of pathogen-specific immune responses. However, if antiretroviral therapy is started in the context of TB treatment, the clinician should be cognizant of potential drug interactions and overlapping toxicities.

Of increasing interest worldwide is the immune reconstitution syndrome, which has been described with the initiation of antiretroviral therapy in patients with advanced HIV disease. Previously unrecognized subclinical opportunistic diseases such as TB may "flare" in this setting. This syndrome has also been described with cryptococcal disease and MAC and CMV infections. In a recent series from Thailand, immune reconstitution syndrome was reported in 13% of patients starting antiretroviral therapy, the majority of whom had disseminated TB. Management includes continuation of both antiretroviral and antituberculous therapies in conjunction with nonsteroidal anti-inflammatory drugs and/or corticosteroids.

Pneumocystis jerovici Pneumonia

In developed countries, PCP has historically been the most common opportunistic infection associated with HIV disease. Prior to the widespread use of trimethoprim-sulfamethoxazole prophylaxis, an estimated 75% of HIV-infected patients would develop PCP in their lifetime. In many developing countries, PCP remains a common opportunistic infection. Early studies, especially from Africa, reported that PCP was an infrequent complication of HIV disease, with prevalence rates ranging from 4% to 22%. However, more recent studies in Africa and elsewhere in the world suggest that PCP now accounts for a greater percentage of opportunistic infections, with prevalence rates ranging from 27% to 55%. It is unknown whether this increased prevalence is the result of better study design or diagnostic techniques or represents a true epidemiologic trend. The few studies that have examined clinical manifestations of PCP in the developing world suggest that it presents in typical fashion, but coinfection with other pathogens such as TB is higher. Treatment of PCP is the same as in developed countries.

Penicillium marneffei Infection

Epidemiology and Pathogenesis

Penicillium marneffei infection is common among HIV-infected patients living or traveling within Southeast Asia. The causative dimorphic fungus was discovered in bamboo rats in 1956. PM infection in humans was first identified in HIV-infected persons in 1988 and has now been reported increasingly throughout Southeast Asia, South China, and Taiwan. It is the third most frequent opportunistic infection after TB and cryptococcal meningitis in northern Thailand. Within Southeast Asia, PM infection is considered an AIDS-defining illness. It occurs late in the course of HIV disease, with patients usually having a CD4 count of less than 50 cells/mm^3. PM appears to infect the lungs initially and then disseminates hematogenously to other organs.

Clinical Manifestations

Penicillium marneffei infection commonly presents with fever, weight loss, lymphadenopathy, hepatosplenomegaly, and characteristic skin lesions. The lesions are papules with central necrotic umbilication distributed predominantly on the face, neck, and trunk and less often on the arms and legs. Lesions may sometimes manifest as pustules, abscesses, nodules, or ulcers. Mucous membrane involvement has also been described. Cutaneous PM lesions need to be distinguished from molluscum contagiosum and lesions associated with other opportunistic infections, including cryptococcosis, blastomycosis, histoplasmosis, and TB.

Diagnosis

Patients with PM infection often have anemia and sometimes lymphopenia, thrombocytopenia, and increased serum transaminase levels. Diagnosis is made by identifying the fungus from a clinical specimen on smear, histopathology, or culture. The organism may be isolated from skin, blood, lymph nodes, bone marrow, liver, or sputum. A rapid presumptive diagnosis can be made by Wright staining of a scraping from a typical skin lesion or of a bone marrow aspirate. Definitive diagnosis is made by growth of the organism in culture.

Management

The mortality rate of patients with PM infection is high without early diagnosis and treatment. Standard treatment consists of amphotericin B 0.6-1 mg/kg/day intravenously for 2 weeks, followed by itraconazole 200 mg orally bid for 10 weeks. Secondary prophylaxis is continued with itraconazole 200 mg/day, but it may be discontinued in patients who become immune reconstituted on antiretroviral therapy. There is no standard rec-ommendation for the use of itraconazole as primary prophylaxis for HIV-infected patients residing in or traveling to endemic areas.

Leishmaniasis

Epidemiology and Pathogenesis
Visceral leishmaniasis is the type of this infection most commonly associ-ated with HIV disease. Although VL has been reported in over 30 countries, the majority of cases originate in the Mediterranean region, where 3% to 7% of patients were affected prior to the introduction of antiretroviral therapy. While cases in Europe are now less frequent, they are being reported in-creasingly in East Africa and India.

Visceral leishmaniasis is caused by intracelluar protozoan of the genus *Leishmania*. Most infections are caused by *L. donovani, L. infantum,* or *L. chagasi.* The parasites commonly infect the human host through a bite from an infected sand fly; however, the majority of cases in Europe have been associated with injection-drug use. VL may also be contracted by blood transfusion and sexual transmission. After the parasites enter the bloodstream, they infect cells of the reticuloendothelial system. When these cells rupture, the parasites widely disseminate.

Clinical Manifestations
Visceral leishmaniasis is the most severe form of the disease and has a mor-tality rate of nearly 100% in the absence of treatment. It usually occurs in HIV-infected patients with a CD4 count of less than 200 cells/mm³. Symptoms and signs of VL include fever, anorexia, weight loss, abdominal pain, diarrhea, hepatosplenomegaly, lymphadenopathy, and nonspecific skin lesions.

Diagnosis
Laboratory findings of VL are nonspecific and may include pancytopenia, increased serum transaminase levels, and hyperbilirubinemia. Biopsy and staining of involved organs may reveal granulomatous inflammation with intracellular amastigotes. Splenic aspiration is the most sensitive diagnostic procedure followed by bone marrow biopsy. Skin biopsy should be per-formed if lesions are present. Parasites may occasionally be found in leuko-cytes on peripheral blood smear, and blood cultures may also be positive.

Management
Pentavalent antimonies (stibogluconate or meglumine antimonate) are the most commonly used drugs to treat VL. Amphotericin B at a dose of 0.7 mg/kg/day intravenously for 28 days is also effective. Treatment should be continued for 28 days, and relapse is common without suppressive therapy. Drugs used for secondary prophylaxis of VL include stibogluconate or meg-

lumine antimonate 20 mg/kg intravenously or intramuscularly once per month or liposomal amphotericin B 3 mg/kg every 21 days.

KEY POINTS

- The rate of progression of HIV infection to AIDS in developing countries is the same as in developed countries. However, survival after the onset of AIDS is shorter in developing countries.
- The differential diagnosis of an HIV-related clinical problem should take into account the immunologic state of the patient, as well as the geographic region of residence or origin. TB, pneumococcal disease, PCP, cryptococcal infection, and non-typhoid *Salmonella* infection are important causes of morbidity and mortality worldwide.
- *Penicillium marneffei* infection is common in Southeast Asia and presents with fever, weight loss, and characteristic skin lesions with central necrotic umbilication.
- Visceral leishmaniasis presents with fever, weight loss, organomegaly, and pancytopenia. It should be considered in patients living in or returning from travel to the Mediterranean region, East Africa, or India.

SUGGESTED READINGS

General
Clezy K, Sirisanthana T, Sirisanthana V, Brew B, Cooper DA. Late manifestations of HIV in Asia and the Pacific. AIDS. 1994;8 Suppl 2:S35-43.
Dal Maso L, Serraino D, Franceschi S. Epidemiology of AIDS-related tumours in developed and developing countries. Eur J Cancer. 2001;37:1188-201.
Gilks CF. HIV care in non-industrialised countries. Br Med Bull. 2001;58:171-86.
Grant AD, Djomand G, De Cock KM. Natural history and spectrum of disease in adults with HIV/AIDS in Africa. AIDS. 1997;11 Suppl B:S43-54.
Orem J, Otieno MW, Remick SC. AIDS-associated cancer in developing nations. Curr Opin Oncol. 2004;16:468-76.
Ruxrungtham K, Brown T, Phanuphak P. HIV/AIDS in Asia. Lancet. 2004;364:69-82.
Sibanda EN, Stanczuk G, Kasolo F. HIV/AIDS in Central Africa: pathogenesis, immunological and medical issues. Int Arch Allergy Immunol. 2003;132:183-95.

Tuberculosis
Aaron L, Saadoun D, Calatroni I, Launay O, Mémain N, Vincent V, et al. Tuberculosis in HIV-infected patients: a comprehensive review. Clin Microbiol Infect. 2004;10:388-98.
Lawn SD, Bekker LG, Miller RF. Immune reconstitution disease associated with mycobacterial infections in HIV-infected individuals receiving antiretrovirals. Lancet Infect Dis. 2005;5:361-73.
Lawn SD, Wood R. Incidence of tuberculosis during highly active antiretroviral therapy in high-income and low-income countries [Editorial]. Clin Infect Dis. 2005;41:1783-6.
Manosuthi W, Kiertiburanakul S, Phoorisri T, et al. Immune reconstitution inflammatory syndrome of tuberculosis among HIV-infected patients receiving antituberculous and anti-retroviral therapy. J Infect 2006;53:357-63.

Murray JF. Pulmonary complications of HIV-1 infection among adults living in Sub-Saharan Africa. Int J Tuberc Lung Dis. 2005;8:826-35.

World Health Organization (WHO). WHO declares TB an emergency in Africa: call for "urgent and extraordinary actions" to halt a worsening epidemic 2 Sept 2005. http://www.who.int/mediacentre/news/2005/africa_emergency/en/.

Pneumocystis jiroveci Pneumonia

Fisk DT, Meshnick S, Kazanjian PH. Pneumocystis carinii pneumonia in patients in the developing world who have acquired immunodeficiency syndrome. Clin Infect Dis. 2003;36:70-8.

Morris A, Lundgren JD, Masur H, Walzer PD, Hanson DL, Frederick T, et al. Current epidemiology of Pneumocystis pneumonia. Emerg Infect Dis. 2004;10:1713-20.

Penicillium marneffei Infection

Chariyalertsak S, Supparatpinyo K, Sirisanthana T, Nelson KE. A controlled trial of itraconazole as primary prophylaxis for systemic fungal infections in patients with advanced human immunodeficiency virus infection in Thailand. Clin Infect Dis. 2002;34:277-84.

Sirisanthana T, Supparatpinyo K. Epidemiology and management of penicilliosis in human immunodeficiency virus-infected patients. Int J Infect Dis. 1998;3:48-53.

Supparatpinyo K, Perriens J, et al. A controlled trial of itraconazole to prevent relapse of Penicillium marneffei infection in patients infected with the human immunodeficiency virus. N Engl J Med. 1998;330:1739-1743.

Vanittanakom N, Cooper CR, et al. Penicillium marneffei infection and recent advances in the epidemiology and molecular biology aspects. Clin Micro Rev. 2006;19(1);95-110.

Leishmaniasis

Desjeux P. Leishmaniasis: current situation and new perspectives. Comp Immunol Microbiol Infect Dis. 2004;27:305-18.

Desjeux P, Alvar J. Leishmania/HIV co-infections; epidemiology in Europe. Ann Trop Med Parasitol. 2002;97 Supp 1:S3-S15.

Russo R, Laguna F, Lopez-Velez R, et al. Visceral leishmaniasis in those infected with HIV: clinical aspects and other opportunistic infections. Ann Trop Med Parasitol. 2002;97 Supp 1:S99-S105.

Chapter 15

Antiretroviral Treatment in Resource-Limited Settings

WILLIAM RODRIGUEZ, MD

Effective combination antiretroviral therapy (ART) has been widely available in the United States and other developed countries since 1996 but remains inaccessible to most HIV-infected patients around the world. In 2006, more than 40 million people were living with HIV infection worldwide. Of those, an estimated 6.5 million had advanced disease and were in need of ART, but only 1.3 million (20%) were receiving treatment. This seemingly bleak situation actually represented significant progress realized over the prior few years.

The natural history and recommended treatment of HIV infection vary little from country to country, though there are a few notable exceptions. There is some evidence that subtype D may be slightly more virulent than other subtypes, and it is associated with more rapid development of nonnucleoside reverse-transcriptase inhibitor (NNRTI) resistance. HIV-2 infection, which has been reported mostly in West Africa, may not be susceptible to all classes of ART. The most important distinction in developing countries is the high prevalence of coinfection with tuberculosis (TB), which complicates the diagnosis and management of HIV infection. This chapter reviews the use of ART in resource-limited settings; Chapter 16 addresses barriers to implementing care.

History of Response to the Global HIV Epidemic

Between 1995 and 2000, global inertia greatly hindered efforts to provide ART to HIV-infected patients worldwide. A general misperception held that, once a person with minimal resources became infected with HIV, nothing could be done to treat his/her disease. Instead, the public health response focused on uninfected people. Educational and behavioral change campaigns were implemented in several countries, most notably Brazil, Thailand, and Uganda. In many nations, even these efforts were limited by stigma, a lack of political will, and a lack of urgency. Although reports filtered out from some countries of a leveling off in HIV prevalence, in general these educational campaigns were unable to reduce the number of new HIV cases, and incidence rates continued to climb. They also had no effect on people already living with and, increasingly, dying from HIV disease. By 2006, the number of new infections (4,900,000 per year) and the number of HIV-related deaths (3,100,000 per year) were both at an all-time high and climbing.

There were exceptions to the widespread indifference to the plight of HIV-infected persons. In some middle-income countries, national HIV treatment campaigns were launched based on standards of care recognized by high-income countries. In Brazil, as in the United States, the HIV epidemic emerged in homosexual men in the 1980s. When effective combination ART became available in 1996, Brazil launched a national program of free, universal access to the drugs for all HIV-infected citizens. Within a year, the HIV-related mortality rate began dropping, and by 1998 the incidence rate had fallen. A few other national governments displayed similar foresight and political will. The Bahamas offered universal access to ART in 2000. In 2001, Thailand started to provide ART through its public health system and scaled up from 3000 to 80,000 patients over five years.

In many countries, pilot programs for delivering ART to HIV-infected patients were initiated outside of the public sector through nongovernmental organizations (NGOs) and private companies, many of which were facing high rates of employee absenteeism and death. Two of the most influential programs were started by Partners In Health (PIH), an NGO based in Boston, and the multinational medical aid agency Médecins Sans Frontières (MSF).

In 1996, PIH and its Haitian partner NGO, Zanmi Lasante (ZL), began treating poor HIV-infected patients with ART. Recognizing that the cost of drugs and the enormous logistical difficulties in procuring them limited their ability to treat the growing number of patients, they launched the HIV Equity Initiative in 1998. The HIV Equity Initiative affirmed the principle that HIV-infected people living in low-income settings had as much right to treatment as anyone else. It also set out to provide universal access to ART for its patients and to demonstrate that quality care was possible in challenging settings such as rural Haiti, beset by poverty, civil strife, and a dysfunctional public health system. Clinical outcomes in the first 100 treated patients were comparable with those in developed countries. Although small, this pilot program helped establish proof of the concept that HIV treatment was possible for all who needed it. Of equal significance was the model PIH and ZL devised to deliver care. It used paid community health workers (referred to locally as "accompagnateurs") to help deliver ART to patients with daily visits for adherence support and symptom monitoring. Community-based health care delivery became the cornerstone of HIV care in Haiti.

By contrast, Médecins Sans Frontières (MSF) is a global organization widely recognized for providing medical services in wars, genocides, and natural disasters. Fresh from its Nobel Peace Prize in 1999, MSF launched its Campaign for Access to Essential Medicines, which was aimed at increasing access to anti-infective drugs and other life-saving medicines in low-income countries. Taking on chronic disease treatment for the first time, MSF included ART in the campaign. By 2000, it had also launched HIV treatment programs at sites in Cameroon, Thailand, and South Africa. Like the HIV Equity Initiative in Haiti, MSF provided universal access to care and reported excellent clinical outcomes, including 93% one-year survival in the sickest AIDS patients and viral suppression in 82% of those treated. MSF's largest South African site, in the township of Khayelitsha near Cape Town, became a flagship treatment program. Within three years, 1700 people were on ART, 70% of whom remained on their initial regimen after three years of treatment. By 2006, MSF was providing ART to more than 57,000 patients in 29 countries.

At the international AIDS conference in Durban, South Africa, in the summer of 2000, the early efforts of PIH, MSF, and dozens of similar, less publicized pilot programs took root. Momentum grew for a truly global campaign to provide ART to all HIV-infected people in need of treatment through the public sector, run by national governments and supported by the international donor community. By the next international AIDS conference in Barcelona in 2002, the tide had largely turned. Reports from these programs showed convincingly that quality HIV care was possible worldwide, even with minimal infrastructure and limited laboratory support. Brazil put forth the argument that ART, while expensive, was actually economical in the long term, with an estimated $2 billion in health expenditure savings from reduced hospitalizations. The international community had also come to realize the economic importance of providing ART worldwide. The Global Fund to Fight AIDS, TB, and Malaria was launched in early 2002, with several billion dollars pledged from developed countries to support HIV treatment.

The small, land-locked, southern African nation of Botswana became the global HIV treatment "canary" in 2002. Because of its location in sub-Saharan Africa and staggeringly high HIV prevalence rate (more than one in three adult Botswanans were HIV-infected), the decision of its government to offer ART to all HIV-infected citizens in need of treatment caught the attention of the world. Although Brazil, Cuba, and Thailand had launched similar programs a few years earlier, Botswana's *Masa* ("new dawn") was the first public ART program in Africa. *Masa* started sluggishly but was supported strongly by the government and philanthropic funding from the Bill & Melinda Gates and Merck Foundations. By late 2004, 30,000 HIV-infected Botswanan adults were on ART, including more than 13,000 people at the largest treatment site in Gabarone. By 2006, 32 public clinics throughout the country were providing HIV care to more than 56,000 infected people. Several sub-Saharan African countries, including Malawi, Rwanda, and Uganda, were quick to follow suit. Even South Africa with its 5 million HIV-infected citizens, long criticized for delayed action,

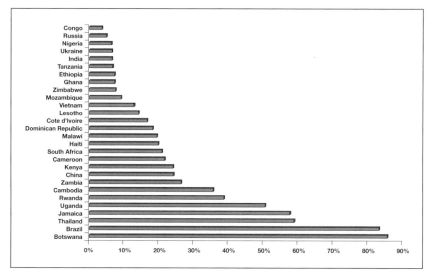

Figure 15-1. Coverage rates of antiretroviral therapy by March 2006.

committed to a national HIV care program in 2004 and brought 200,000 people into treatment within three years.

The launch of the World Health Organization's (WHO's) "3 by 5" Initiative on World AIDS Day 2003 marked a shift in the argument from whether HIV treatment should be provided worldwide to how it should be done and how quickly could it be accomplished. WHO advocated strongly for the enrollment of 3 million HIV-infected people into ART-based care by the end of 2005. Although efforts fell short of this target, radical change had occurred in just five years. By 2006, national programs had been launched in every country in the world, 1.3 million people were on ART, and $8.3 billion was being spent on HIV care annually. Still, this progress marked only the first steps of an effective global response to the epidemic. The number of deaths and new infections continues to rise, only 20% coverage has been achieved with 5 million people still in need of care, and available funding is $10 billion per year short of the projected need (Figure 15-1).

HIV Care in Resource-Limited Settings

Resource constraints and the prevalence of TB impose a modified approach to clinical care of HIV-infected patients in developing countries. Ironically, the premium on resources means that evidence-based care is even more critical. The earliest treatment programs generally adhered to United States Department of Health and Human Services (DHHS) guidelines. Preferred first-line regimens included two nucleoside reverse-transcriptase inhibitors (NRTIs) given with an NNRTI or a protease inhibitor (PI). Eligibility was determined by a combination of clinical staging and CD4 cell count; some programs, such as Botswana's *Masa*, also incorporated viral load measurements into the eligibility criteria. No limitations were put on drug regimen choices or laboratory monitoring, although in reality many drugs and tests were not readily available. However, as additional national programs were launched in Sub-Saharan countries with fewer resources than Botswana and as MSF, PIH, and other NGOs expanded their efforts, local protocols emerged that reflected existing limitations.

Three resource challenges predominated. First, few antiretroviral drugs were economically priced. MSF's access campaign, along with efforts by the Clinton Foundation to build a rational market for ART working directly with government ministries and generic drug manufacturers to create market efficiencies, paved the way for prices to drop precipitously. By 2006, the annual per-patient cost of first-line treatment with stavudine (d4T), lamivudine (3TC), and nevirapine (NVP) was below $150. Substituting zidovudine (ZDV) for d4T raised the price to $230 per patient-year, and substituting efavirenz (EFV) for NVP raised the price to more than $500 per person-year. PIs remained prohibitively expensive. In addition, a consortium of five branded companies joined with the WHO and others to create the *Accelerating Access Initiative*, which brought the price of brand-name, NNRTI-based treatment down to roughly $300 per patient-year in parts of West Africa and the Caribbean. Funding restrictions from some donors required certain programs to purchase higher-priced regimens. Despite the more attractive prices from generic companies and the *Accelerating Access Initiative*, availability was also limited by logistical difficulties, including regulatory approval, supply chain management, and drug procurement challenges. As a result of cost and availability considerations, most low-income countries opted for a single first-line regimen, usually d4T, 3TC, and NVP. Second-line regimens proved more problematic as no low-cost option was available.

A second key constraint was laboratory infrastructure. Public health laboratories in most low-income countries were extremely limited in both capacity and scope. Outside of national reference laboratories in capital cities, little was offered beyond malaria and TB microscopy, basic immunoassays, and a limited number of chemistries. Even some national reference laboratories lacked the ability to perform HIV viral loads or other complex diagnostics. As with ART, donor-supported price reductions negotiated by the Clinton Foundation began to expand laboratory capacity starting in 2003. HIV antibody testing and CD4 counts became more readily available. However, most national treatment protocols did not incorporate viral load or resistance testing because of cost and availability considerations.

Third, the general shortage of trained health professionals, including physicians, nurses, laboratory technicians, and pharmacists, complicated treatment and monitoring protocols. Expert HIV clinicians was a luxury few countries could support given the lack of health workers and the need to enroll tens of thousands of new patients rapidly into care. Based on the encouraging results on community-based care from pilot programs, efforts were made to decentralize routine monitoring, adherence support, prevention, and counseling away from physicians and toward nurses and other less expensive health care workers.

Treatment Guidelines from the World Health Organization

The affordability of only a limited number of antiretroviral drugs, the difficulties in their procurement, the modest laboratory capacity, and the health care worker limitations in resource-limited countries were recognized by the WHO when it released, *Scaling up Antiretroviral Therapy in Resource-Limited Settings: Treatment Guidelines for a Public Health Approach*, in 2003. This document represented the consensus of a panel of HIV treatment experts from around the world and, for the first time, established international standards by which national treatment protocols could be assessed. Thereafter, most countries adhered closely to WHO recommendations, which encompassed adult treatment, pediatric treatment, prevention of mother-to-child transmission (PMTCT), and opportunistic infection (OI) prophylaxis.

As treatment programs expanded throughout sub-Saharan Africa, Asia, Eastern Europe, and Latin America, as more antiretroviral drugs became available in both generic and branded forms, and as data accumulated, the WHO recognized the need to update these guidelines. In 2006, they were revised and released as three separate documents covering adult treatment, pediatric treatment, and PMTCT. Key components of adult treatment are outlined below, with reference as to how they differ from guidelines used in developed countries.

When to Start Antiretroviral Therapy

WHO guidelines and most national protocols base treatment eligibility primarily on clinical and immunologic (e.g., CD4 count) criteria; viral load measurements are not readily available in most settings and, therefore, not included. To establish clinical criteria for treatment initiation, the WHO categorizes HIV disease into four clinical stages, which bear a loose resemblance to the 1993 Revised Classification System developed by the Centers for Disease Control and Prevention (CDC) for surveillance purposes (Table 15-1). Treatment eligibility is determined by a combination of clinical stage and CD4 count when available and clinical stage alone when the latter is not available (Table 15-2).

Table 15-1. WHO Clinical Staging of HIV/AIDS for Adults and Adolescents

WHO Clinical Stage I

• Asymptomatic	• Generalized lymphadenopathy

WHO Clinical Stage II

• Moderate unexplained weight loss (<10% of presumed or measured body weight)

• Recurrent respiratory tract infections (e.g., as sinusitis, bronchitis, otitis media, pharyngitis)

• Herpes zoster

• Recurrent oral ulcerations

• Papular pruritic eruptions

• Angular cheilitis

• Seborrheic dermatitis

• Fungal finger nail infections

WHO Clinical Stage III

Conditions where a presumptive diagnosis can be made on the basis of clinical signs or simple investigations:

• Unexplained chronic diarrhea for longer than one month

• Unexplained persistent fever (intermittent or constant for longer than one month)

• Severe weight loss (>10% of presumed or measured body weight)

• Oral candidiasis

• Oral hairy leukoplakia

• Pulmonary tuberculosis diagnosed in last two years

• Severe presumed bacterial infections (e.g. pneumonia, empyema, meningitis, bacteremia, pyomyositis, bone or joint infection)

• Acute necrotizing ulcerative stomatitis, gingivitis. or periodontitis

Conditions where confirmatory diagnostic testing is necessary:

• Unexplained anemia (< 8.0 mg/dl) and/or neutropenia (<500 cells/μl) and/or thrombocytopenia (<50,000/μl) for more than one month)

WHO Clinical Stage IV

Conditions where a presumptive diagnosis can be made on the basis of clinical signs or simple investigations:

• HIV wasting syndrome

• *Pneumocystis jiroveci* pneumonia

• Recurrent severe bacterial pneumonia

• Chronic herpes simplex infection (orolabial, genital, or anorectal of more than one month's duration)

• Esophageal candidiasis

• Extrapulmonary tuberculosis

• Kaposi's sarcoma

• Central nervous system toxoplasmosis

• HIV encephalopathy

• Extrapulmonary cryptococcosis including meningitis

Conditions where confirmatory diagnostic testing is necessary:

• Disseminated non-tuberculous mycobacterial infection

• Progressive multifocal leukoencephalopathy

• Chronic cryptosporidiosis

• Chronic isosporiasis

• Any disseminated mycosis

• Recurrent non-typhoidal *Salmonella* septicemia

• Lymphoma

• Invasive cervical carcinoma

• Visceral leishmaniasis

• HIV-associated nephropathy

• HIV-associated cardiomyopathy

Table 15-2.   2006 WHO Recommendations for Initiating Antiretroviral Therapy

WHO Clinical Stage	If CD4 count is available:	If CD4 count is not available:
I	CD4-guided treatment (below)	Do not treat
II	CD4-guided treatment (below)	Consider treatment
III	CD4-guided treatment (below); consider treatment regardless of CD4 count	Treat
IV	Treat regardless of CD4 count	Treat

Absolute CD4 Count	Recommendation
<200 cells/mm³	Treat regardless of clinical stage
200–500 cells/mm³	Consider treatment; initiate before count drops below 200 cells/mm³
>500 cells/mm³	Do not treat

Table 15-3.   Cost of Common First-Line Antiretroviral Regimens

First-line Regimen						Cost in 2006 (per person-year)
d4T	+	3TC	+	NVP		$140
ZDV	+	3TC	+	NVP		$240
d4T	+	3TC	+	EFV		$430
ZDV	+	3TC	+	EFV		$540

d4T = stavudine; EFV = efavirenz; NVP = nevirapine; 3TC = lamivudine; ZDV = zidovudine.

Recommended Regimens

The most notable difference between the WHO treatment guidelines for resource-limited settings and the DHHS guidelines is the restricted number of recommended regimens. The 2003 WHO guidelines included only four regimens as first-line treatment: ZDV/3TC/NVP, d4T/3TC/NVP, ZDV/3TC/EFV, and d4T/3TC/EFV. In addition to simplifying national protocols, provider training, and disease management, the limited number of recommended regimens allowed generic manufacturers to focus production on a small number of drugs and to develop fixed-dose combinations of two or three drugs in a single pill. Fixed-dose combinations are available for ZDV/3TC, d4T/3TC, and d4T/3TC/NVP (the last two in both 30 and 40 mg forms of d4T).

Many national programs initially chose generic versions of d4T/3TC/NVP as the standard first-line regimen for patients treated in the public health system. The rationale was clear: Generic regimens were generally half the price of branded regimens; d4T-based regimens were nearly 50% less expensive than ZDV-based regimens; and NVP-based regimens were 65% cheaper than EFV-based regimens (Table 15-3). Thus, by early 2006, except for Brazil, nearly 60% of HIV-infected patients receiving ART in low- and middle-income countries were on d4T/3TC/NVP.

Balancing Price, Availability, and Toxicity

As programs matured and as new drugs became available, the global HIV treatment community recognized the need to support *high-quality* treatment in a *sustained* manner. Several issues, including the long-term toxicity of d4T, the simplicity of once-daily regimens, the development of heat-stable boosted PI therapy, and the increasing availability of competitively priced drugs, led the WHO to revise its 2003 guidelines in 2006, expanding the list of recommended regimens. Notable changes from 2003 include additional first-line regimens with tenofovir (TDF) or abacavir (ABC) in place of d4T or ZDV, using emtricitabine (FTC) interchangeably with 3TC, the emphasis on boosted PIs in second-line regimens, and a clear sequencing from first-line to second-line regimens (Table 15-4).

As the WHO guidelines for resource-limited settings begin to look more like those in developed countries, it is important to remember that key constraints will continue to limit the drug-regimen choice in most settings. First, although the 2006 WHO recommendations for first-line regimens are broad, individual countries have generally continued to commit to a single regimen, with limited substitution allowed for special circumstances, such as drug toxicity, pregnancy, or TB coinfection. In principle, commitment to a single regimen simplifies recordkeeping, procurement, provider training, and monitoring protocols. Second, boosted PIs as the cornerstone for second-line regimens remain problematic because of the lack of refrigeration required to keep them stable in tropical heat. Finally, as discussed later,

Table 15-4. 2006 WHO Recommendations for First-Line and Second-Line Antiretroviral Therapy Regimens

First-Line Regimens	Second-Line Regimens	
	RTI Component	*PI Component*
(ZDV or d4T) + (3TC or FTC) + (EFV or NVP)	ABC + ddI *or* ABC + TDF *or* TDF + ZDV + (3TC or FTC)	ATV/RTV *or* FPV/RTV *or* IDV/RTV *or* LPV/RTV *or* SQV/RTV
TDF + (3TC or FTC) + (EFV or NVP)	ABC + ddI *or* ddI + ZDV + (3TC or FTC)	Same regimen as above
ABC + (3TC or FTC) + (EFV or NVP)	TDF + ZDV + (3TC or FTC) *or* ddI + ZDV + (3TC or FTC)	Same regimen as above
(ZDV or d4T) + (3TC or FTC) + (ABC or TDF)*	(EFV or NVP) + ddI *or* (EFV or NVP) + 3TC	Same regimen as above

*Alternative regimen where NNRTI options would be associated with unacceptable toxicity.
ABC = abacavir; ATV = atazanavir; ddI = didanosine; d4T = stavudine; EFV = efavirenz; FPV = fosamprenavir; FTC = emtricitabine; IDV = indinavir; LPV = lopinavir; NVP = nevirapine; RTV = ritonavir; SQV = saquinavir; TDF = tenofovir; 3TC = lamivudine; ZDV = zidovudine.

defining treatment failure and sequencing regimens are extremely difficult in settings where viral load testing is not available and where only a single second-line option exists. For these reasons, many patients in resource-limited settings have remained on first-line regimens significantly longer than their counterparts in developed countries.

Adherence Support

With the benefit of experience gleaned from developed countries, as well as widespread fears of drug resistance, many HIV programs in resource-limited settings and provide appropriate adherence support. As an added incentive, the budgetary implications of switching from first- to second-line regimens are significant, and every patient on a second-line regimen means ten fewer patients enrolled into care. Adherence support interventions in resource-limited settings may include preparedness classes, regular counseling, and directly observed therapy (DOT). Many HIV programs require patients to undergo an ART preparedness class over 2 to 4 weeks before initiating therapy, where basic disease management is taught and adherence is emphasized. Programs do not generally dispense more than a 1-month supply of ART to patients, ensuring frequent contact with health care providers.

The most ambitious HIV programs assign each patient to an identified community health worker. Individual protocols vary, but essentially the health worker is responsible for making sure that patients are adherent to their regimen and serving as an "early warning system" for drug toxicity, clinical progression, or other problems. The success of community health worker-based adherence support has been demonstrated by the improved clinical outcomes in some programs. The minimal additional costs have been justified on the basis of the savings obtained by reducing the number of people who switch to expensive second-line regimens.

Patient Monitoring and Treatment Failure

In the United States and other developed countries, "treatment failure" is generally divided into three components: virologic failure, immunologic failure, and clinical disease progression. Pathophysiologically, virologic failure occurs first, with low-level viremia and the gradual, stepwise emergence of drug-resistance mutations. Loss of CD4 cells and immunologic failure follows, and ultimately clinical treatment failure ensues. Monitoring strategies and decisions about when to switch from a failing regimen in the United States are driven by our understanding of this sequence of events and strong interest in changing a failing regimen before a significant number of resistance mutations have emerged. Implicit in this approach is the ready availability of second-line, third-line, and even salvage ART regimens. Thus, HIV viral load measurements have been the cornerstone of patient monitoring in the United States, and the decision to switch to a new regimen is made before clinical and immunologic endpoints become apparent.

In most resource-limited settings, regular viral load monitoring is not possible, and multiple second-line regimens may not be readily available. The constraints on viral load monitoring include the high cost of reagents, the limited laboratory capacity, the shortage of trained technicians, and the lack of laboratory information systems to get results back to clinicians in a meaningful time frame. A few better-resourced countries, including Botswana, Brazil, and South Africa, have incorporated routine viral load monitoring for patients on treatment. However, in general, treatment monitoring protocols and the definition of treatment failure in resource-limited settings are based on immunologic and clinical grounds in most instances and less often on clinical grounds alone.

Clinical monitoring consists of symptom identification by a health worker supplemented by monthly evaluations by a nurse or doctor. The most important marker of disease progression is weight loss. Laboratory monitoring generally consists of hemoglobin and liver enzyme measurements during the first few months of ART and CD4 counts every 3 to 6 months. Immunologic triggers for switching to second-line regimens vary but typically include a 50% or greater drop in the CD4 count or its return to pretreatment baseline. As more affordable and simpler methods for measuring the viral load and CD4 count become available in the next several years, the approach to patient monitoring and the definition of treatment failure in resource-limited settings will likely move closer to the current practice in developed countries.

Treatment Outcome

In general, clinical outcomes and, where studied, virologic outcomes in the first few years of ART in resource-limited settings were similar to, and in some instances better than, outcomes in the United States and Europe. Early data came from MSF's global programs. In Khayelitsha, follow-up was available on the first 1700 patients enrolled in care since 2001. In this group of patients, 70% were women, the median baseline CD4 count was 76 cells/mm^3, and the median baseline viral load was 5.2 log$_{10}$ copies/mL, reflecting the advanced state of disease at presentation. At 2 years follow-up, 92% of patients remained on their first-line regimen allowing for single-drug substitutions for toxicity; for those few patients with 3 years follow-up, 90% remained on their first-line regimen.

The most worrisome finding in Khayelitsha, which has been confirmed in several other sites, was the unsurprisingly high cumulative rate of d4T toxicity. At 1 year, 7.2% of patients had evidence of neuropathy, lipodystrophy, or lactic acidosis; this rate increased to 16% at 3 years. In addition, alarmingly high rates of lactic acidosis have been reported in South Africa. Given this information, the WHO has begun to encourage programs to consider minimizing the use of d4T despite its cost advantage.

In other countries, including Botswana, Cambodia, Rwanda, Thailand, and Uganda, some themes have emerged from the first few years of experience:

- More women than men are accessing ART.
- Death rates are higher in the first months of treatment than in developed countries, likely reflecting the advanced stage at which HIV infection is diagnosed in patients entering care.
- Universal access to free care is associated with fewer treatment interruptions and better clinical outcomes.
- Gains in weight and CD4 counts following the initiation of ART are comparable to those seen in developed countries.
- Loss to follow-up is a critical challenge to ART delivery and has been reported to be as high as 25% in some programs in Africa, particularly those without community health worker support.
- Sixty percent to 90% of patients have undetectable viral loads (where available) after 1 to 2 years of treatment.
- As in the United States, failure of NNRTI-based therapy is associated with the K103N mutation.

Pediatric Care

There are 2.3 million HIV-infected children worldwide, most of whom are in developing countries. Without access to treatment and orphaned by parents succumbing to AIDS, 50% of HIV-infected infants die before reaching the age of 2. In 2005, 550,000 children succumbed to AIDS, and another 560,000 were in need of treatment. Pediatric formulations have been slow to be added to the list of drugs manufactured generically, and pediatric drugs still cost roughly twice as much as adult drugs. Also, diagnosing infants younger than 18 months of age remains problematic in the developing world because viral load measurements are necessary. In addition, there is a general shortage of pediatricians globally. Nonetheless, efforts by UNICEF, MSF, Columbia University's MTCT-Plus Program, Baylor University, the Elizabeth Glaser Pediatric AIDS Foundation, the Clinton Foundation's Pediatric HIV Initiative, and other organizations have recently highlighted the difficult circumstances of HIV-infected children worldwide and the need to do more for this population.

HIV Infection and Tuberculosis

The high prevalence of TB in most resource-limited settings adds a significant challenge to the management of HIV-infected patients. The global HIV epidemic has fueled an extraordinary increase in active TB cases, particularly in Sub-Saharan Africa, where the incidence rate of TB increased from 146 per 100,000 in 1990 to 345 per 100,000 in 2003. In some African countries, over 70% of patients with active TB are coinfected with HIV. A similar resurgence is occurring in Eastern Europe, India, and Southeast Asia.

Four issues complicate the care of HIV/TB coinfected patients in resource-limited settings. First, infection-control systems are not reliably in place; thus, HIV-infected patients without TB are often exposed to patients with active TB presenting for care. Second, the diagnosis of TB remains problematic. With higher rates of extrapulmonary and smear-negative pulmonary TB in HIV-infected patients and limited tools to diagnose such cases, management is difficult. Third, there are significant drug interactions between TB therapy and ART, particularly NVP, which is the key component in most first-line regimens. Fourth, and perhaps most important, the management of HIV/TB coinfected patients is often fragmented, with little coordination of care. Typically, HIV and TB programs have separate administrative structures, funding, personnel, and facilities. Integrating the management of these two diseases has proven extraordinarily difficult worldwide.

The Future of Antiretroviral Therapy in Resource-Limited Settings

Through 2006, significant progress had been made in delivering HIV care in resource-limited settings. More than 5100 treatment facilities had been opened around the world in three years. Prices for first-line antiretroviral drugs and for HIV diagnostics had plummeted as much as 90%. Fifty thousand patients were starting ART each month. Still, much remains to be done.

From a distance, HIV infection in resource-limited settings appears remarkably similar to the disease in the United States and other developed countries. Nonetheless, providing ART to the millions of people living in resource-limited settings represents an entirely different undertaking. Decisions about which drugs to use, when to start treatment, how to monitor patients, how to define treatment failure, and when to switch to a new regimen have important worldwide public health and social implications. Funding, long thought to be the critical barrier to the delivery of effective care, is now less important than some of the other limitations described in this chapter and Chapter 16. Collectively, the Global Fund to Fight AIDS, TB, and Malaria, the United States Government's President's Emergency Plan for AIDS Relief (PEPFAR), and bilateral and multilateral funding sources have contributed more than $8.3 billion per year to the global HIV treatment and prevention campaign. While this funding represents a sizable investment, projections indicate that $16 to $20 billion per year will eventually be needed to combat the HIV epidemic.

Key Points

- The devastating impact of HIV infection in resource-limited countries has brought overdue attention to the plight of those affected. The number of people receiving ART increased from 400,000 to close to 2 million in the past few years; however, 4.5 million more people are still in need of treatment.
- Global efforts have had a major impact on the cost of ART and other resources needed for HIV care. Comprehensive care in resource-limited settings is now below $1000 per person per year. Sustained external funding remains important, but the lack of public health infrastructure, shortage of health care professionals, and limited management expertise have become more critical issues in the short term.
- Decisions on when to start treatment, how to monitor patients, and when to switch from failing therapies are based on the same principles as in the developed world. However, resource constraints require more of a "public health approach," where the choices of first-line regimens and the frequency and type of monitoring are limited, and the trigger for switching to more expensive second-line regimens is delayed.
- In most of the world, HIV infection is and will remain a primary care disease. Providing HIV treatment cannot be separated from addressing malnutrition, treating malaria and tuberculosis, providing prenatal, maternal and family care, and building sustainable health programs.
- Community-based adherence support is critical, given the need to leverage the available health infrastructure and the financial and logistical consequences of first-line regimen failure.
- Clinical and virologic outcomes from ART programs in resource-limited countries have been comparable to care sites in the developed world. Fear of the development of widespread drug resistance has proven unfounded. Whether similarly high success rates can be sustained as programs scale up remains a challenge.

SUGGESTED READINGS

Antiretroviral Therapy in Lower Income Countries (ART-LINC) Collaboration. Mortality of HIV-1-infected patients in the first year of antiretroviral therapy: comparison between low-income and high-income countries. Lancet. 2006;367:817-24.

Calmy A, Klement E, Teck R, Berman D, Pécoul B, Ferradini L. Simplifying and adapting antiretroviral treatment in resource-poor settings: a necessary step to scaling-up [Editorial]. AIDS. 2004;18:2353-60.

Carpenter CC. Universal access to antiretroviral therapy: when, not if [Editorial]. Clin Infect Dis. 2006;42:260-1.

Koenig SP, Léandre F, Farmer PE. Scaling-up HIV treatment programmes in resource-limited settings: the rural Haiti experience. AIDS. 2004;18 Suppl 3:S21-5.

Wools-Kaloustian K, Kimaiyo S, Diero L, Siika A, Sidle J, Yiannoutsos CT, et al. Viability and effectiveness of large-scale HIV treatment initiatives in sub-Saharan Africa: experience from western Kenya. AIDS. 2006; 20:41–48

World Health Organization. Progress on Global Access to HIV Antiretroviral Therapy: A Report on "3 by 5" and Beyond. March 2006.

Chapter 16

Barriers to Implementing Care in Resource-Limited Settings

LOUISE IVERS, MD, MPH

In 2003, the World Health Organization (WHO) announced the "3 by 5" initiative for global AIDS care with the goal of having 3 million HIV-infected patients in low- and middle-income countries on antiretroviral therapy by the end of 2005. Although the initiative did not meet this numeric target, it was successful on many levels (see Chapter 15). At the time of writing, over 1 million people with HIV infection in developing countries are being managed with combination antiretroviral therapy; dozens of countries have received grants from the Global Fund to Fight AIDS, TB, and Malaria to support HIV testing and care; and the cost of antiretroviral drugs has fallen dramatically. The "3 by 5" initiative invigorated a previously complacent international community and encouraged efforts to provide treatment to all patients who needed it based on their right to medical care and not on their ability to pay. However, despite these advances, barriers to providing effective care for HIV-infected patients in the developing world persist. In 2003, approximately 3 million people, three-quarters from Sub-Saharan Africa, died of AIDS. An additional 5 million people were newly HIV-infected. Only 5% to 8% of HIV-infected persons worldwide are currently aware of their serostatus, and only 5% of those who need treatment have access to it.

Some barriers to AIDS care in the developing world are the same as those in rich countries. These include differential access to care, social stigma, and personal health beliefs. Other barriers, including lack of infrastructure and inadequate public health funds, are unique to the developing world. This chapter addresses both structural and individual barriers in this setting. Programs in resource-limited countries have proven that, despite obstacles, with appropriate advocacy and funding it is possible to treat patients successfully, with results that are at least equivalent, if not superior, to those in rich countries.

The provision of quality HIV care requires several infrastructure and programmatic components to be in place (Box 16-1) and barriers to their implementation to be overcome (Box 16-2). Each impediment has its own set of challenges. For example, challenges in HIV education include a rapidly changing and incomplete knowledge base, different training requirements of learners, and social and cultural issues related to health care.

Box 16-1.   Components of Quality HIV Care

- Screening for HIV infection
- Trained health care providers
- Health care facilities
- Diagnostic testing

- Therapeutic interventions
- Medication adherence
- Follow-up care
- Patient support

Structural Barriers to Care

In much of the developing world, medical care in the public sector is extremely limited or unavailable. Overworked and understaffed clinics are often insufficient to deal with even routine primary health care needs. Morbidity and mortality from common conditions such as malaria, tuberculosis, measles, and malnutrition are high. In this context, the implementation of treatment programs for a complicated disease such as AIDS requires a commitment to overcome both the barriers to regular medical care and those that are unique to HIV infection.

Poverty, Migration, and Displacement

Over 1 billion people worldwide live below the poverty line, earning less than $1 per day. Millions more live in destitution, without access to clean water, shelter, and adequate nutrition. Poverty has a profound impact on one's ability to access and receive medical care. User fees, transportation fees, and medication costs are all barriers to care for persons whose first priority is securing a meal or shelter for the day. HIV clinic service fees and required payments for antiretroviral therapy have been shown to be associated with worse treatment outcomes. Migration and displacement to search for work or to avoid political violence not only puts individuals at

---

Box 16-2.   Barriers to Care in Resource-Limited Settings

Structural Barriers
- Poverty, migration, and displacement
- Lack of infrastructure
- Social status of women
- Food insecurity
- International debt

Individual Barriers
- Delay in diagnosis
- Delay in presentation for care
- Lack of engagement in care

increased risk of HIV infection but also affects their ability to receive health care. In the case of antiretroviral therapy, continuity of care is essential to maximize the likelihood of medication adherence.

Individual poverty is compounded by poverty at the country level. Low- and middle-income countries with the highest HIV burdens struggle to provide resources necessary to combat the epidemic. However, success stories can be found across the globe. Uganda, Botswana, and Thailand are a few examples of countries where government efforts have been instrumental in developing and supporting effective HIV prevention and treatment programs.

Lack of Infrastructure

Lack of physical infrastructure is a significant barrier to medical care. Poor roads and absence of public transportation makes getting to and from clinics difficult, especially in the rainy season. Electricity and water supply may be limited, intermittent, or nonexistent. Sensitive laboratory equipment, such as flow cytometers for CD4 cell count testing, are in short supply and vulnerable to heat, dust, and humidity. Reagents for laboratory tests and consumables such as blood vacutainers may not be stored appropriately.

Many individuals, especially the rural poor, in resource-limited settings do not have documentation (e.g., birth certificate, national identification card) of their personal identity, and the illiteracy rate is often high. These two issues affect HIV program development in important ways. Medication record keeping is a challenge without identification cards, counseling must be appropriate for the level of patient education, and accounting practices may be questioned when programs receiving international monies cannot provide authorized signatures. Inventive approaches are often needed to overcome these problems.

System decentralization is another barrier to health care in the developing world. Private sector clinics, non-profit organizations, and government programs often work independently, creating parallel systems that are not coordinated and have little exchange of knowledge or resources. Vertical programs can create similar problems, and horizontal integration with other health care initiatives (e.g., primary care, tuberculosis, nutrition) is of key importance. HIV treatment programs in Haiti and Rwanda are two successful examples where public health systems, in partnership with private nonprofit organizations, have led to important advances in patient care. Although some aspects of HIV care may benefit from targeted approaches, providing counseling and testing in the context of general medical care and combining prevention and treatment efforts have had highly favorable outcomes.

A lack of skilled health care workers is an additional important barrier. The HIV epidemic has had a large impact on staffing as a result of mortality from the disease. In Malawi and Zambia, the death rate of health care workers increased six-fold between the early 1990s and 2000s. Further attrition of staff occurs as they leave lower paying government positions to work in private sector or university research facilities.

Social Status of Women

Addressing the social status of women, especially in areas of the world characterized by gender inequity, is a critical component to their care. At the end of 2003, half of the 40 million adults with HIV infection globally were women, with an increase in the prevalence in almost every region. Fifty-seven percent of HIV-infected persons in Sub-Saharan Africa are women. In the United States, the prevalence is disproportionately high in women of color.

HIV infection in women is often sexually acquired. Saying "no" to sex or insisting that a partner uses condoms is not a realistic option for many women around the world regardless of their marital status. Commercial sex work and trafficking of women are prevalent, as is sexual assault, especially in times of armed conflict. Women may avoid HIV testing or avoid disclosure of their results for fear of alerting their male partner. As opportunities are lost for care of this population, so too are those for the prevention of mother-to-child transmission of HIV infection.

Food Insecurity

HIV-infected persons who are largely dependent on agriculture for sustenance lose productivity, income, and often their personal food supply when they are ill. The goal of reducing hunger by half by 2015, which was established in 1996 and reinforced at the Millennium Development Summit in 2000, will likely miss the target. Fully 852 million people, the vast majority in developing countries, were chronically undernourished in 2000 to 2002. This figure does not include those suffering from transitory food shortages, which affects an additional 5% to 10% of the world population.

The impact of hunger on medical care cannot be overestimated. For a hungry family, food becomes the priority. Travel to clinics may become impossible because of weakness and lethargy. Skills and knowledge of farming are lost as family members die of AIDS, leading them into worsening cycles of poverty and hunger. Evidence exists that HIV infection has resulted in decreased agricultural production at the level of individual households.

International Debt

The costs of attempting to overcome the structural barriers to HIV care are many and, in the case of resource-limited countries, often impossible to pay from national budgets. In the context of multilateral debt payments, even well-intentioned governments may be crippled by lack of resources for health care and education. African nations, for example, spend $13 billion per year on debt payments, whereas The Joint United Nations Programme on HIV/AIDS (UNAIDS) estimated in 2002 that $10 billion per year would be required in annual spending to provide a basic package of HIV prevention, treatment, and care and support services. The financial support of the international community is essential in the effort to scale-up HIV care in conjunction with the elimination of global poverty. In 2005, the International Monetary Fund cancelled all debt of 19 nations in an effort to make resources available for those countries to fight poverty. International agencies such as the Global Fund to Fight AIDS, TB, and Malaria have played a critical role in supplying funds for HIV treatment and prevention programs. In 2005, $729 million was made available to treat the three diseases, with 40% of the funds for HIV care and 6% for strengthening health systems. However, there remains a funding shortfall of $1.1 billion for 2006 and $2.6 billion for 2007. Individual governments and private, nonprofit organizations have also been part of the effort to secure funds for treatment. Nonetheless, current global spending on HIV treatment and prevention is only $4 billion per year, which is well below the $15 billion estimated to be required annually by 2007.

Individual Barriers to Care

Access to HIV care in resource-limited settings is subject not only to the structural barriers discussed above but also by barriers at the level of the patient. In many instances, these individual barriers to health care are no different from those in developed countries. However, little research has been carried out in poor countries to determine which factors are most important. Individual barriers to care include delay in diagnosis, delay in presentation for care, and lack of engagement in care. Understanding these barriers is the first step toward their remediation.

Delay in Diagnosis

Since antiretroviral therapy was not available until recently in the developing world, one might argue that there was little motivation for asymptomatic persons to be tested for HIV infection. In addition, the separation of HIV testing from primary care (e.g., performed by a counselor often in another setting) has been another impediment to early diagnosis. In 1993 the Centers for Disease Control and Prevention (CDC) recommended that clinics and hospitals in the United States in areas of high HIV prevalence offer routine voluntary HIV testing to all patients aged 15 to 54. These recommendations have recently been broadened to include all healthy adults. Studies have demonstrated that HIV infection may be diagnosed at an earlier stage of disease by "mainstreaming" counseling and testing activities. In 2003, the WHO recommended routine voluntary testing for HIV infection in general outpatient medical clinics in the developing world where the prevalence rate is high. However, few such programs have been implemented to date.

Delay in Presentation for Care

Since the diagnosis of early HIV infection is associated with lower morbidity and mortality, researchers have tried to identify factors responsible for delay in presentation for care. One study found ethnicity to be associated with later presentation and female gender to be associated with earlier presentation. Competing financial needs and fear of discrimination have also been identified as barriers to HIV care in the developed world. Economic choices appear to play an even more important role in patients of a lower socioeconomic status. Another study found that lack of education and poor housing were associated with low enrollment rates in a program for subsidized HIV treatment in Côte D'Ivoire. A recent meta-analysis showed better program outcomes in resource-limited settings where services and medications were free compared with programs where payment was required.

HIV-related social stigma, an important barrier to prevention and care efforts, is a complex phenomenon that is difficult to measure quantitatively. Experience with other diseases has shown that stigma may diminish with time as they are better understood and as treatment becomes available. Surveys revealed a decrease in stigmatizing attitudes towards HIV infection in the United States between 1991 and 1997. HIV-related stigma is also likely to decrease over time in the developing world.

Personal health beliefs are another important component of health-seeking behavior. For example, if an individual does not believe himself to be at risk for HIV infection, then he is less likely to seek care and to accept testing if it is offered. Lack of perceived personal risk has been shown to be a factor in pregnant women who have declined to be tested in the United States.

Lack of Engagement in Care

Engagement in care and adherence to medical therapies are essential after the diagnosis of HIV infection is made. Structural factors, such as distance from the clinic and cost of care, are important, but more research is needed into the individual factors that affect engagement in care in the developing world. Studies in Botswana and Senegal have shown that financial constraints, migration, stigma, and drug side effects are the major barriers to adherence.

KEY POINTS

- The barriers to implementing HIV care in resource-limited settings are both structural and individual in nature. Each barrier has its own set of challenges and potential solutions.
- Structural barriers are unique to the developing world and include: 1) poverty, migration, and displacement; 2) lack of infrastructure; 3) social status of women; 4) food insecurity; and 5) international debt.
- Individual barriers are similar to those in the developed word and include: 1) delay in diagnosis; 2) delay in presentation for care; and 3) lack of engagement in care.
- HIV advocacy, funding, and treatment are part of the greater struggle for improved health care in resource-limited settings around the world.

SUGGESTED READINGS

Castro A, Farmer P. Understanding and addressing AIDS-related stigma: from anthropological theory to clinical practice in Haiti. Am J Public Health. 2005;95:53-9.

Cunningham WE, Andersen RM, Katz MH, Stein MD, Turner BJ, Crystal S, et al. The impact of competing subsistence needs and barriers on access to medical care for persons with human immunodeficiency virus receiving care in the United States. Med Care. 1999;37: 1270-81.

Eastwood JB, Conroy RE, Naicker S, West PA, Tutt RC, Plange-Rhule J. Loss of health professionals from sub-Saharan Africa: the pivotal role of the UK. Lancet. 2005;365:1893-900.

Gillespie, Stuart. 2006. AIDS, poverty, and hunger: challenges and responses. Washington, D.C.: International Food Policy Research Institute.

Ivers LC, Kendrick D, Doucette K. Efficacy of antiretroviral therapy programs in resource-poor settings: a meta-analysis of the published literature. Clin Infect Dis. 2005;41:217-24.

Mukherjee JS, Farmer PE, Niyizonkiza D, McCorkle L, Vanderwarker C, Teixcira P, et al. Tackling HIV in resource poor countries. BMJ. 2003;327:1104-6.

Ojikutu BO, Stone VE. Women, inequality, and the burden of HIV. N Engl J Med. 2005; 352:649-52.

Petti CA, Polage CR, Quinn TC, Ronald AR, Sande MA. Laboratory medicine in Africa: a barrier to effective health care. Clin Infect Dis. 2006;42:377-82.

Porter K, Wall PG, Evans BG. Factors associated with lack of awareness of HIV infection before diagnosis of AIDS. BMJ. 1993;307:20-3.

Royce RA, Walter EB, Fernandez MI, et al. Barriers to universal prenatal HIV testing in 4 US locations in 1997. Am J Public Health. 2001;91:727-33.

Samet JH, Freedberg KA, Savetsky JB, Sullivan LM, Stein MD. Understanding delay to medical care for HIV infection: the long-term non-presenter. AIDS. 2001;15:77-85.

Weiser S, Wolfe W, Bangsberg D, Thior I, Gilbert P, Makhema J, et al. Barriers to antiretroviral adherence for patients living with HIV infection and AIDS in Botswana. J Acquir Immune Defic Syndr. 2003;34:281-8.

Appendix I

HIV Drug Glossary

HOWARD LIBMAN, MD

Antiretroviral Therapy

Nucleoside and Nucleotide Reverse-Transcriptase Inhibitors (NRTIs)*

Abacavir (ABC, Ziagen)

<u>Indications</u>:   Treatment of HIV infection in combination with other agents.

<u>Contraindications</u>:   Known or suspected hypersensitivity.

<u>Dosage</u>:   300 mg PO bid. Also available as Trizivir, a fixed-dose combination of ZDV 300 mg, 3TC 150 mg, and ABC 300 mg; and Epzicom, a fixed-dose combination of 3TC 300 mg and ABC 600 mg.

<u>Toxicity</u>:   Four percent of patients develop a hypersensitivity reaction, usually within 6 weeks of initiating therapy, manifested by fever, constitutional or respiratory symptoms, gastrointestinal intolerance, and/or rash. Stopping the drug leads to rapid resolution of symptoms. *Never rechallenge a patient thought to have had a hypersensitivity reaction to abacavir; severe reactions and death have been reported.*

Other side effects include gastrointestinal intolerance, headache, malaise.

Pregnancy category C. (See pregnancy category abbreviations at end of Appendix.)

---

*Lactic acidosis, rarely with hepatomegaly and steatosis, has been associated with all drugs in this class.

Didanosine (ddI, Videx)

Indications: Treatment of HIV infection in combination with other agents.

Contraindications: Known hypersensitivity; history of pancreatitis or significant peripheral neuropathy.

Dosage: Enteric-coated formulation: 400 mg PO qd for weight ≥60 kg and 250 mg PO qd for weight <60 kg.

Also available in buffered powder: ≥60 kg → 250 mg PO bid; <60 kg → 167 mg PO bid.

Both formulations are taken on an empty stomach (>30 minutes before a meal or >2 hours after a meal).

Toxicity: Peripheral neuropathy, acute pancreatitis, gastrointestinal intolerance, abnormal liver function tests. Not recommended for co-administration with d4T or TDF.

Pregnancy category B.

Emtricitabine (FTC, Emtriva)

Indications: Treatment of HIV infection in combination with other agents. Also has activity against hepatitis B virus.

Contraindications: Known hypersensitivity.

Dosage: 200 mg PO qd. Also available as Truvada, a fixed-dose combination of TDF 300 mg and FTC 200 mg; and Atripla, a fixed-dose combination of TDF 300 mg, FTC 200 mg, and EFV 600 mg.

Toxicity: Hyperpigmentation of palms and soles. Flares of chronic hepatitis B infection have been reported with discontinuation of FTC in co-infected patients.

Pregnancy category B.

Lamivudine (3TC, Epivir)

Indications: Treatment of HIV infection in combination with other agents. Also has activity against hepatitis B virus.

Contraindications: Known hypersensitivity.

Dosage: 150 mg PO bid or 300 mg PO qd. Also available as Combivir, a fixed-dose combination of ZDV 300 mg with 3TC 150 mg; Trizivir, a fixed-dose combination of ZDV 300 mg, 3TC 150 mg, and ABC 300 mg; and Epzicom, a fixed-dose combination of 3TC 300 mg and ABC 600 mg.

Toxicity: Uncommon. Headache, gastrointestinal intolerance, and insomnia have been reported. Flares of chronic hepatitis B infection have been reported with discontinuation of 3TC in co-infected patients.

Pregnancy category C.

Stavudine (d4T, Zerit)

Indications: Treatment of HIV infection in combination with other agents.

Contraindications: Known hypersensitivity; concurrent ZDV use because of pharmacologic antagonism; history of significant peripheral neuropathy.

Dosage: Immediate-release formulation: $\geq$60 kg $\rightarrow$ 40 mg PO bid; <60 kg $\rightarrow$ 30 mg PO bid. Dose adjustment for peripheral neuropathy: 20 mg PO bid.

Toxicity: Peripheral neuropathy, acute pancreatitis, abnormal liver function tests. Not recommended for co-administration with ddI.

Pregnancy category C.

Tenofovir (TDF, Viread)

Indications: Treatment of HIV infection in combination with other agents. Also has activity against hepatitis B virus.

Tenofovir is a nucleotide agent.

Contraindications: Known hypersensitivity.

Dosage: 300 mg PO qd with food. Also available as Truvada, a fixed-dose combination of TDF 300 mg and FTC 200 mg; and Atripla, a fixed-dose combination of TDF 300 mg, FTC 200 mg, and EFV 600 mg.

Toxicity: Gastrointestinal intolerance, renal dysfunction. Not recommended for co-administration with ddI. Flares of chronic hepatitis B infection have been reported with discontinuation of TDF in co-infected patients.

Pregnancy category B.

Zalcitabine (ddC, HIVID)

Indications: Treatment of HIV infection in combination with other agents.

Contraindications: Known hypersensitivity; history of significant peripheral neuropathy.

Dosage: 0.75 mg PO tid.

Toxicity: Peripheral neuropathy, aphthous ulcers of mouth and esophagus, acute pancreatitis, abnormal liver function tests.

Pregnancy category C.

Zidovudine (ZDV, AZT, Retrovir)

Indications: Treatment of HIV infection in combination with other agents. In addition, ZDV may have specific benefits for patients who have HIV-related thrombocytopenia or encephalopathy.

Prevention of perinatal transmission when given prenatally and during delivery to HIV-infected mother and to infant postpartum. Combination antiretroviral therapy should be administered in this setting.

Contraindications: Known hypersensitivity.

Dosage: Treatment of HIV infection in adults: 300 mg PO bid. Also available as Combivir, a fixed-dose combination of ZDV 300 mg with 3TC 150 mg; and Trizivir, a fixed-dose combination of ZDV 300 mg, 3TC 150 mg, and ABC 300 mg.

Prevention of perinatal transmission: Pregnancy weeks 14-34 → 300 mg PO bid; during labor → 2 mg/kg IV loading dose over 30 minutes to 1 hour, then 1 mg/kg/hr IV through delivery; and infant → 2 mg/kg syrup q6h for 6 weeks.

Toxicity: Gastrointestinal intolerance, headache, fingernail discoloration, myopathy, anemia, leukopenia, macrocytosis, abnormal liver function tests.

Pregnancy category C.

Non-Nucleoside Reverse-Transcriptase Inhibitors (NNRTIs)

Delavirdine (Rescriptor)

Indications: Treatment of HIV infection in combination with other agents.

Contraindications: Known hypersensitivity.

Dosage: 400 mg PO tid. Two tablets must be dissolved in ≥3 oz of water to produce a slurry. Antacids and ddI should not be taken one hour before or after the dose. *There are many potential drug interactions, some of which may require dosage modification or preclude its co-administration with other agents; see Physicians' Desk Reference or package insert for more information.*

Toxicity: Rash is common and does not require discontinuation of the drug unless accompanied by fever, mucous membrane involvement, or other systemic manifestations. Stevens-Johnson syndrome has been reported infrequently.

Pregnancy category C.

Efavirenz (EFV, Sustiva)

Indications: Treatment of HIV infection in combination with other agents.

Contraindications: Known hypersensitivity; pregnancy.

Dosage: 600 mg PO qhs. Avoid taking with high fat meals. Also available as Atripla, a fixed-dose combination of TDF 300 mg, FTC 200 mg, and EFV 600 mg. *There are many potential drug interactions, some of which may require dosage modification or preclude its co-administration with other agents; see Physicians' Desk Reference or package insert for more information.*

Toxicity: Rash is common and does not require discontinuation of the drug unless accompanied by fever, mucous membrane involvement, or other systemic manifestations. Other side effects include vivid dreams or nightmares, neurocognitive dysfunction, hyperlipidemia, abnormal liver function tests.

Pregnancy category D; teratogenic in non-human primates. Not recommended for use in first trimester of pregnancy or in sexually active women with child-bearing potential who are not using effective contraception.

Nevirapine (NVP, Viramune)

Indications: Treatment of HIV infection in combination with other agents.

Contraindications: Known hypersensitivity. Because of a high incidence of significant hepatic dysfunction in women with CD4 count $> 250/mm^3$ and in men with CD4 count $> 400/mm^3$, NVP should be avoided in these settings unless the benefit clearly outweighs the risk.

Dosage: 200 mg PO qd $\times$ 2 weeks; 200 mg PO bid thereafter. Patients who develop rash during the first two weeks should not increase the dose until the rash resolves. *There are many potential drug interactions, some of which may require dosage modification or preclude its co-administration with other agents; see Physicians' Desk Reference or package insert for more information.*

Toxicity: Rash is common (about 17% of patients, although fewer with dose escalation regimen) and does not require discontinuation of the drug unless accompanied by fever, mucous membrane involvement, or other systemic manifestations. Stevens-Johnson syndrome has been reported infrequently. Other side effects include nausea, headache, abnormal liver function tests.

Pregnancy category C.

Protease Inhibitors (PIs)**

Atazanavir (Reyataz)

<u>Indications</u>:   Treatment of HIV infection in combination with other agents.

<u>Contraindications</u>:   Known hypersensitivity.

<u>Dosage</u>:   400 mg PO qd. When co-administered with TDF or EFV, dose is 300 mg PO qd with ritonavir 100 mg PO qd. *There are many potential drug interactions, some of which require dosage modification; see Physicians' Desk Reference or package insert for more information.*

<u>Toxicity</u>:   Gastrointestinal intolerance, hyperbilirubinemia. Unlike other protease inhibitors, this drug does not appear to be associated with hyperlipidemia.

Pregnancy category B.

Darunavir (Prezista)

<u>Indications</u>:   Treatment of HIV infection in combination with other agents.

<u>Contraindications</u>:   Known hypersensitivity.

<u>Dosage</u>:   600 mg PO bid co-administered with ritonavir 100 mg PO bid as pharmacologic booster. *There are many potential drug interactions, some of which may require dosage modification or preclude its co-administration with other agents; see Physicians' Desk Reference or package insert for more information.*

<u>Toxicity</u>:   Gastrointestinal intolerance, rash, headache, abnormal liver function tests.

Pregnancy category B.

**Hyperlipidemia, glucose intolerance/diabetes mellitus, and body fat redistribution have been associated with combination antiretroviral therapy, especially regimens containing protease inhibitors.

Fosamprenavir (Lexiva)

<u>Indications</u>:   Treatment of HIV infection in combination with other agents.

<u>Contraindications</u>:   Known hypersensitivity.

<u>Dosage</u>:   1400 mg PO bid. When co-administered with ritonavir (100 mg PO bid) as pharmacologic booster, dose is 700 mg PO bid. *There are many potential drug interactions, some of which may require dosage modification or preclude its co-administration with other agents; see Physicians' Desk Reference or package insert for more information.*

<u>Toxicity</u>:   Gastrointestinal intolerance, rash, headache, oral paresthesias.

Pregnancy category C.

Indinavir (Crixivan)

<u>Indications</u>:   Treatment of HIV infection in combination with other agents.

<u>Contraindications</u>:   Known hypersensitivity.

<u>Dosage</u>:   800 mg PO q8h on an empty stomach or with a non-fat meal. Patients should drink at least 48 oz of fluid a day. When co-administered with ritonavir (100-200 mg PO bid) as pharmacologic booster, dose is 800 mg PO bid without food restrictions. *There are many potential drug interactions, some of which may require dosage modification or preclude its co-administration with other agents; see Physicians' Desk Reference or package insert for more information.*

<u>Toxicity</u>:   Nephrolithiasis, gastrointestinal intolerance, hyperbilirubinemia.

Pregnancy category C.

Lopinavir/Ritonavir (Kaletra)

<u>Indications</u>:   Treatment of HIV infection in combination with other agents.

Lopinavir is a protease inhibitor combined with ritonavir, which significantly augments its blood level.

<u>Contraindications</u>:   Known hypersensitivity; concurrent use of ritonavir.

<u>Dosage</u>:   Two tablets (each 200 mg lopinavir/50 mg ritonavir) PO bid; four tablets PO qd has been approved in treatment-naïve patients. *There are many potential drug interactions, some of which may require dosage modification or preclude its co-administration with other agents; see Physicians' Desk Reference or package insert for more information.*

Toxicity: Gastrointestinal intolerance, weakness, headache.

Pregnancy category C.

Nelfinavir (Viracept)

Indications: Treatment of HIV infection in combination with other agents.

Contraindications: Known hypersensitivity.

Dosage: 1250 mg PO bid or 750 mg PO tid with food. *There are many potential drug interactions, some of which may require dosage modification or preclude its co-administration with other agents; see Physicians' Desk Reference or package insert for more information.*

Toxicity: Diarrhea.

Pregnancy category B.

Ritonavir (Norvir)

Indications: Treatment of HIV infection in combination with other agents (infrequently used in this manner because of gastrointestinal toxicity and drug interactions). Often co-administered as pharmacologic booster with other protease inhibitors.

Contraindications: Known hypersensitivity.

Dosage: 600 mg PO q12h with food following two week dose escalation regimen (day 1 and 2: 300 mg PO bid; days 3-5: 400 mg PO bid; days 6-13: 500 mg PO bid). When co-administered as pharmacologic booster, dosage is reduced. *There are many potential drug interactions, some of which may require dosage modification or preclude its co-administration with other agents; see Physicians' Desk Reference or package insert for more information.*

Toxicity: Gastrointestinal intolerance, circumoral paresthesias, abnormal liver function tests.

Pregnancy category B.

Saquinavir (Invirase)

Indications: Treatment of HIV infection in combination with other agents.

Contraindications: Known hypersensitivity.

Dosage: 1200 mg PO tid with food. When co-administered with ritonavir (400 mg PO bid or 100 mg PO bid) as pharmacologic booster, dose is 400 or 1000 mg PO bid respectively. *There are many potential drug interactions, some of which may require dosage modification or preclude its co-administration with other agents; see Physicians' Desk Reference or package insert for more information.*

Toxicity: Gastrointestinal intolerance, abnormal liver function tests.

Pregnancy category B.

Tipranavir (Aptivus)

Indications: Treatment of HIV infection in combination with other agents.

Contraindications: Known hypersensitivity. Administration is generally not recommended in patients with chronic hepatitis because of the risk of severe hepatic toxicity.

Dosage: 500 mg PO bid co-administered with ritonavir 200 mg PO bid as pharmacologic booster. *There are many potential drug interactions, some of which may require dosage modification or preclude its co-administration with other agents; see Physicians' Desk Reference or package insert for more information.*

Toxicity: Gastrointestinal intolerance, abnormal liver function tests, intracranial hemorrhage (rare).

Pregnancy category C.

Entry Inhibitors

Enfuvirtide (Fuzeon)

Indications: Treatment of HIV infection in combination with other agents. Enfuvirtide is the first of a class of entry.

Contraindications: Known hypersensitivity.

Dosage: 90 mg SC bid.

Toxicity: Injection site reactions.

Pregnancy category B.

Pneumocystis jiroveci (carinii) Pneumonia (PCP): Treatment and Prophylaxis

Atovaquone (Mepron)

Indications: Treatment (mild-to-moderate infection) and prophylaxis of PCP in patients unable to tolerate trimethoprim-sulfamethoxazole (TMP-SMX) or dapsone.

Contraindications: Known hypersensitivity.

Dosage: 750 mg of suspension PO bid with food $\times$ 3 weeks for treatment. Same dosing regimen for prophylaxis.

Toxicity: Gastrointestinal intolerance, rash, headache, fever.

Pregnancy category C.

Clindamycin/Primaquine

Indications: Treatment of PCP in patients unable to tolerate TMP-SMX.

Contraindications: Known hypersensitivity; glucose 6-phosphate dehydrogenase (G6PD) deficiency is contraindication to primaquine use.

Dosage: Clindamycin 600-900 mg IV q6-8h (or 300-450 mg PO qid) and primaquine 15 mg base PO qd $\times$ 3 weeks.

Toxicity: Clindamycin: diarrhea, nausea, rash. Primaquine: nausea, dyspepsia, hemolytic anemia (G6PD deficiency).

Pregnancy categories B (clindamycin) and C (primaquine).

Dapsone

Indications: Treatment of PCP (mild-to-moderate infection) in combination with trimethoprim; prophylaxis of PCP in patients unable to tolerate TMP-SMX; primary prophylaxis of toxoplasmosis in combination with pyrimethamine.

Contraindications: Known hypersensitivity; G6PD deficiency.

Dosage: PCP treatment: dapsone 100 mg qd and trimethoprim 15 mg/kg/day $\times$ 3 weeks.

PCP prophylaxis: 100 mg PO qd; toxoplasmosis prophylaxis: add pyrimethamine 50 mg weekly with folinic acid 25 mg.

Toxicity: Rash, fever, gastrointestinal intolerance, neutropenia, methemo-globinemia.

Pregnancy category C.

Pentamidine (Aerosol [NebuPent], Intravenous [Pentam])

Indications: Treatment and prophylaxis of PCP in patients unable to tolerate TMP-SMX or dapsone.

Contraindications: Known hypersensitivity; severe asthma or bronchospasm; active pulmonary tuberculosis (aerosol preparation).

Dosage: Treatment: 3-4 mg/kg IV qd for up to three weeks.

Prophylaxis: aerosol 300 mg via Respirgard II nebulizer once a month.

Toxicity: Aerosol: bronchospasm, particularly in patients with history of asthma or chronic obstructive pulmonary disease; pharyngeal irritation; metallic taste. Intravenous: hypotension, nephrotoxicity, hypoglycemia, hyperglycemia, leukopenia, thrombocytopenia, hypokalemia, hypocalcemia.

Pregnancy category C.

Trimethoprim-sulfamethoxazole (TMP-SMX, Bactrim, Septra)

Indications: Treatment and prophylaxis of PCP; primary prophylaxis of toxoplasmosis.

Contraindications: Known hypersensitivity to trimethoprim or sulfonamides; megaloblastic anemia.

Dosage: Treatment of PCP: 5 mg/kg PO/IV q8h of trimethoprim component (equivalent to 2 tabs PO tid of DS for 65 kg patient) × 3 weeks.

Prophylaxis of PCP: one DS or SS tablet PO qd. Prophylaxis of toxoplasmosis: one DS tablet PO qd.

Toxicity: Side effects are common in HIV-infected patients and include gastrointestinal intolerance; rash, urticaria, photosensitivity, Stevens-Johnson syndrome; fever; leukopenia, thrombocytopenia, hemolytic anemia; abnormal liver function tests; renal dysfunction, interstitial nephritis; aseptic meningitis.

Patients with history of mild-to-moderate drug toxicity should be given retrial of TMP-SMX or desensitized using an established protocol.

Pregnancy category C; avoid use at term because of risk of kernicterus in newborn.

Toxoplasmosis: Treatment and Prophylaxis[†]

Clindamycin

Indications: Treatment of toxoplasmic encephalitis (for patients unable to tolerate sulfadiazine) in combination with pyrimethamine.

Contraindications: Known hypersensitivity.

Dosage: Initial therapy: 600 mg IV or PO qid × 6 weeks.

Maintenance therapy (secondary prophylaxis): 300-450 mg PO q6h.

Toxicity: Diarrhea, nausea, rash.

Pregnancy category B.

Dapsone.   *See section on PCP Treatment and Prophylaxis.*

Pyrimethamine

Indications: Treatment of toxoplasmic encephalitis in combination with sulfadiazine or clindamycin.

Primary prophylaxis of toxoplasmosis in combination with dapsone.

Contraindications: Known hypersensitivity.

Dosage: Initial therapy: 100-200 mg PO loading dose, followed by 50-75 mg PO qd × 6 weeks in conjunction with folinic acid 10-25 mg PO qd.

Maintenance therapy (secondary prophylaxis): 25-50 mg PO with folinic acid 10-25 mg PO qd.

Prophylaxis: 50 mg weekly with folinic acid 25 mg.

Toxicity: Reversible bone marrow suppression, gastrointestinal intolerance.

Pregnancy category C; teratogenic in animals.

[†]For primary prophylaxis, see PCP Treatment and Prophylaxis section.

Sulfadiazine

Indications: Treatment of toxoplasmic encephalitis in combination with pyrimethamine.

Contraindications: Known hypersensitivity to sulfonamides.

Dosage: Initial therapy: 1-2 g PO qid × 6 weeks.

Maintenance therapy (secondary prophylaxis): 0.5-1 g PO qid.

Toxicity: Fever, rash, pruritus, bone marrow suppression.

Pregnancy category C; avoid use at term because of risk of kernicterus in newborn.

Trimethoprim-Sulfamethoxazole. *See section on PCP Treatment and Prophylaxis.*

Mycobacterium avium Complex (MAC) Infection and Tuberculosis (TB): Treatment and Prophylaxis***

Amikacin (Amikin)

Indications: Treatment of MAC infection in combination with other agents.

Contraindications: Known hypersensitivity to aminoglycoside antibiotics.

Dosage: 7.5-15 mg/kg/day IV for first four weeks of MAC therapy.

Toxicity: Ototoxicity, especially with larger total dose and longer duration (more auditory than vestibular and usually irreversible); nephrotoxicity.

Pregnancy category D.

Azithromycin (Zithromax)

Indications: Treatment of MAC infection in combination with other agents; prophylaxis of MAC infection.

***Drugs for TB can also be administered as directly observed therapy (DOT) in different dosage regimens. Consultation with an expert clinician in this area is recommended.

Contraindications: Known hypersensitivity to macrolide antibiotics.

Dosage: MAC treatment: 600 mg PO qd; prophylaxis: 1200 mg PO weekly.

Toxicity: Gastrointestinal intolerance.

Pregnancy category B.

Ciprofloxacin (Cipro)

Indications: Treatment of MAC infection in combination with other agents; treatment of TB in combination with other agents.

Contraindications: Known hypersensitivity.

Dosage: 500-750 mg PO bid.

Toxicity: Gastrointestinal intolerance, central nervous system dysfunction, rash.

Pregnancy category C.

Clarithromycin (Biaxin)

Indications: Treatment of MAC infection in combination with other agents; prophylaxis of MAC infection.

Contraindications: Known hypersensitivity to macrolide antibiotics.

Dosage: MAC treatment and prophylaxis: 500 mg PO bid.

Toxicity: Gastrointestinal intolerance, abnormal liver function tests.

Pregnancy category C; teratogenic in animals.

Ethambutol (Myambutol)

Indications: Treatment of MAC infection in combination with other agents; treatment of TB in combination with other agents.

Contraindications: Known hypersensitivity; history of optic neuritis.

Dosage: 25 mg/kg/day PO for one to two months, followed by 15 mg/kg/day.

Toxicity: Optic neuritis, rash, gastrointestinal intolerance, hepatotoxicity.

Pregnancy category C; teratogenic in animals.

Isoniazid (INH)

Indications: Treatment of TB in combination with other agents; prophylaxis of TB in context of positive PPD.

Contraindications: Known hypersensitivity; significant hepatic disease.

Dosage: Treatment: 300 mg PO qd (or 900 mg twice a week [DOT]); prophylaxis: 300 mg PO qd for nine months. Pyridoxine should be given concurrently for prevention of peripheral neuropathy.

Toxicity: Rash, hepatotoxicity, especially in alcoholics and persons older than 50; fever; peripheral neuropathy.

Pregnancy category C.

Pyrazinamide

Indications: Treatment of TB in combination with other agents.

Contraindications: Known hypersensitivity; significant hepatic disease.

Dosage: 25 mg/kg PO qd.

Toxicity: Rash, abnormal liver function tests, hyperuricemia.

Pregnancy category C.

Rifabutin (Mycobutin)

Indications: Treatment of MAC infection in combination with other agents; treatment of TB in combination with other agents; prophylaxis of MAC infection in patients unable to tolerate clarithromycin or azithromycin.

Contraindications: Known hypersensitivity.

Dosage: Treatment and prophylaxis: 300 mg PO qd (or 600 mg 2-3 times a week [DOT]). *There are many potential drug interactions, some of which may require dosage modification or preclude its co-administration with other agents; see Physicians' Desk Reference or package insert for more information.*

Toxicity: Rash, orange discoloration of body secretions, gastrointestinal intolerance, abnormal liver function tests. Acute uveitis has been reported when used in association with clarithromycin.

Pregnancy category C.

Rifampin

Indications: Treatment of TB in combination with other agents.

Contraindications: Known hypersensitivity; significant hepatic disease.

Dosage: 600 mg PO qd. *There are many potential drug interactions, some of which may require dosage modification or preclude its co-administration with other agents; see Physicians' Desk Reference or package insert for more information.*

<u>Toxicity</u>: Rash, orange discoloration of body secretions, gastrointestinal intolerance, abnormal liver function tests.

Pregnancy category C.

Streptomycin

<u>Indications</u>: Treatment of TB in combination with other agents.

<u>Contraindications</u>: Known hypersensitivity to aminoglycoside antibiotics.

<u>Dosage</u>: 15 mg/kg IM qd.

<u>Toxicity</u>: Ototoxicity, vestibular toxicity.

Pregnancy category D.

Cytomegalovirus (CMV) Infection: Treatment and Prophylaxis

Cidofovir (Vistide)

<u>Indications</u>: Treatment of CMV infection, including ganciclovir-resistant strains.

<u>Contraindications</u>: Known hypersensitivity; significant renal dysfunction; use of other nephrotoxic medications.

<u>Dosage</u>: Initial therapy: 5 mg/kg IV once a week × 2.

Maintenance therapy (secondary prophylaxis): 5 mg/kg IV once every other week.

Probenecid 2 g PO 3 hr before infusion, and 1 g PO 2 hr before and 8 hr after infusion, should be administered to prevent nephrotoxicity; 1 L normal saline is also given before cidofovir dosing.

<u>Toxicity</u>: Nephrotoxicity, neutropenia. Probenecid is associated with fever, chills, headache, rash, nausea.

Pregnancy category C.

Fomivirsen (Vitravene)

<u>Indications</u>: Treatment of relapsing CMV retinitis.

<u>Contraindications</u>: Known hypersensitivity.

<u>Dosage</u>: Initial therapy: 300 μg intravitreally every other week × 2.

Maintenance therapy (secondary prophylaxis): 330 μg intravitreally every 4 weeks.

Toxicity: Blurred vision, iritis, vitreitis.

Pregnancy category C.

Foscarnet (Foscavir)

Indications: Treatment of CMV infection, including ganciclovir-resistant strains.

Contraindications: Known hypersensitivity; significant renal dysfunction.

Dosage: Initial therapy: 60 mg/kg IV q8h or 90 mg/kg IV q12h × 14 days.

Maintenance therapy (secondary prophylaxis): 90-120 mg/kg IV qd.

Toxicity: Nephrotoxicity, hypocalcemia, hypophosphatemia, hypokalemia, headache, fatigue, nausea, anemia, seizures.

Pregnancy category C.

Ganciclovir (Cytovene)

Indications: Treatment and prophylaxis of CMV infection.

Contraindications: Known hypersensitivity; neutropenia; thrombocytopenia.

Dosage: Initial therapy: 5 mg/kg IV q12h × 14-21 days.

Maintenance therapy (secondary prophylaxis): 5 mg/kg IV qd.

Also available as vitreal implant requiring ophthalmologic surgery.

Toxicity: Neutropenia, thrombocytopenia, anemia, nausea, abdominal pain, headache, confusion.

Pregnancy category C; teratogenic in animals.

Valganciclovir (Valcyte)

Indications: Treatment and prophylaxis of CMV infection.

Contraindications: Known hypersensitivity; neutropenia; thrombocytopenia.

Dosage: Initial therapy: 900 mg PO bid × 3 weeks.

Maintenance therapy (secondary prophylaxis): 900 mg PO qd.

Toxicity: Neutropenia, thrombocytopenia, anemia, nausea, abdominal pain, headache, confusion.

Pregnancy category C.

Herpes Simplex Virus (HSV) and Varicella-Zoster Virus (VZV) Infections: Treatment and Prophylaxis[††]

Acyclovir (Zovirax)

Indications: Treatment and prophylaxis of HSV and VZV infections.

Contraindications: Known hypersensitivity.

Dosage: HSV treatment: 400 mg PO tid × 7 days; secondary prophylaxis: 400 mg PO bid is standard dose, but larger doses may be necessary in advanced HIV disease. For extensive or disseminated disease, intravenous therapy (5 mg/kg q8h) is given.

VZV treatment: 800 mg PO 5×/day for 7 days. For disseminated zoster or ophthalmic involvement, intravenous therapy (10 mg/kg q8h) is given. Secondary prophylaxis generally is not indicated.

Toxicity: Nausea, renal dysfunction.

Pregnancy category C.

Famciclovir (Famvir)

Indications: Treatment and prophylaxis of HSV and VZV infections.

Contraindications: Known hypersensitivity.

Dosage: HSV treatment: 250-500 mg PO bid × 7 days; secondary prophylaxis: 250 mg PO bid.

VZV treatment: 500 mg PO tid × 7 days. Secondary prophylaxis generally is not indicated.

Toxicity: Headache, nausea.

Pregnancy category B.

[††]Cidofovir and forcarnet also have activity against HSV and VZV and may have a role in the treatment of resistant strains. Valacyclovir, an acyclovir analog, has been associated with cases of thrombotic thrombocytopenic purpura (TTP) in patients with advanced HIV disease.

Fungal Infections: Treatment and Prophylaxis

Amphotericin B

<u>Indications</u>:   Pharmacist-prepared suspension for treatment of oral candidiasis; intravenous drug for treatment of systemic fungal infections.

<u>Contraindications</u>:   Known hypersensitivity.

<u>Dosage</u>:   Oral candidiasis: 1-5 mL suspension PO qid × 14 days.

Systemic fungal infections: intravenous doses range from 0.3-1.0 mg/kg/day depending on the pathogen and type of infection. Lipid complex preparations are less toxic but very expensive.

<u>Toxicity</u>:   Oral suspension: nausea, vomiting, diarrhea, rash; intravenous drug: infusion-related fever, chills, phlebitis, hypotension, nausea, vomiting, nephrotoxicity, hypokalemia, hypomagnesemia, hypocalcemia, anemia.

Pregnancy category B.

Caspofungin (Cancidas)

<u>Indications</u>:   Treatment of resistant oroesophageal candidiasis.

<u>Contraindications</u>:   Known hypersensitivity.

<u>Dosage</u>:   50 mg IV qd × 2 weeks.

<u>Toxicity</u>:   Rash, gastrointestinal intolerance, abnormal liver function tests. *There are many potential drug interactions, some of which may require dosage modification or preclude its co-administration with other agents; see Physicians' Desk Reference or package insert for more information.*

Pregnancy category C.

Clotrimazole

<u>Indications</u>:   Treatment of mucosal candidiasis.

<u>Contraindications</u>:   Known hypersensitivity.

<u>Dosage</u>:   Oral candidiasis: 10 mg lozenge dissolved in the mouth 5 times a day; vaginal candidiasis: 100 mg tablet per vagina bid × 3 days.

<u>Toxicity</u>:   Nausea, abnormal liver function tests.

Pregnancy category C.

Fluconazole (Diflucan)

Indications: Treatment and secondary prophylaxis of mucosal candidiasis; secondary prophylaxis of cryptococcal infection.

Contraindications: Known hypersensitivity.

Dosage: Treatment of oral candidiasis: 100 mg PO qd × 7-14 days; esophageal candidiasis: 200 mg PO qd × 14-21 days; vaginal candidiasis: 150 mg PO × one. Secondary prophylaxis of mucosal candidiasis: 50-200 mg PO qd. *There are many potential drug interactions, some of which may require dosage modification or preclude its co-administration with other agents; see Physicians' Desk Reference or package insert for more information.*

Cryptococcal infection maintenance therapy (secondary prophylaxis): 200 mg PO qd. Most experts recommend initial treatment of cryptococcal infection with amphotericin B; if using fluconazole, dose 400 mg PO qd × 8 weeks.

Toxicity: Nausea, headache, hepatotoxicity.

Pregnancy category C.

Nystatin

Indications: Treatment of mucosal candidiasis.

Contraindications: Known hypersensitivity.

Dosage: Oral candidiasis: 5 ml suspension to be gargled and swallowed 5 times a day × 7-14 days; vaginal candidiasis: 100,000 U tab intravaginally 1-2 times a day × 7-14 days.

Toxicity: Nausea, vomiting, diarrhea

Pregnancy category C.

Posaconazole (Noxafil)

Indications: Treatment of resistant oroesophageal candidiasis.

Contraindications: Known hypersensitivity.

Dosage: 400 mg PO bid.

Toxicity: Gastrointestinal intolerance, abnormal liver function tests. *There are many potential drug interactions, some of which may require dosage modification or preclude its co-administration with other agents; see Physicians' Desk Reference or package insert for more information.*

Pregnancy category C.

Voriconazole (Vfend)

<u>Indications</u>:   Treatment of resistant oroesophageal candidiasis.

<u>Contraindications</u>:   Known hypersensitivity.

<u>Dosage</u>:   200 mg PO bid.

<u>Toxicity</u>:   Rash, gastrointestinal intolerance, peripheral edema, abnormal liver function tests. *There are many potential drug interactions, some of which may require dosage modification or preclude its co-administration with other agents; see Physicians' Desk Reference or package insert for more information.*

Pregnancy category D.

Miscellaneous Therapeutic Agents

Dronabinol (Marinol)

<u>Indications</u>:   Appetite stimulant for treatment of AIDS wasting syndrome.

<u>Contraindications</u>:   Known hypersensitivity; significant cognitive dysfunction.

<u>Dosage</u>:   2.5 mg PO bid.

<u>Toxicity</u>:   Neuropsychiatric symptoms, gastrointestinal intolerance.

Pregnancy category C.

Erythropoietin (Procrit)

<u>Indications</u>:   Treatment of HIV- or ZDV-associated anemia (HCT $\leq$ 30) in patients with serum erythropoietin levels $\leq$ 500 mU/mL.

<u>Contraindications</u>:   Known hypersensitivity to mammalian cell-derived products or human albumin; uncontrolled hypertension.

<u>Dosage</u>:   40,000 U SC once a week; response usually seen between 2 and 6 weeks.

<u>Toxicity</u>:   Headache, nausea, arthralgia, hypertension, seizures.

Pregnancy category C; teratogenic in animals.

Granulocyte-Colony Stimulating Factor (G-CSF, Filgrastim)

Indications: Treatment of neutropenia, defined as ANC < 500-750/mm^3, as a result of HIV disease, chemotherapy, or other drugs (ganciclovir, ZDV, TMP-SMX).

Contraindications: Known hypersensitivity to drug or *Escherichia coli*-derived products.

Dosage: 5-10 µg/kg/day SC × 2-4 weeks.

Toxicity: Bone pain.

Pregnancy category C.

Human Growth Hormone (Somatropin, Serostim)

Indications: Hormonal treatment of AIDS wasting syndrome.

Contraindications: Known hypersensitivity; presence of an actively growing intracranial tumor.

Dosage: For patients > 55 kg, dose is 6 mg SC qd; for patients 45-55 kg, dose is 5 mg SC qd; for patients 35-45 kg, dose is 4 mg SC qd.

Toxicity: Arthralgia, edema, hypertension, hyperglycemia.

Pregnancy category B.

Megestrol Acetate (Megace)

Indications: Appetite stimulant for treatment of AIDS wasting syndrome.

Contraindications: Known hypersensitivity; pregnancy.

Dosage: 400-800 mg of suspension PO qd.

Toxicity: Hypogonadism, adrenal insufficiency, diarrhea, impotence, rash, hyperglycemia.

Pregnancy category D.

Oxandrolone (Oxandrin)

Indications: Anabolic steroid for treatment of AIDS wasting syndrome.

Contraindications: Known hypersensitivity; history of breast or prostate cancer; significant hepatic dysfunction; nephrosis; pregnancy.

Dosage: 5-10 mg PO bid.

Toxicity: Edema, hypertension, virilization, glucose intolerance, hyperlipidemia, abnormal liver function tests.

Pregnancy category X.

Pegylated Interferon (PEGASYS, PEG-Intron)

Indications: Treatment of chronic hepatitis C infection in combination with ribavirin.

Contraindications: Known hypersensitivity.

Dosage: Pegylated interferon alfa-2a (PEGASYS) 180 μg SC weekly with ribavirin 400 mg PO bid.

Pegylated interferon alfa-2b (PEG-Intron) 1.5 μg/kg SC weekly with ribavirin 400 mg PO bid.

Toxicity: Constitutional symptoms; depression; anemia; leukopenia.

Pregnancy categories C (PEGASYS) and X (PEG-Intron).

Ribavirin

Indications: Treatment of chronic hepatitis C infection in combination with pegylated interferon.

Contraindications: Known hypersensitivity; severe anemia; pregnancy.

Dosage: 400 mg PO bid with pegylated interferon regimen as above. A higher dose of ribavirin may be necessary with genotype 1 infection. *There are many potential drug interactions, some of which require dosage modification or preclude its co-administration with other agents; see Physicians' Desk Reference or package insert for more information.*

Toxicity: Rash, hemolytic anemia.

Pregnancy category X.

Testosterone

Indications: Treatment of hypogonadism; treatment of AIDS wasting syndrome.

Contraindications: Known hypersensitivity; history of male breast or prostate cancer; pregnancy.

Dosage: 200-400 mg IM q 2 weeks. Topical treatment is also available: gel preparation (Androgel) 5 g topically qd; and transdermal systems via non-scrotal patch including Androderm and Testoderm.

<u>Toxicity</u>:   Coagulopathy, cholestatic jaundice, increased libido, edema, flushing, priapism, local reaction with patches.

Pregnancy category X.

Thalidomide (Thalomid)

<u>Indications</u>:   Treatment of refractory aphthous ulcers; treatment of refractory AIDS wasting syndrome.

<u>Contraindications</u>:   Known hypersensitivity; pregnancy.

<u>Dosage</u>:   50-200 mg PO qd. Physicians and pharmacists must be registered in the STEPS program (System for Thalidomide Education and Prescribing Safety at 1-888-4-Celgene) to prescribe thalidomide. Female patients must have a negative pregnancy test within 24 hours of starting therapy, weekly pregnancy tests in the first month of therapy, monthly pregnancy tests thereafter, and agree to use two forms of contraception. Male patients must use a condom for contraception.

<u>Toxicity</u>:   Peripheral neuropathy, drowsiness, orthostatic hypotension, fever, rash, neutropenia.

Pregnancy category X.

Pregnancy Categories

A   Controlled studies show no risk
B   No evidence of risk in humans
C   Risk cannot be excluded
D   Evidence of risk
X   Contraindicated in pregnancy

Appendix II

Update of the Drug Resistance Mutations in HIV-1: Fall 2006

VICTORIA A. JOHNSON, MD
FRANÇOISE BRUN-VÉZINET, MD, PhD
BONAVENTURA CLOTET, MD, PhD
DANIEL R. KURITZKES, MD
DEENAN PILLAY, MD, PhD
JONATHAN M. SCHAPIRO, MD
DOUGLAS D. RICHMAN, MD

The International AIDS Society–USA (IAS–USA) Drug Resistance Mutations Group is marking 6 years as an independent volunteer panel of experts focused on identifying key HIV-1 drug resistance mutations. The goal of the effort is to quickly deliver accurate and unbiased information on these mutations to HIV clinical practitioners.

This version of the IAS–USA Drug Resistance Mutations Figures replaces the version published in this journal in October/November 2005.[1] The IAS–USA Drug Resistance Mutations Figures are designed for use in identifying mutations associated with viral resistance to antiretroviral drugs and in making therapeutic decisions. Care should be taken when using this list of mutations for surveillance or epidemiologic studies of transmission of drug-resistant virus. A number of amino acid substitutions, particularly minor mutations, represent polymorphisms that in isolation may not reflect prior drug selective pressure or reduced drug susceptibility.

In the context of making clinical decisions regarding antiretroviral therapy, evaluating the results of HIV genotypic testing includes: (1) assessing whether the pattern or absence of a pattern in the mutations is consistent with the patient's antiretroviral history; (2) recognizing that in the absence of drug (selection pressure), resistant strains may be present at levels below the limit of detection of the test (analyzing stored samples, collected under selection pressure, could be useful in this setting); and (3) recognizing that virologic failure of the first regimen typically involves HIV-1 isolates with resistance to only 1 or 2 of the drugs in the regimen (in this setting, resistance

Reprinted from Top HIV Med. 2006;14:125-30; with permission.

most commonly develops to lamivudine or the nonnucleoside reverse transcriptase inhibitors [NNRTIs]).[2-6] The absence of detectable drug resistance following treatment failure may result from the presence of drug-resistant minority viral populations, patient medication nonadherence, laboratory error, drug-drug interactions leading to subtherapeutic drug levels, and possibly compartmental issues, indicating that drugs may not reach optimal levels in specific cellular or tissue reservoirs.

Revisions to the Figures for the August/September 2006 Update

Nucleoside (or Nucleotide) Reverse Transcriptase Inhibitors

Among the changes in the August/ September 2006 version of the figures and user notes, user note 1 has updates about NNRTI hypersusceptibility. On the nucleoside (or nucleotide) reverse transcriptase inhibitor (nRTI) bars, the K70E mutation has been added to tenofovir. User note 4 discusses mutations outside of the reverse transcriptase gene region depicted on the figure bars. These mutations may prove to be important for HIV drug resistance. Also on the nRTI bars, the E44D and V118I mutations have been removed from stavudine and zidovudine because the significance of E44D or V118I when each occurs in isolation is unknown (see user note 5).

Nonnucleoside Reverse Transcriptase Inhibitors

The multi-NNRTI resistance bars have been removed because the presence of 2 or more of the NNRTI mutations depicted on these bars may lead to poorer long-term virologic response (see user note 12).

Protease Inhibitors

In the protease inhibitor (PI) category, the ritonavir bar has been removed because ritonavir is now used only for pharmacologic purposes, not as monotherapy, as discussed in user note 15. The "/ritonavir" designation has been added to atazanavir, fosamprenavir, darunavir, indinavir, and saquinavir to indicate boosting with low-dose ritonavir. User note 16 provides an update on how HIV-1 Gag cleavage site changes can cause PI resistance in vitro.

Based on new data (see user note 17), the following minor mutations have been added to atazanavir with or with out ritonavir: L10C, K20T/V, E34Q, F53L/Y, I54A, I64L/M/V, V82F/I, and I93M. A darunavir/ritonavir bar has been added for the fully approved drug formerly known as TMC-114 (see user note 18). The darunavir/ritonavir major mutations on the bar are I50V, I54M, L76V, and I84V and the minor mutations are V11I, V32I, L33F, I47V, I54L, G73S, and L89V. Minor mutations added to saquinavir/ritonavir are: L24I, I62V, and V82F/T/S.

List of Mutations

The International AIDS Society–USA Drug Resistance Mutations Group reviews new data on HIV drug resistance in order to maintain a current list of mutations associated with clinical resistance to HIV. This list includes mutations that may contribute to a reduced virologic response to a drug.

The mutations listed have been identified by 1 or more of the following criteria: (1) in vitro passage experiments or validation of contribution to resistance by using site-directed mutagenesis; (2) susceptibility testing of laboratory or clinical isolates; (3) genetic sequencing of viruses from patients in whom the drug is failing; (4) correlation studies between genotype at baseline and virologic response in patients exposed to the drug. In addition, the group only reviews data that have been published or have been presented at a scientific conference. Drugs that have been approved by the US Food and Drug Administration (FDA) are included (listed in alphabetical order by drug class). User notes provide additional information as necessary. Although the Drug Resistance Mutations Group works to maintain a complete and current list of these mutations, it cannot be assumed that the list presented here is exhaustive. Readers are encouraged to consult the literature and experts in the field for clarification or more information about specific mutations and their clinical impact.

Comments?

The IAS–USA Drug Resistance Mutations Group welcomes comments on the mutations figures and user notes. Please send your evidence-based comments, including relevant reference citations, to the IAS–USA at resistance2006@iasusa.org or by fax at 415-544-9401. Please include your name and institution.

Reprint Requests

The Drug Resistance Mutations Group welcomes interest in the mutations figures as an educational resource for practitioners and encourages dissemination of the material to as broad an audience as possible. However, we require that permission to reprint the figures be obtained and that no alternations in the content be made. If you wish to reprint the mutations figures, please send your request to the IAS–USA via e-mail (see above) or fax. Requests to reprint the material should include the name of the publisher or sponsor, the name or a description of the publication in which you wish to reprint the material, the funding organization(s), if applicable, and the intended audience of the publication. Requests to make any minimal adaptations of the material should include the former, plus a detailed explanation of how the adapted version will be changed from the original version and, if possible, a copy of the proposed adaptation. In order to ensure the integrity of the mutations figures, it is the policy of the IAS–USA to grant permission for only minor preapproved adaptations of the figures (eg, an adjustment in size). Minimal adaptations only will be considered; no alterations of the content of the figures or user notes will be permitted. Please note that permission will be granted only for requests to reprint or adapt the most current version of the mutations figures as they are posted on the Web site (www.iasusa.org). Because scientific understanding of HIV drug resistance is evolving quickly and the goal of the Drug Resistance Mutations Group is to maintain the most up-to-date compilation of mutations for HIV clinicians and researchers, the publication of out-of-date figures is counterproductive. If you have any questions about reprints or adaptations, please contact us.

Financial Disclosures
The authors disclose the following affiliations with commercial organizations that may have interests related to the content of this article: Dr Brun-Vézinet has received grant support from Bayer, bioMérieux, Bristol-Myers Squibb, GlaxoSmithKline, and PE Biosystems and has served as a consultant to Abbott, Bayer, Boehringer Ingelheim, GlaxoSmithKline, Gilead, Roche, and Tibotec; Dr Clotet has served as a consultant and received grant support from Abbott, Boehringer Ingelheim, Bristol-Myers Squibb, Gilead Sciences, GlaxoSmithKline, Pfizer, and Roche; Dr Johnson has served as a consultant to GlaxoSmithKline, Bristol-Myers Squibb, Virco, and ViroLogic and as a speaker or on a speakers bureau for Abbott, Bayer, Boehringer Ingelheim/Roxanne, Bristol-Myers Squibb, Chiron, GlaxoSmithKline, Merck, Roche, Vertex, and ViroLogic, and has received grant support from Boehringer Ingelheim, Bristol-Myers Squibb, Glaxo-SmithKline, and Bayer; Dr Kuritzkes has served as a consultant to Abbott, Anormed, Avexa, Bayer, Boehringer Ingelheim, Bristol-Myers Squibb, Chiron, Gilead, Glaxo-SmithKline, Merck, Monogram Biosciences, Panacos, Pfizer, Roche/Trimeris, Schering-Plough, Tanox, Tibotec, and VirXsys, and has received honoraria from Abbott, Anormed, Avexa, Bayer, Boehringer Ingelheim, Bristol-Myers Squibb, Gilead, GlaxoSmithKline, Human Genome Sciences, Merck, Monogram Biosciences, Panacos, Pfizer, Roche/Trimeris, and VirXsys, and grant support from Bayer, Boehringer Ingelheim, Bristol-Myers Squibb, Glaxo-SmithKline, Human Genome Sciences, Merck, Roche/Trimeris, Schering-Plough, and Tibotec; Dr Pillay has served as a consultant to and has received research grants from GlaxoSmithKline, Gilead, Bristol-Myers Squibb, Roche, and Tibotec-Virco; Dr Richman has served as a consultant to Achillion, Anadys, Bristol-Myers Squibb, Gilead, GlaxoSmithKline, Idinex, Merck, Monogram, Pfizer, Roche, and Tibotec; Dr Schapiro has served as a scientific advisor to Bayer and Roche and on the speakers bureau for Abbott, Bristol-Myers Squibb, and Roche, and has received other financial support from GlaxoSmithKline and Virology Education.

Funding/Support

This work was funded by IAS–USA. No private sector or government funding contributed to this effort. Panel members are not compensated.

Author Affiliations

Dr Johnson (Group Chair), Birmingham Veterans Affairs Medical Center and the University of Alabama at Birmingham School of Medicine, Birmingham, AL; Dr Brun-Vézinet, Hôpital Bichat-Claude Bernard, Paris, France; Dr Clotet, Fundacio irsiCAIXA and HIV Unit, Hospital Universitari Germans Trias i Pujol, Barcelona, Spain; Dr Kuritzkes, Brigham and Women's Hospital, Harvard Medical School, Boston, MA; Dr Pillay, Royal Free and University College Medical School, London, England; Dr Schapiro, National Hemophilia Center, Sheba Medical Center, Tel Aviv, Israel; Dr Richman (Group Vice Chair), Veterans Affairs San Diego Healthcare System and the University of California San Diego, La Jolla, CA.

References

1. Johnson VA, Brun-Vézinet F, Clotet B, et al. Update of the drug resistance mutations in HIV-1: Fall 2005. Top HIV Med. 2005;13:125-131.

2. Descamps D, Flandre P, Calvez V, et al. Mechanisms of virologic failure in previously untreated HIV-infected patients from a trial of induction-maintenance therapy. Trilege (Agence Nationale de Recherches sur le SIDA 072) Study Team. JAMA. 2000;283:205-211.

3. Havlir DV, Hellmann NS, Petropoulos CJ, et al. Drug susceptibility in HIV infection after viral rebound in patients receiving indinavir-containing regimens. JAMA. 2000;283:229-234.

4. Maguire M, Gartland M, Moore S, et al. Absence of zidovudine resistance in antiretroviral-naive patients following zidovudine/ lamivudine/protease inhibitor combination therapy: virological evaluation of the AVANTI 2 and AVANTI 3 studies. AIDS. 2000;14:11951201.

5. Gallego O, Ruiz L, Vallejo A, et al. Changes in the rate of genotypic resistance to antiretroviral drugs in Spain. AIDS. 2001;15:1894-1896.

6. Walmsley S, Bernstein B, King M, et al. Lopinavir-ritonavir versus nelfinavir for the initial treatment of HIV infection. N Engl J Med. 2002;346:2039-2046.

MUTATIONS IN THE REVERSE TRANSCRIPTASE GENE ASSOCIATED WITH RESISTANCE TO REVERSE TRANSCRIPTASE INHIBITORS

Nucleoside and Nucleotide Reverse Transcriptase Inhibitors (nRTIs)[1]

Multi-nRTI Resistance: 69 Insertion Complex[2] (affects all nRTIs currently approved by the US FDA)

M	A	▼	K					L	T	K
41	**62**	**69**	**70**					**210**	**215**	**219**
L	V	Insert	R					W	Y	Q
									F	E

Multi-nRTI Resistance: 151 Complex[3] (affects all nRTIs currently approved by the US FDA except tenofovir)

	A			V	F		F	Q	
	62		**75**	**77**			**116**	**151**	
	V		I	L			Y	M	

Multi-nRTI Resistance: Thymidine Analogue-associated Mutations[4,5] (TAMs; affect all nRTIs currently approved by the US FDA)

M		D	K					L	T	K
41		**67**	**70**					**210**	**215**	**219**
L		N	R					W	Y	Q
									F	E

Abacavir[6]

	K		L			Y		M	
	65		**74**			**115**		**184**	
	R		V			F		V	

Didanosine[7,8]

	K		L
	65		**74**
	R		V

Emtricitabine

	K		M
	65		**184**
	R		V
			I

Lamivudine

	K		M
	65		**184**
	R		V
			I

Stavudine[4,5,9,10]

M		D	K					L	T	K
41		**67**	**70**					**210**	**215**	**219**
L		N	R					W	Y	Q
									F	E

Tenofovir[11]

	K		K
	65		**70**
	R		E

Zidovudine[4,5,9,10]

M		D	K					L	T	K
41		**67**	**70**					**210**	**215**	**219**
L		N	R					W	Y	Q
									F	E

Nonnucleoside Reverse Transcriptase Inhibitors (NNRTIs)[1,12]

Delavirdine

	K	V			Y		Y		P
	103	**106**			**181**		**188**		**236**
	N	M			C		L		L

Efavirenz

L	K	V	V		Y	Y	G		P
100	**103**	**106**	**108**		**181**	**188**	**190**		**225**
I	N	M	I		C	L	S		H
					I		A		

Nevirapine

L	K	V	V		Y	Y	G
100	**103**	**106**	**108**		**181**	**188**	**190**
I	N	A	I		C	C	A
		M			I	L	
						H	

MUTATIONS IN THE PROTEASE GENE ASSOCIATED WITH RESISTANCE TO PROTEASE INHIBITORS[13,14,15,16]

Atazanavir +/- ritonavir[17]

Position	10	16	20	24	32	33	34	36	46	48	50	53	54	60	62	64	71	73	82	84	85	88	90	93
Wild-type	L	G	K	L	V	L	E	M	M	G	**I**	F	I	D	I	I	A	G	V	**I**	I	N	L	I
Mutations	E	R	I	I	I	Q		I	V	L	L	Y	L	E	V	L	C	A	V	V	V	S	M	L
	F		M					L	L				E			V	I	S	T		S	M		M
	V		I			F		V					M				V	T	F					
	C		T			V							T				T	T	I					
			V										A				L	A						

Fosamprenavir/ritonavir

Position	10	32	46	47	50	54	73	82	84	90
Wild-type	L	V	M	I	**I**	I	G	V	I	L
Mutations	F	I	I	V	V	L	S	A	V	M
	I		L			V		V		
	R					M		F		
	V							S/T		

Darunavir/ritonavir[18]

Position	11	32	33	47	50	54	73	76	84	89
Wild-type	V	V	L	I	**I**	I	G	L	I	L
Mutations	I	I	F	V	V	M	S	V	V	V
						L				

Indinavir/ritonavir

Position	10	20	24	32	36	46	54	71	73	77	82	84	90
Wild-type	L	K	L	V	M	**M**	I	A	G	V	V	I	L
Mutations	I	M	I	I	I	I	V	V	A	I	A	V	M
	R	R				L		T			F		
	V										T		

Lopinavir/ritonavir[19]

Position	10	20	24	32	33	46	47	50	53	54	63	71	73	82	84	90
Wild-type	L	K	L	V	L	M	**I**	I	F	I	L	A	G	**V**	I	L
Mutations	F	M	I	I	F	I	V	V	L	V	P	V	S	A	V	M
	I	R				L	A			L		T		F		
	R									A				T		
	V									M				S		
										T						
										S						

Nelfinavir[20]

Position	10	30	36	46	71	77	82	84	88	90
Wild-type	L	**D**	M	M	A	V	V	I	N	**L**
Mutations	F	N	I	I	V	I	A	V	D	M
	I			L	T		F		S	
							T			
							S			

Saquinavir/ritonavir

Position	10	24	48	54	62	71	73	77	82	84	90
Wild-type	L	L	**G**	I	I	A	G	V	V	I	**L**
Mutations	I	I	V	V	V	V	S	I	A	V	M
	R			L		T			F		
	V								T		
									S		

Tipranavir/ritonavir[21]

Position	10	13	20	33	35	36	43	46	47	54	58	69	74	82	83	84	90
Wild-type	L	I	K	L	E	M	K	M	I	I	Q	H	T	V	N	**I**	L
Mutations	V	V	M	F	G	I	T	L	V	A	E	K	P	L	D	V	M
			R							M				T			
										V							

MUTATIONS IN THE GP41 ENVELOPE GENE ASSOCIATED WITH RESISTANCE TO ENTRY INHIBITORS

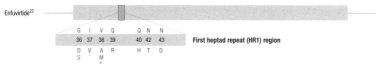

Enfuvirtide[22]

Position	36	37	38	39	40	42	43
Wild-type	G	I	V	Q	Q	N	N
Mutations	D	V	A	R	H	T	D
	S		M				
			E				

First heptad repeat (HR1) region

Amino acid abbreviations: A, alanine; C, cysteine; D, aspartate; E, glutamate; F, phenylalanine; G, glycine; H, histidine; I, isoleucine; K, lysine; L, leucine; M, methionine; N, asparagine; P, proline; Q, glutamine; R, arginine; S, serine; T, threonine; V, valine; W, tryptophan; Y, tyrosine.

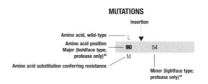

MUTATIONS

Insertion

Amino acid, wild-type — L

Amino acid position / Major (boldface type; protease only)[14] — 90

Amino acid substitution conferring resistance — M

Minor (lightface type; protease only)[14] — 54

User Notes

1. Numerous nucleoside (or nucleotide) reverse transcriptase inhibitor (nRTI) mutations, such as the M41L, L210W, and T215Y mutations, may lead to viral hypersusceptibility to the nonnucleoside reverse transcriptase inhibitors (NNRTIs) in nRTI-treated individuals. The presence of these mutations may improve subsequent virologic response to NNRTI-containing regimens in NNRTI treatment-naive individuals (Shulman et al, *AIDS,* 2004; Demeter et al, 11th CROI, 2004; Haubrich et al, *AIDS,* 2002; Tozzi, *J Infect Dis,* 2004; Katzenstein et al, *AIDS,* 2003). NNRTI hypersusceptibility can be conferred by 2 distinct phenotypes: increased enzyme susceptibility to NNRTI (eg, V118I/T215Y) or decreased virion associated levels of reverse transcriptase (eg, H208Y/T215Y and V118I/H208Y/T215Y). The viruses that contained less reverse transcriptase replicated less efficiently than those with wild-type levels of reverse transcriptase. (Clark et al, *Antivir Ther,* 2006). The clinical relevance of all these mutations has not been assessed.

2. The 69 insertion complex consists of a substitution at codon 69 (typically T69S) and an insertion of 2 or more amino acids (S-S, S-A, S-G, or others). The 69 insertion complex is associated with resistance to all nRTIs currently approved by the US FDA when present with 1 or more thymidine analogue-associated mutations (TAMs) at codons 41, 210, or 215 (Miller et al, *J Infect Dis,* 2004). Some other amino acid changes from the wild-type T at codon 69 without the insertion may also be associated with broad nRTI resistance.

3. Tenofovir retains activity against the Q151M complex of mutations (Miller et al, *J Infect Dis,* 2004).

4. Multi-nRTI resistance mutations, also known as nucleoside analogue-associated mutations (NAMs), are associated with resistance to numerous nRTIs. The M41L, D67N, K70R, L210W, T215Y/F, and K219Q/E are known as TAMs. TAMs are a subset of NAMs that are selected by the thymidine analogues zidovudine and stavudine and are associated with cross-resistance to all nRTIs currently approved by the US FDA (Larder et al, Science, 1989; Kellam et al, *Proc Natl Acad Sci USA,* 1992; Calvez et al, *Antivir Ther,* 2002; Kuritzkes et al, *J Acquir Immune Defic Syndr,* 2004). Mutations at the C-terminal reverse transcriptase domains (amino acids 293–560) outside of regions depicted on the figure bars may prove to be important for HIV drug resistance. Mutations in the connection (A371V) and RNase H (Q509L) domains of reverse transcriptase are coselected on the same genome as TAMs and increase significantly zidovudine resistance when combined with TAMs. They also increase, although to a much lesser extent, cross-resistance to lamivudine, abacavir, and tenofovir but not to stavudine or didanosine (Brehm et al. *Antiviral Ther,* 2006). In zidovudine-exerienced patients, it has been shown by drug susceptibility testing that, in the C-terminal domain, the mutations G335C, N348I, and A360I exhibited 30-, 35-, and 30-fold increases in zidovudine resistance, respectively. (Nikolenko et al, *Antiviral Ther,* 2006.) Three mutations (N348I, T369I, and E399D) in the reverse transcriptase C-terminus are associated with the increased resistance to zidovudine and to NNRTIs. Mutations at this level could modulate NNRTI resistance by affecting dimerization of p66/p51 heterodimers (Gupta et al. *Antivir Ther,* 2006). The clinical relevance of these mutations has not been assessed.

5. The E44D and the V118I mutations increase the level of resistance to zidovudine and stavudine in the setting of TAMs, and correspondingly increase cross-resistance to the other nRTIs. The significance of E44D or V118I when each occurs in isolation is unknown (Romano et al, *J Infect Dis,* 2002; Walter et al, *Antimicrob Agents Chemother,* 2002; Girouard et al, *Antivir Ther,* 2002).

6. The M184V mutation alone does not appear to be associated with a reduced virologic response to abacavir in vivo (Harrigan et al, *J Infect Dis,* 2000; Lanier et al, *Antivir Ther,* 2004). When present with 2 or 3 TAMs, M184V contributes to reduced susceptibility to abacavir and is associated with impaired virologic response in vivo (Lanier et al, *Antivir*

Ther, 2004). The M184V plus 4 or more TAMs resulted in no virologic response to abacavir in vivo (Lanier et al, *Antivir Ther,* 2004).

7. The K65R mutation may be selected by didanosine and is associated in vitro with decreased susceptibility to the drug (Winters et al, *Antimicrob Agents Chemother,* 1997). The impact of the K65R mutation in vivo is unclear.

8. The presence of 3 of the following—M41L, D67N, L210W, T215Y/F, and K219Q/E—has been associated with resistance to didanosine (Marcelin et al, *Antimicrob Agents Chemother,* 2005). The K70R and M184V mutations are not associated with a decreased virologic response to didanosine in vivo (Molina et al, *J Infect Dis,* 2005).

9. The presence of the M184V mutation appears to delay or prevent emergence of TAMs (Kuritzkes et al, *AIDS,* 1996). This effect may be overcome by an accumulation of TAMs or other mutations. The clinical significance of this effect of M184V is not known.

10. The T215A/C/D/E/G/H/I/L/N/S/V substitutions are revertant mutations at codon 215, conferring increased risk of virologic failure of zidovudine or stavudine in antiretroviral-naive patients (Riva et al, *Antivir Ther,* 2002; Chappey et al, *Antivir Ther,* 2003; Violin et al, *AIDS,* 2004). In vitro studies and preliminary clinical studies suggest that the T215Y mutant may emerge quickly from one of these mutations in the presence of zidovudine or stavudine (Garcia-Lerma et al, *J Virol,* 2004; Lanier et al, *Antivir Ther,* 2002; Riva et al, *Antivir Ther,* 2002).

11. The K65R mutation is associated with a reduced virologic response to tenofovir in vivo (Miller et al, *J Infect Dis,* 2004). A reduced response occurs in the presence of 3 or more TAMs inclusive of either M41L or L210W (Miller et al, *J Infect Dis,* 2004). Slightly increased treatment responses to tenofovir in vivo were observed if M184V was present (Miller et al, *J Infect Dis,* 2004).

12. The long-term virologic response to sequential NNRTI use is poor, particularly when 2 or more mutations are present (Antinori et al, *AIDS Res Hum Retroviruses,* 2002; Lecossier et al, *J Acquir Immune Defic Syndr,* 2005). The K103N or Y188L mutation alone prevents the clinical utility of all NNRTIs currently approved by the US FDA (Antinori et al, *AIDS Res Human Retroviruses,* 2002). The V106M mutation is more common in HIV-1 subtype C than in subtype B, and confers cross-resistance to all currently approved NNRTIs (Brenner et al, *AIDS,* 2003; Cane et al, *J Clin Micro,* 2001).

13. The same mutations usually emerge whether or not PIs are boosted with low-dose ritonavir, although the relative frequency of mutations may differ. Data on the selection of mutations in antiretroviral-naive patients in whom a boosted PI is failing are very limited. Numerous mutations are often necessary to significantly impact virologic response to a boosted PI. Although numbers vary for the different drugs, 3 or more mutations are often required.

14. Resistance mutations in the protease gene are classified as either "major" or "minor," if data are available.

Major mutations in the protease gene are defined in general either as those selected first in the presence of the drug; or those shown at the biochemical or virologic level to lead to an alteration in drug binding or an inhibition of viral activity or viral replication. Major mutations have an effect on drug susceptibility phenotype. In general, these mutations tend to be the primary contact residues for drug binding.

Minor mutations generally emerge later than major mutations, and by themselves do not have a significant effect on phenotype. In some cases, their effect may be to improve replicative fitness of the virus containing major mutations. However, some minor mutations are present as common polymorphic changes in HIV-1 nonsubtype B clades, such as K20I/R and M36I in protease.

15. Ritonavir is not listed separately as it is currently used at therapeutic doses as a pharmacologic booster of other PIs. At higher doses tested previously in humans, ritonavir administered as monotherapy produces mutations similar to those produced by indinavir (Molla, *Nature Med,* 1996).

16. HIV-1 Gag cleavage site changes can cause PI resistance in vitro. It has been observed that mutations in the N-terminal part of *gag* (MA: E40K; L75R; K113E and CA: M200I; A224A/V), outside the cleavage site, contribute directly to PI resistance by enhancing the overall Gag processing by wild-type protease. (Nijhuis et al. *Antivir Ther*, 2006). The clinical relevance of these mutations has not been assessed.

17. In most patients in whom an atazanavir/ritonavir-containing regimen was failing virologically, accumulations of the following 13 mutations were found (L10F/I/V, G16E, L33F/I/V, M46I/L, I54L/V/M/T, D60E, I62V, A71I/T/L, V82A/T, I84V, I85V, L90M, and I93L). Seven mutations were retained in an atazanavir score (L10F/I/V, G16E, L33F/I/V, M46I/L, D60E, I84V, I85V); the presence of 3 or more of these mutations predicts a reduced virologic response at 3 months, particularly when L90M was present (Vora, et al, *Antivir Ther*, 2005). A different report (Bertoli et al, *Antivir Ther*, 2006) found that the presence of 0, 1, 2, or greater than or equal to 3 of the following mutations were associated with 92%, 93%, 75%, and 0% virologic response to atazanavir/ritonavir: L10C/I/V, V32I, E34Q, M46I/L, F53L, I54A/M/V, V82A/F/I/T, I84V; presence of I15E/G/L/V, H69K/M/N/Q/R/T/Y, and I72M/T/V improved the chances of response. For unboosted atazanavir, the presence of 0, 1, 2, or greater than or equal to 3 of the following mutations was associated with 83%, 67%, 6%, and 0% response rates: G16E, V32I, K20I/M/R/T/V, L33F/I/V, F53L/Y, I64L/M/V, A71I/T/V, I85V, I93L/M.

18. Darunavir (formerly TMC-114), boosted with ritonavir, was approved by the US FDA in June 2006. Resistance data are therefore still preliminary and limited. HIV RNA response to boosted darunavir correlated with baseline susceptibility and the presence of multiple specific PI mutations. Reductions in response were associated with increasing numbers of the mutations indicated in the bar. Some of these mutations appear to have a greater effect on susceptibility than others (eg, I50V versus V11I). Further study and analysis in other populations are required to refine and validate these findings.

19. In PI-experienced patients, the accumulation of 6 or more of the mutations indicated on the bar is associated with a reduced virologic response to lopinavir/ritonavir (Masquelier et al, *Antimicrob Agents Chemother*, 2002; Kempf et al, *J Virol*, 2001). The product information states that accumulation of 7 or 8 mutations confers resistance to the drug. In contrast, in those in whom lopinavir/ritonavir is their first PI used, resistance to this drug at the time of virologic rebound is rare. However, there is emerging evidence that specific mutations, most notably I47A (and possibly I47V) and V32I are associated with high-level resistance (Mo et al, *J Virol*, 2005; Friend et al, *AIDS* 2004; Kagan et al, *Protein Sci*, 2005).

20. In some nonsubtype-B HIV-1, D30N is selected less frequently than other PI mutations (Gonzalez et al, *Antivir Ther*, 2004).

21. Accumulation of more than 2 mutations at positions 33, 82, 84, and 90 correlate with reduced virologic response to tipranavir/ritonavir, although an independent role for L90M was not found. Detailed analyses of data from phase II and III trials in PI-experienced patients identified mutations associated with reduced susceptibility or virologic response. These include: L10V, I13V, K20M/R, L33F, E35G, M36I, K43T, M46L, I47V, I54A/M/V, Q58E, H69K, T74P, V82L/T, N83D, and I84V. Accumulation of these mutations is associated with reduced response. Subsequent genotype-phenotype and genotype-virologic response analyses determined some mutations have a greater effect than others (eg, I84V versus I54M). Refinement and clinical validation of these findings are pending (Schapiro et al, CROI, 2005; Kohlbrenner et al, DART, 2004; Mayers et al, *Antivir Ther*, 2004; Hall et al, *Antivir Ther*, 2003; McCallister et al, *Antivir Ther*, 2003; Parkin et al, CROI, 2006; Bacheler et al, European HIV Drug Resistance Workshop, 2006).

22. Although resistance to enfuvirtide is associated primarily with mutations in the first heptad repeat (HR1) region of the gp41 envelope gene, wild-type viruses in the depicted HR1 region vary 500-fold in susceptibility. Such pretreatment susceptibility differences were not associated with differences in clinical responses (Labrosse et al, *J Virol*, 2003).

Furthermore, mutations or polymorphisms in other regions in the envelope (eg, the HR2 region or those yet to be identified) as well as coreceptor usage and density may affect susceptibility to enfuvirtide (Reeves et al, *Proc Natl Acad Sci USA,* 2002; Reeves et al, *J Virol,* 2004; Xu et al, *Antimicrob Agents Chemother,* 2005). Thus, testing to detect only the depicted HR1 mutations may not be adequate for clinical management of suspected failure (Reeves et al, *J Virol,* 2004; Menzo et al, *Antimicrob Agents Chemother,* 2004; Poveda et al, *J Med Virol,* 2004; Sista et al, *AIDS,* 2004; Su, *Antivir Ther,* 2004).

Index

Color Plates

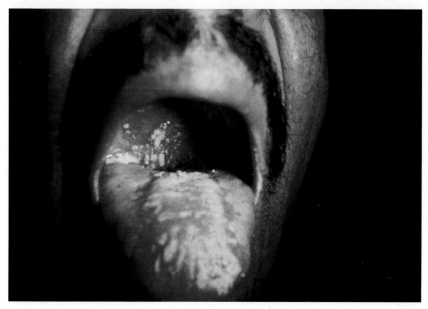

Plate 1 Pseudomembranous variant of oral candidiasis. For further information, see discussion of Figure 9-2, *A,* in Chapter 9 text (where Plate 1 is reproduced in black and white).

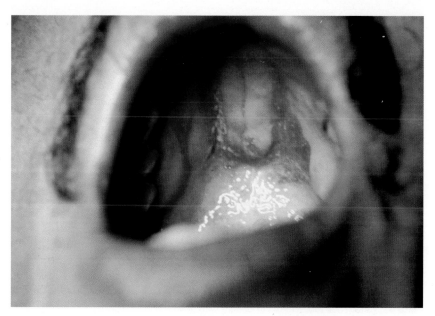

Plate 2 Atrophic variant of oral candidiasis. For further information, see discussion of Figure 9-2, *B,* in Chapter 9 text (where Plate 2 is reproduced in black and white).

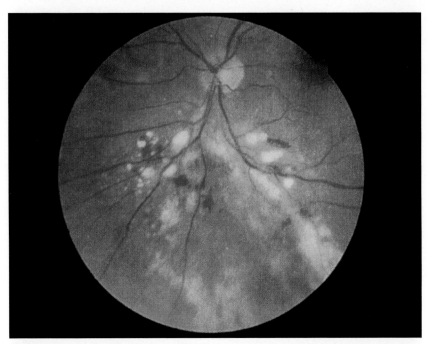

Plate 3 Retinal photograph of patient with cytomegalovirus retinitis. For further information, see discussion of Figure 9-4 in Chapter 9 text (where Plate 3 is reproduced in black and white).

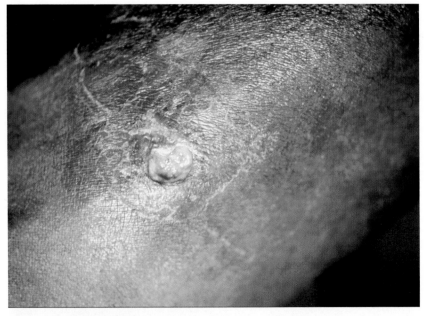

Plate 4 Cutaneous tuberculosis in patient with advanced HIV disease. For further information, see discussion of Figure 9-11 in Chapter 9 text (where Plate 4 is reproduced in black and white).

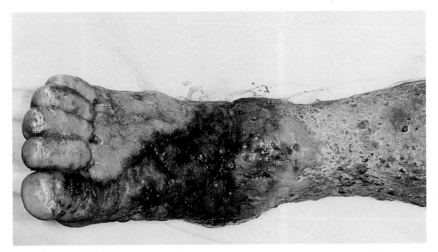

Plate 5 Plaque-like lesion on foot with breakdown of overlying skin in an AIDS patient with Kaposi's sarcoma. (Reprinted with permission from van den Brink MR, Dezube BJ. AIDS-related Kaposi's sarcoma. *J Clin Oncol.* 1997;15:1283.) For further information, see discussion of Figure 10-2, *A,* in Chapter 10 text (where Plate 5 is reproduced in black and white).

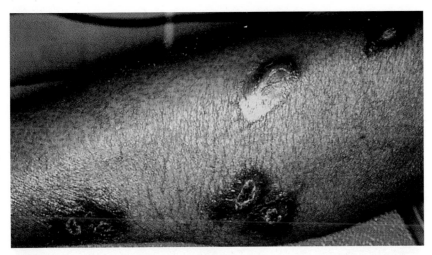

Plate 6 Multiple colored lesions on leg in an AIDS patient with Kaposi's sarcoma. (Reprinted with permission from van den Brink MR, Dezube BJ. AIDS-related Kaposi's sarcoma. *J Clin Oncol.* 1997;15:1283.) For further information, see discussion of Figure 10-2, *B,* in Chapter 10 text (where Plate 6 is reproduced in black and white).

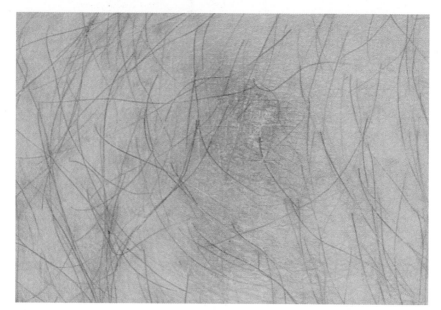

Plate 7 Yellow perilesional halo in an AIDS patient with Kaposi's sarcoma. (Reprinted with permission from van den Brink MR, Dezube BJ. AIDS-related Kaposi's sarcoma. *J Clin Oncol.* 1997;15:1283.) For further information, see discussion of Figure 10-2, *C,* in Chapter 10 text (where Plate 7 is reproduced in black and white).

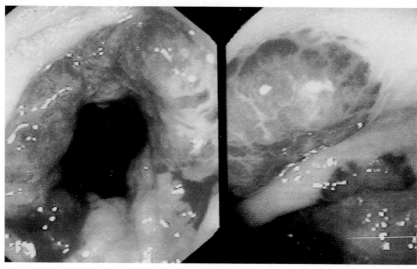

Plate 8 Kaposi's sarcoma can appear as large annular masses with circumferential infiltration and luminal obstruction in the colon and rectum. (Reprinted with permission from van den Brink MR, Dezube BJ. AIDS-related Kaposi's sarcoma. *J Clin Oncol.* 1997;15:1283.) For further information, see discussion of Figure 10-3 in Chapter 10 text (where Plate 8 is reproduced in black and white).